Women's Imaging

Guest Editors

VIKRAM S. DOGRA, MD
DENIZ AKATA, MD

ULTRASOUND CLINICS

www.ultrasound.theclinics.com

July 2008 • Volume 3 • Number 3

SAUNDERS an imprint of ELSEVIER, Inc.

W.B. SAUNDERS COMPANY
A Division of Elsevier Inc.

1600 John F. Kennedy Boulevard • Suite 1800 • Philadelphia, Pennsylvania 19103-2899

http://www.theclinics.com

ULTRASOUND CLINICS Volume 3, Number 3
July 2008 ISSN 1556-858X, ISBN-13: 978-1-4377-0316-0, ISBN-10: 1-4377-0316-X

Editor: Barton Dudlick
Developmental Editor: Donald Mumford

Ultrasound Clinics (ISSN 1556-858X) is published quarterly by W.B. Saunders, 360 Park Avenue South, New York, NY 10010-1710. Months of publication are January, April, July, and October. Business and editorial offices: 1600 John F. Kennedy Boulevard, Suite 1800, Philadelphia, Pennsylvania 19103-2899. Accounting and circulation offices: 6277 Sea Harbor Drive, Orlando, FL 32887-4800. Periodicals postage paid at New York NY, and additional mailing offices. Subscription prices are $189 per year for (US individuals), $274 per year for (US institutions), $94 per year for (US students and residents), $215 per year for (Canadian individuals), $306 per year for (Canadian institutions), $229 per year for (international individuals), $306 per year for (international institutions), and $114 per year for (Canadian and foreign students/residents). To receive student/resident rate, orders must be accompanied by name of affiliated institution, date of term, and the signature of program/residency coordinator on institution letterhead. Orders will be billed at individual rate until proof of status is received. Foreign air speed delivery is included in all Clinics subscription prices. All prices are subject to change without notice. **POSTMASTER:** Send address changes to *Ultrasound Clinics*, Elsevier Periodicals Customer Service, 11830 Westline Industrial Drive, St. Louis, MO 63146. **Customer Service: 1-800-654-2452 (US). From outside the United States, call 1-314-453-7041. Fax: 1-314-453-5170. E-mail: JournalsCustomerService-usa@elsevier.com (for print support) or JournalsOnlineSupport-usa@elsevier.com (for online support).**

Reprints: For copies of 100 or more, of articles in this publication, please contact the Commercial Reprints Department, Elsevier Inc., 360 Park Avenue South, New York, NY 10010-1710. Tel.: (+1) 212-633-3812; Fax: (+1) 212-462-1935; E-mail: reprints@elsevier.com.

Printed in the United States of America.

Contributors

GUEST EDITORS

VIKRAM S. DOGRA, MD
Professor of Radiology, Urology and
Biomedical Engineering, Director of
Ultrasound, Department of Radiology, and
Associate Chair for Education and Research,
University of Rochester School of Medicine
and Dentistry, Rochester, New York

DENIZ AKATA, MD
Professor, Department of Radiology,
Hacettepe University Medical School, Sıhhiye,
Ankara, Turkey

AUTHORS

DENIZ AKATA, MD
Professor, Department of Radiology,
Hacettepe University Medical School, Sıhhiye,
Ankara, Turkey

CARRIE BETEL, MD
Lecturer, Department of Medical Imaging,
University of Toronto, Ontario, Canada

SHWETA BHATT, MD
Department of Radiology, University of
Rochester School of Medicine and Dentistry,
Rochester, New York

FIGEN BAŞARAN DEMIRKAZIK, MD
Professor of Radiology, Faculty of Medicine,
Hacettepe University, Sıhhiye, Ankara,
Turkey

VIKRAM S. DOGRA, MD
Professor of Radiology, Urology and
Biomedical Engineering, Director of
Ultrasound, Department of Radiology,
and Associate Chair for Education and
Research, University of Rochester School
of Medicine and Dentistry, Rochester,
New York

ELIF ERGUN, MD
Instructor of Radiology, Department of
Radiology, Ankara Training and Research
Hospital, Ankara, Turkey

GUL ESEN, MD
Professor, Department of Radiology, Istanbul
University, Cerrahpasa Medical School,
Istanbul, Turkey

KARTHIK GANESAN, DNB
Dr. Joshi's Imaging Clinic, Dadar T.T, Mumbai,
Maharashtra, India

SUBRAMANIA GANESAN, MD
Dr. Joshi's Imaging Clinic, Dadar T.T, Mumbai,
Maharashtra, India

PHYLLIS GLANC, MD
Assistant Professor, Department of Medical
Imaging, and Department of Obstetrics &
Gynecology, University of Toronto,
Sunnybrook Health Sciences Center, Toronto,
Ontario, Canada

SAFIYE GUREL, MD
Associate Professor, Department of Radiology,
Izzet Baysal University, School of Medicine,
Golkoy, Bolu, Turkey

MUKUND JOSHI, MD, FAMS
Dr. Joshi's Imaging Clinic, Dadar T.T, Mumbai,
Maharashtra, India

FATIH KANTARCI, MD
Department of Radiology, Istanbul University,
Cerrahpasa Medical Faculty, Istanbul, Turkey

DENIZ KARCAALTINCABA, MD
Instructor, Etlik Women's Hospital, Ankara, Turkey

MUSTURAY KARCAALTINCABA, MD
Associate Professor of Radiology, Department of Radiology, Hacettepe University School of Medicine, Ankara, Turkey

ERCAN KOCAKOC, MD
Associate Professor of Radiology, Department of Radiology, Faculty of Medicine, Firat University, Elazig, Turkey

ASHWIN LAWANDE, DNB
Dr. Joshi's Imaging Clinic, Dadar T.T, Mumbai, Maharashtra, India

ANNA LEV-TOAFF, MD
Professor of Radiology, Department of Radiology, University of Pennsylvania, Hospital of the University of Pennsylvania, Philadelphia, Pennsylvania

ISMAIL MIHMANLI, MD
Department of Radiology, Istanbul University, Cerrahpasa Medical Faculty, Istanbul, Turkey

HARSHA NAVANI MUNSHI, DNB
Dr. Joshi's Imaging Clinic, Dadar T.T, Mumbai, Maharashtra, India

AYSENUR OKTAY, MD
Professor, Department of Radiology, Medical School of Ege University, Izmir, Turkey

DENIZ CEBI OLGUN, MD
Assistant Professor of Radiology, Department of Radiology, Istanbul University, Cerrahpasa Medical School, Istanbul, Turkey

RAJ M. PASPULATI, MD
Assistant Professor in Radiology, Department of Radiology, University Hospitals, Case Medical Center, Case Western Reserve, University, Cleveland, Ohio

MUSTAFA SECIL, MD
Professor of Radiology, Faculty of Medicine, Department of Radiology, Dokuz Eylul University, Izmir, Turkey

AHMET T. TURGUT, MD
Instructor of Radiology, Department of Radiology, Ankara Training and Research Hospital; and Karakusunlar, Ankara, Turkey

Contents

Palpable and Nonpalpable Breast Masses   277

Figen Başaran Demirkazik

> Breast ultrasonography (US) is not only useful in identifying the cystic content of breast masses but also in characterization of the solid masses. BI-RADS US lexicon, like the mammography lexicon, provides a standard terminology and assessment for breast US reports. In this article, the author examines the different types of cysts and solid lesions and examines how they should be treated. He focuses on categories 2 through 6 of the BI-RADS ultrasonography final assessment categories in American College of Radiology Imaging Network 6666 protocol, which indicate how and if cysts and lesions should be treated by biopsy or aspiration.

Ultrasound-Guided Breast Biopsies and Aspirations   289

Aysenur Oktay

> Ultrasonography is an efficient modality for guidance in interventional procedures in the breast. It is inexpensive and well tolerated by patients, and the risks are rare. Ultrasonographically guided breast core biopsy is commonly used in many centers as an accurate alternative to surgical biopsy for suspicious lesions. The advantages include decreased cost, absence of surgical scarring, no need for general anesthesia, and speed of the procedure. A good imaging–histologic correlation is necessary to decrease false-negative results. Other interventional procedures like cyst aspiration and needle localization can also be performed easily under ultrasound guidance.

Ultrasonography of the Postsurgical Breast Including Implants   295

Gul Esen

> Surgical interventions lead to alterations in breast tissue causing difficulty in interpretation of clinical and radiologic findings. Radiologists must detect and recognize these alterations to diagnose recurrent tumor while there is a chance for curative surgery. It is important to avoid overdiagnosis so as not to lead to unnecessary biopsies. Ultrasonography is an adjunct to mammography in evaluating post-treatment changes. Changes in the breast can be visualized clearly and directly without superimposition of structures. This article reviews sonographic findings in operated breasts, with a focus on the conservatively treated breast, and findings associated with excisional biopsies, breast implants, augmentation, and reduction mammoplasties.

vi Contents

Ectopic pregnancy (EP) is a challenging obstetrical entity in terms of diagnosis both for the clinican and the radiologist. It is still the leading cause of pregnancyrelated morbidity and mortality and fallopian tube is the commonest site of ectopic pregnancy. Incidence of rare forms of EP such as heterotopic and C-section scar EP is increasing because of the high rate of C-section surgeries and increased use of in vitro fertilization. Ultrasonography, combined with serum β-hCG level, is still the most effective radiologic modality in diagnosing EP. Ultrasound and color flow Doppler features of fallopian tube ectopic pregnancy and other rare types of ectopic pregnancies are reviewed and addressed in this article.

Vaginal bleeding is the most common cause of emergency care in the first trimester of pregnancy and accounts for the majority of premenopausal bleeding cases. Ultrasound evaluation combined with a quantitative beta human chorionic gonadotropin test is an established diagnostic tool to assess these patients. Spontaneous abortion because of genetic abnormalities is the most common cause of vaginal bleeding; ectopic pregnancy and gestational trophoblastic disease are other important causes and in all patients presenting with first trimester bleeding, ectopic pregnancy should be suspected and excluded, as it is associated with significant maternal morbidity and mortality. A thorough knowledge of the normal sonographic appearance of intrauterine gestation is essential to understand the manifestations of an abnormal gestation. Arteriovenous malformation of the uterus is a rare but important cause of vaginal bleeding in the first trimester, as it has to be differentiated from the more common retained products of conception, with which it is often mistaken.

Transabdominal sonography combined with high-frequency endovaginal ultrasound is considered the community standard for the performance of pelvic ultrasound for evaluation of an adnexal mass. Subjective evaluation of ovarian masses based on pattern recognition can achieve a sensitivity of 88% to 100% and specificity of 62% to 96%. Addition of color and power Doppler to grayscale imaging for pelvic mass evaluation increases the specificity in the range of 82% to 97% and increases the positive predictive value to 63% to 91%, aiding in subsequent evaluation and management. Pelvic sonography can confidently diagnose most of the benign adnexal masses and helps with triage of patients for surgical management in collaboration with tumor markers.

Postmenopausal bleeding (PMB) may be defined as recurrent vaginal bleeding in a menopausal woman at least 1 year after cessation of cycles. In postmenopausal bleeding, transvaginal ultrasonography (TVUS) is preferred over endometrial biopsy as an initial diagnostic tool. The use of TVUS decreases the need for invasive diagnostic procedures for women without abnormalities, and ultrasound increases the sensitivity of detecting abnormalities in women with postmenopausal bleeding. It is a less invasive procedure, is generally painless, has no complications, and may be more sensitive for detecting carcinoma than blind biopsy. Sonohysterography allows reliable differentiation between focal and diffuse endometrial and subendometrial lesions, with the most common being polyps and submucosal fibroids.

Endometriosis   399

Ercan Kocakoc, Shweta Bhatt, and Vikram Dogra

Ultrasound is the initial imaging modality for the assessment of endometriosis. Ovarian endometrioma, bladder endometriosis, and scar endometriosis are diagnosed reliably using ultrasound. The presence of hyperechoic wall foci and low-level echoes are very specific for endometriomas. Bilateral and multiple lesions may favor the diagnosis of endometriosis. Diagnosing deep endometriosis and adhesions is difficult with ultrasound, and laparoscopy is performed for diagnosis and staging. Endometriosis should be considered in the differential diagnosis of any woman of reproductive age who has pelvic pain or infertility.

Pelvic Congestion Syndrome   415

Musturay Karcaaltincaba, Deniz Karcaaltincaba, and Vikram S. Dogra

Radiologic imaging plays an important role in the diagnosis of pelvic congestion syndrome in patients with chronic pelvic pain. Pelvic congestion syndrome is a diagnosis of exclusion and differential diagnosis includes endometriosis, pelvic inflammatory disease, and ovarian cysts. In this syndrome, ovarian and pelvic veins are dilated owing to incompetence and venous reflux or to reversed venous flow associated with renal vein or ovarian vein stenosis. Ovarian vein venography is the gold standard for the definite diagnosis, which is usually performed before treatment. In this review, radiologic findings of pelvic congestion syndrome are discussed with their advantages and limitations. Role of interventional radiology and other treatment options including medical and surgical treatments are reviewed.

Sonohysterography: Technique and Clinical Applications   427

Phyllis Glanc, Carrie Betel, and Anna Lev-Toaff

This article examines the role of sonohysterography as an extension of the transvaginal ultrasound examination. This technique is used to improve visualization of the endometrial cavity and its relationship to the uterus. The authors find that it is well tolerated and causes few complications. The improved anatomic resolution increases diagnostic confidence and helps direct the patient to appropriate therapeutic options, potentially decreasing the need for more costly or invasive examinations. The addition of three-dimensional ultrasound makes the examination quicker and expands the utility of the procedure. The authors conclude that it will play a growing role in the evaluation of common gynecologic problems and in defining uterine pathology.

Ovarian Torsian and Its Mimics   451

Deniz Akata

During routine clinical practice, radiologists must often evaluate a wide range of cases with acute abdominal and pelvic pain. Although ultrasound is the primary imaging modality of choice for the evaluation of pelvic pain in the female patient, MR imaging has proven to be a valuable adjunct to characterize the adnexal mass. Computed tomography is mostly performed if ultrasound findings are equivocal or if the abnormality extends beyond the field of view achievable with the endovaginal probe. This article reviews the radiologic evaluation of ovarian torsion and its mimics. The complementary roles of ultrasound, CT, and MR imaging in the evaluation of various acute pelvic disorders is also discussed.

Color flow Doppler (CFD) imaging provides valuable information about the vascularity of tissue, organs, or systems. CFD imaging is commonly used during the evaluation of uterus and ovaries in addition to gray-scale imaging and is a helpful imaging modality in the diagnosis of various pathologic conditions in gynecology and obstetrics. The main limitation of CFD imaging is its user dependency that may lead to misdiagnosis owing to the artifacts or pitfalls derived from improper technique, incorrect use of imaging parameters, and unawareness of physical properties of the modality by the user. This article summarizes the CFD imaging technique, the optimization of imaging parameters, and the useful findings in the evaluation of uterus and ovaries.

Ultrasound Clinics

THE CLINICS ARE NOW AVAILABLE ONLINE!

Access your subscription at:
www.theclinics.com

GOAL STATEMENT

The goal of the *Ultrasound Clinics* is to keep practicing radiologists and radiology residents up to date with current clinical practice in ultrasound by providing timely articles reviewing the state of the art in patient care.

ACCREDITATION

The *Ultrasound Clinics* is planned and implemented in accordance with the Essential Areas and Policies of the Accreditation Council for Continuing Medical Education (ACCME) through the joint sponsorship of the University of Virginia School of Medicine and Elsevier. The University of Virginia School of Medicine is accredited by the ACCME to provide continuing medical education for physicians.

The University of Virginia School of Medicine designates this educational activity for a maximum of 15 *AMA PRA Category 1 Credits*™. Physicians should only claim credit commensurate with the extent of their participation in the activity.

The American Medical Association has determined that physicians not licensed in the US who participate in this CME activity are eligible for 15 *AMA PRA Category 1 Credits*™.

Credit can be earned by reading the text material, taking the CME examination online at http://www.theclinics.com/home/cme, and completing the evaluation. After taking the test, you will be required to review any and all incorrect answers. Following completion of the test and evaluation, your credit will be awarded and you may print your certificate.

FACULTY DISCLOSURE/CONFLICT OF INTEREST

The University of Virginia School of Medicine, as an ACCME accredited provider, endorses and strives to comply with the Accreditation Council for Continuing Medical Education (ACCME) Standards of Commercial Support, Commonwealth of Virginia statutes, University of Virginia policies and procedures, and associated federal and private regulations and guidelines on the need for disclosure and monitoring of proprietary and financial interests that may affect the scientific integrity and balance of content delivered in continuing medical education activities under our auspices.

The University of Virginia School of Medicine requires that all CME activities accredited through this institution be developed independently and be scientifically rigorous, balanced and objective in the presentation/discussion of its content, theories and practices.

All authors/editors participating in an accredited CME activity are expected to disclose to the readers relevant financial relationships with commercial entities occurring within the past 12 months (such as grants or research support, employee, consultant, stock holder, member of speakers bureau, etc.). The University of Virginia School of Medicine will employ appropriate mechanisms to resolve potential conflicts of interest to maintain the standards of fair and balanced education to the reader. Questions about specific strategies can be directed to the Office of Continuing Medical Education, University of Virginia School of Medicine, Charlottesville, Virginia.

The faculty and staff of the University of Virginia Office of Continuing Medical Education have no financial affiliations to disclose.

The authors/editors listed below have identified no professional or financial affiliations for themselves or their spouse/partner:

Deniz Akata, MD (Guest Editor); Matthew J. Bassignani, MD (Test Author); Carrie Betel, MD, FRCP(C); Shweta Bhatt, MD; Figen Başaran Demirkazik, MD; Vikram S. Dogra, MD (Guest Editor); Barton Dudlick (Acquisitions Editor); Elif Ergun, MD; Gul Esen, MD; Karthik Ganesan, DNB; Subramania Ganesan, MD; Phyllis Glanc, MD; Safiye Gurel, MD; Mukund Joshi, MD, FAMS; Fatih Kantarci, MD; Deniz Karcaaltincaba, MD; Musturay Karcaaltincaba, MD; Ercan Kocakoc, MD; Ashwin Lawande, DNB; Ismail Mihmanli, MD; Harsha Navani Munshi, DNB; Aysenur Oktay, MD; Deniz Cebi Olgun, MD; Raj Mohan Paspulati, MD; Mustafa Secil, MD; and Ahmet Tuncay Turgut, MD.

The authors/editors listed below have identified the following professional or financial affiliations for themselves or their spouse/partner:

Disclosure of Discussion of Non-FDA Approved Uses for Pharmaceutical Products and/or Medical Devices.
The University of Virginia School of Medicine, as an ACCME provider, requires that all faculty presenters identify and disclose any off-label uses for pharmaceutical and medical device products. The University of Virginia School of Medicine recommends that each physician fully review all the available data on new products or procedures prior to clinical use.

TO ENROLL

To enroll in the Ultrasound Clinics Continuing Medical Education program, call customer service at 1-800-654-2452 or visit us online at www.theclinics.com/home/cme. The CME program is available to subscribers for an additional fee of $205.00.

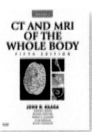 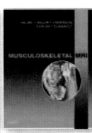 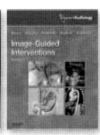 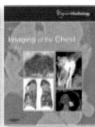 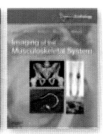
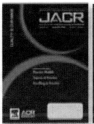 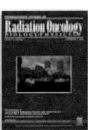 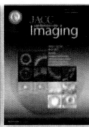 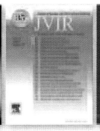 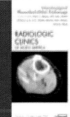 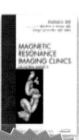
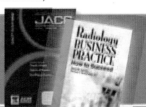

Preface

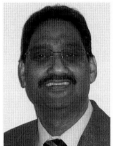
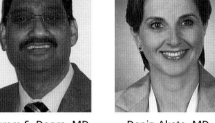

Vikram S. Dogra, MD   Deniz Akata, MD
Guest Editors

This issue of *Ultrasound Clinics* takes a close look at women's imaging, a subspecialty of radiology that focuses on the diagnosis and treatment of diseases and conditions unique to women, such as infertility, pregnancy, breast abnormalities, and genitourinary problems.

Ultrasound is one of the most frequently used diagnostic tools in women's imaging; it is safe, noninvasive, and affordable. The most well-known application of ultrasound for women is fetal imaging. However, in this issue of *Ultrasound Clinics*, we examine ultrasound's effectiveness in detecting palpable and nonpalpable breast masses, ectopic pregnancy, pregnancy-related genitourinary diseases, postmenopausal bleeding, endometriosis, pelvic congestion syndrome, saline sonohysterography, and ovarian torsion and its mimics. We also look at how ultrasound is used to guide breast biopsies and aspirations, and how color-flow Doppler techniques aid in evaluating the uterus and ovaries.

We have assembled a group of leading radiologists to provide information about the latest advances and newest developments in women's imaging. This information will be beneficial for obstetricians, gynecologists, sonographers, radiologists, and residents.

It is our privilege to be the guest editors for this issue of *Ultrasound Clinics*. We wish to thank Barton Dudlick at Elsevier, and our contributors for their outstanding work and cooperation.

Vikram S. Dogra, MD
Department of Imaging Sciences
University of Rochester Medical Center
601 Elmwood Avenue, Box 648
Rochester, NY 14642-8648, USA

Deniz Akata, MD
Department of Radiology
Hacettepe University Medical School
Sıhhiye 06100
Ankara
Turkey

E-mail addresses:
Vikram_Dogra@URMC.Rochester.edu
(V.S. Dogra)
dakata@hacettepe.edu.tr
(D. Akata)

Ultrasound Clin 3 (2008) xiii
doi:10.1016/j.cult.2008.10.003
1556-858X/08/$ – see front matter © 2008 Elsevier Inc. All rights reserved.

Palpable and Nonpalpable Breast Masses

Figen Başaran Demirkazık, MD

KEYWORDS

- Breast ultrasonography • BI-RADS • Palpable breast mass
- Nonpalpable breast mass • Breast cancer

Breast ultrasonography (US) has been used as an adjunct to clinical palpation and mammography for about 30 years. Although its main role in breast imaging had been to differentiate cysts from solid masses, improvements in equipment quality and software have enabled breast US to become a valuable imaging modality in the differential diagnosis of solid breast masses.[1,2] It may affect management in 64% of patients who have palpable masses or with mammographically detected masses and prevent unnecessary biopsies in 12.7% of solid masses.[3]

SONOGRAPHIC TECHNIQUE AND ANATOMY

Breast US should be performed with a linear array, high-frequency transducer of 7.5 MHz or higher. The patient should be placed in a supine oblique position to minimize the thickness of the breast portion being evaluated.[1] The patient's ipsilateral arm should be above the arm. The breast should be scanned in two perpendicular projections, either in radial and antiradial planes or in transverse and sagittal planes. Focal zone and gain settings should be adjusted to obtain high-quality images.

The breast skin is visualized on US as a hyperechoic line of less than 3 mm, except at the areola. Beneath the skin, subcutaneous hypoechoic fat lobules are found. In adults, breast parenchyma appears as a hyperechoic tissue between the subcutaneous and retromammary fat layers. Glandular tissue may be homogeneously echogenic or heterogeneous because of the hypoechoic ducts. Fat lobules may be interspersed. Cooper ligaments appear as fine curvilinear structures surrounding the subcutaneous fat lobules and supporting the

parenchyma. They may produce acoustic shadowing that should be distinguished from pathologic shadowing. The ribs and chest wall are recognized beneath the retromammary fat layer. The appropriate indications of breast US are summarized in **Box 1**.[4]

In addition to these accepted indications, some other areas are being researched:

- Supplemental screening of breast US after mammography in high-risk patients who have dense breasts[5]
- Preoperative evaluation of patients who have breast cancer for multicentric and multifocal disease, particularly when breast conserving surgery is planned[2]
- Evaluation of the axilla for occult lymph node metastasis in patients who have newly diagnosed breast cancer[6]

US findings should be correlated with mammographic features and clinical signs and symptoms.[2] If the patient has had breast US previously, the current findings should be compared with prior findings.

NONPALPABLE BREAST MASSES

Breast US is mostly used for the evaluation of palpable masses or nonpalpable masses that are detected on screening mammography. However, many unexpected masses may be found on targeted or whole-breast US. Screening US may detect small nonpalpable invasive breast cancers without mammographic findings. The American College of Radiology Imaging Network (ACRIN) has designed a multicenter randomized trial to

Department of Radiology, Hacettepe University, 06100, Sıhhiye, Ankara, Turkey
E-mail address: fdemirka@hacettepe.edu.tr

Ultrasound Clin 3 (2008) 277–287
doi:10.1016/j.cult.2008.08.003

determine whether screening whole-breast US is useful in the detection of cancers occult to mammography in high-risk women.[7]

After the worldwide acceptance of the Breast Imaging Reporting and Data System (BI-RADS) mammography lexicon, the American College of Radiology developed the US lexicon in 2003.[8] It provides a standardized terminology in reporting and classification of the lesions detected on breast US. Its use may improve the sonographic evaluation of the breast masses and clarify the indication for biopsy of suspicious lesions.[8]

Simple Cysts

US is highly accurate in differentiating cysts from solid masses. However, Berg and colleagues[9] reported that cysts smaller than 5 mm may not be characterized accurately. Use of lower-frequency transducers and tissue harmonic imaging may improve the characterization of a lesion as a cyst.[10] A thin-walled, anechoic mass with sharp borders and posterior acoustic enhancement is defined as a simple cyst (**Fig. 1**). Simple cysts are accepted as benign lesions and categorized as BI-RADS 2 (**Box 2**).[8]

Complicated Cysts

If a cyst has a fluid-debris layer or mobile internal echoes without a mural solid nodule, it should be

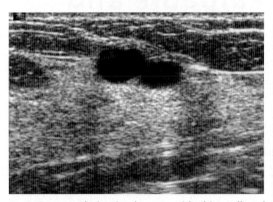

Fig. 1. Two anechoic, simple cysts with thin wall and posterior enhancement.

defined as a complicated cyst according to BI-RADS US lexicon (**Fig. 2**). If aspirated, the cyst fluid may be a clear yellow or turbid green color. Complicated cysts do not contain solid mural nodules. In the series of Kolb and colleagues,[11] fine needle aspiration was performed on 30 complicated cysts and all of the specimens were benign. None of the complicated cysts in 96 patients proved to be malignant. In another series, Buchberger and colleagues[12] reported that all of the 133 complex cysts were benign. Only one of the 308 complicated cysts in the series of Venta and colleagues[13] turned out to be malignant. In the series of Berg and colleagues,[10] all of the 38 complicated cysts were benign. The malignancy rate was 0.2% cumulatively in these studies. In ACRIN 6666 protocol, nonpalpable round or oval masses with imperceptible wall, posterior enhancement, and mobile internal echoes or mobile fluid-debris level with no evidence of intracystic mass, thick wall, or thick septations are defined as category 2 and dismissed as benign.[5,7]

Sometimes, it may be difficult to define a circumscribed, hypoechoic, oval lesion with homogeneous low-level internal echoes and with acoustic enhancement or no posterior features as a cystic or solid mass (**Fig. 3**). Also, a small simple cyst may look like solid nodules or complicated cysts. These nonpalpable, indeterminate lesions may be considered as probably benign (category 3) and a short-interval follow-up (at 6, 12, and 24 months) may be recommended.[7,9] Multiple and bilateral complicated cysts accompanied by simple cysts may be reevaluated in 1 year.[5] Any abnormal interval change should prompt biopsy.

Clustered Microcysts

With the improvement of high-resolution US equipment and software, pure clusters of microcysts without a solid component are detected more frequently than before in asymptomatic patients (**Fig. 4**). These microcysts are often due to apocrine metaplasia and other fibrocystic changes. Berg[14] reported that none of the 79 lesions characterized as clustered microcysts turned out to be malignant. Asymptomatic microlobulated or oval masses composed entirely of clustered microcysts with or without layering microcalcifications can be considered as probably benign (category 3) and followed up sonographically at 6, 12, and 24 months.[7]

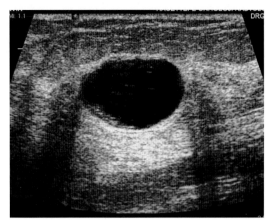

Fig. 2. Complicated cyst with mobile internal echoes (BI-RADS category 2).

Complex Masses

In BI-RADS US lexicon, lesions with anechoic (cystic) and echogenic (solid) components are defined as complex masses (**Fig. 5**). These lesions may have solid mural nodules or thick septations (≥ 5 mm). Berg and colleagues[14] reported that 7 of 23 cysts with a thick wall or thick septations were malignant (30%), whereas 4 of 18 cysts with a solid component proved to be malignant (22%). Abscesses, inflamed or ruptured cysts, or ducts and hematomas may manifest as a cystic mass with a thick wall or thick septations (**Fig. 6**). Fat necrosis may present as a thick-walled cystic lesion or a complex mass with cystic and solid components. It would be appropriate to follow up a thick-walled cystic lesion until resolution (2–3

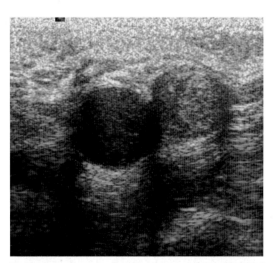

Fig. 3. Two round, circumscribed nodules (BI-RADS category 3); one is hypoechoic with homogeneous internal echoes (probably a complicated cyst) and the other is isoechoic.

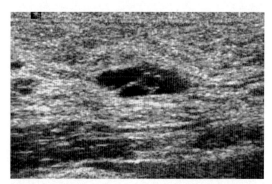

Fig. 4. Cluster of microcysts (BI-RADS category 3).

months) if the patient has a history of trauma or signs of infection. Biopsy should be performed if such a lesion enlarges.[14]

Berg and colleagues[10] indicated that complex masses with solid components require biopsy. These masses may be defined as category 4b (see **Box 2**). Benign and malignant papillary lesions may present as intracystic or intraductal solid masses. Central solitary papilloma present as an intraductal hypoechoic mass in an isolated duct. Although papillary lesions account for 4% to 5% of the lesions evaluated by biopsy, malignant papillary lesions are rare.[15] Percutaneous biopsy may underestimate papillary lesions. Liberman and colleagues[16] and Rosen and colleagues[15] reported that when percutaneous core biopsy reveals benign papillary lesions that are concordant with imaging findings, these lesions may be followed with imaging. However, surgical excision is necessary when the core biopsy reveals atypical papillary lesion or papillary ductal carcinoma in

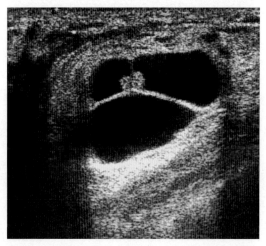

Fig. 5. Complex mass with a mural solid nodule (BI-RADS category 4b). Excision showed intracystic papilloma.

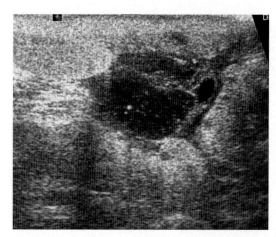

Fig. 6. Complex mass with thick wall and septations, and internal echoes (BI-RADS category 4a). Abscess was diagnosed with clinical findings and aspiration material.

situ or when the imaging findings are discordant with histologic findings.

Solid Masses

In the BI-RADS US lexicon, a mass is a space-occupying lesion that is seen on at least two projections.[8] It should be defined by its shape, orientation, margin, boundary, echo pattern, and posterior acoustic features. In addition, the effect of a mass on surrounding tissue is evaluated.

The shape of a mass may be round, oval, or irregular. The orientation of a mass is defined with reference to skin line. If the long axis of a mass parallels the skin line, its orientation is parallel and it is "wider than tall" (**Fig. 7**). If the anterior-posterior or vertical dimension is greater than the transverse or horizontal dimension, the mass has "not parallel" orientation (**Fig. 8**). Vertical orientation and "taller-than-wide" orientation are used as synonyms. Not parallel orientation can suggest spread of the lesion thorough tissue-plane boundaries, whereas parallel orientation indicates that the lesion is contained in one tissue plane.[17] A parallel or wider-than-tall orientation is a property of some benign masses; however, many carcinomas may also have this orientation.[8]

A circumscribed margin is one that is well defined or sharp, with an abrupt transition between the lesion and the surrounding tissue. Most circumscribed lesions have round or oval shapes (see **Fig. 7**). Circumscribed margins and oval shape shows uniform growth without involvement of surrounding tissue.[17] Fibroadenomas are typically oval, circumscribed masses with parallel orientation. They may have a few lobulations. A

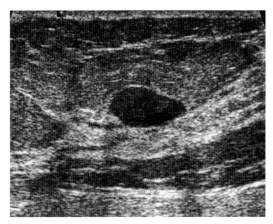

Fig. 7. Circumscribed, oval, hypoechoic, solid mass with parallel orientation (BI-RADS category 3). Core-needle biopsy confirmed fibroadenoma.

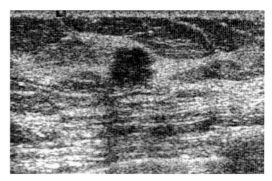

Fig. 9. Hypoechoic, round, nonpalpable mass with indistinct margins (BI-RADS category 4b). Pathology: invasive ductal carcinoma.

medullary carcinoma may also appear as a well-defined solid mass and resemble a fibroadenoma.[1]

If the margin of a mass is not circumscribed, it may be described as indistinct, angular, microlobulated, or spiculated (see **Fig. 8; Figs. 9–11**). A spiculated margin suggests an invasive nature of the lesion into the surrounding tissue.[17,18] Stavros and colleagues[18] reported that an ellipsoid shape (wider-than-tall) and well-circumscribed undulations are characteristics of benign lesions, whereas angular or spiculated margins and taller-than-wide orientation are features of malignant lesions. Hong and colleagues[17] reported that sonographic BI-RADS descriptors showing high predictive value for malignancy include spiculated margin (86%), irregular shape (62%), and nonparallel orientation (69%). In their series, the most common malignancy was invasive ductal carcinoma (120 of the 141 cancers). Sonographic

BI-RADS descriptors highly predictive of benign lesions include circumscribed margin (90%), parallel orientation (78%), and oval shape (84%).

Another sonographic feature is lesion boundary, which describes the transition zone between the mass and the surrounding tissue. Abrupt interface defines the sharp transition zone that can be imperceptible or a distinct, well-defined echogenic rim of any thickness. An echogenic halo defines a wide echogenic transition zone between the mass and the surrounding tissue (**Fig. 12**). This feature is associated with some carcinomas and abscesses.[8] In the series of Hong and colleagues,[17] an abrupt interface was more common in benign lesions than in malignant lesions, whereas an echogenic halo was more common in malignant lesions.

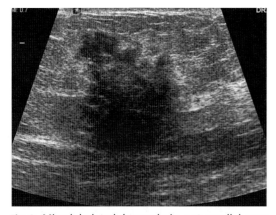

Fig. 8. Microlobulated, hypoechoic, not parallel mass with slight posterior shadowing (BI-RADS category 4c). Biopsy revealed invasive ductal carcinoma.

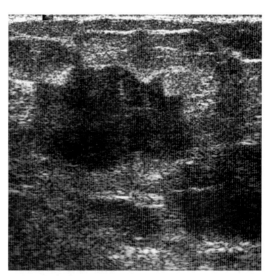

Fig. 10. Hypoechoic mass with angular margins (BI-RADS category 5). Core-needle biopsy revealed invasive ductal carcinoma.

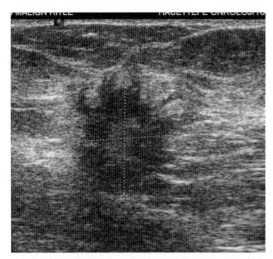

Fig. 11. Spiculated, hypoechoic mass (BI-RADS category 5). Pathology: invasive ductal carcinoma.

Uniformly hyperechogenic masses are uncommon lesions that may be lipomas or focal fibrosis (Fig. 13). Such lesions are considered as benign in the absence of any suspicious findings.[5,13,18] Hyperechoic masses with central hypoechoic to anechoic components suggesting fat necrosis are classified as probably benign in ACRIN 6666 study.[7]

In BI-RADS US lexicon, the posterior acoustic features of a mass are defined as no posterior acoustic features, enhancement, or shadowing. Enhancement may be detected not only behind cysts but also behind benign lesions and some malignant lesions. Shadowing is the result of posterior attenuation of the acoustic transmission

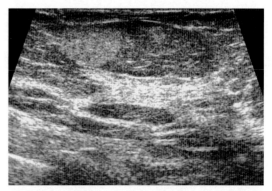

Fig. 13. Hyperechogenic lipoma in the subcutaneous fat (BI-RADS category 2).

as a result of fibrosis (see Fig. 8; Figs. 14, 15). Benign lesions, such as postsurgical scars, fibrous mastopathy, or cancers with desmoplastic reaction, may have posterior shadowing.[8] Stavros and colleagues[18] reported this finding as a sign of malignancy and indicated that low-grade infiltrating carcinomas and tubular carcinomas growing slowly enough to allow shadowing desmoplastic reaction, whereas highly cellular special-type tumors, such as papillary and medullary tumors, mucinous carcinomas, and necrotic infiltrating carcinomas, have normal or enhanced through-transmission of sound. In the series of Hong and colleagues,[17] benign and malignant lesions had posterior shadowing. Some fibroadenomas, even those without calcification, may have posterior shadowing; a mass with otherwise benign features may be categorized as category 3 (see Fig. 14). In contrast, if the margins of a mass with shadowing are not well defined, malignancy should be considered. Sometimes, shadowing may be the primary sign of malignancy without a discrete mass (see Fig. 15).[1]

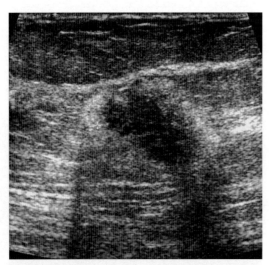

Fig. 12. Solid, not parallel mass with indistinct margins and echogenic halo (BI-RADS category 5). Surgical biopsy confirmed mixed invasive ductal and lobular carcinoma.

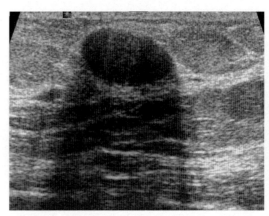

Fig. 14. Circumscribed, parallel, oval mass with posterior shadowing. It was classified as BI-RADS category 3 and remained stable during follow up.

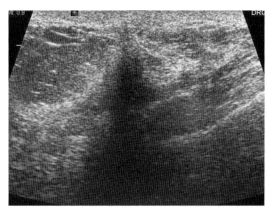

Fig.15. Intense shadowing of a mass without a discrete mass (BI-RADS category 5). Pathology: invasive ductal carcinoma.

Identification of surrounding tissue effects such as edema, architectural distortion, or changes to the Cooper's ligaments is infrequent. Lazarus and colleagues[19] reported that identification of surrounding tissue effects had a high predictive value for malignancy.

Although poorly characterized with US, calcifications can be recognized as echogenic foci in a mass, in fibroglandular tissue, or in fat (**Fig. 16**).[8] Microcalcifications, with or without a mass, found on breast US should always be categorized after full mammographic workup.

Vascularity is another sonographic feature that may be applied to evaluation of a mass. Vascularity may or may not be present in a mass, may be present immediately adjacent to a lesion, or diffusely increased vascularity may be evident in surrounding tissue. If a mass is avascular and has other features, it may be a cyst. Although no specific pattern is useful in differentiating benign

masses from malignant ones,[8] benign lesions may be avascular with poor and peripheral vascularity or may have one vascular pole with color Doppler US.[20] Malignant tumors may be hypervascular with irregular and abundant vascularization and more than one vascular pole (**Fig. 17**). However, musinous and in situ carcinomas and small invasive ductal carcinomas may be avascular, whereas some benign lesions such as phylloid tumors and fibroadenomas may be hypervascular. Spectral Doppler imaging is less useful than color Doppler US in differential diagnosis because of a wide overlap of parameters.[2]

Multiple and bilateral circumscribed lesions detected on mammographies have been shown to present a low risk for malignancy. Leung and Sickles[21] reported that the interval cancer rate associated with multiple masses (0.14%) detected on screening mammographies is much lower than the approximately 1% incident cancer rate reported for solitary, probably benign, lesions. Their interval cancers were low-grade and early-stage cancers. Thus, they concluded that short-term follow-up would be an overaggressive management and although their experience was limited, omission of short-term follow-up would probably not affect the patient's prognosis.

In the series of Graf and colleagues,[22] 7.6% of the women had multiple solid masses with similar, probably benign, sonographic features. Because all of them proved to be benign on follow-up, they suggested that multiplicity, especially if bilateral, increases the level of confidence in probably benign assessment.

The probably benign assessment (category 3)
The safety and efficacy of short-term follow-up for nonpalpable, probably benign lesions are accepted after several clinical studies.[18,22–24] Stavros and

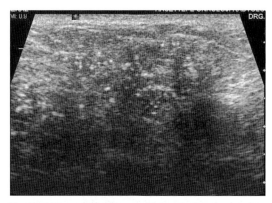

Fig. 16. Microcalcifications with posterior shadowing, defined as BI-RADS category 5 after full mammographic workup. Pathology: mixed invasive lobular and ductal carcinoma.

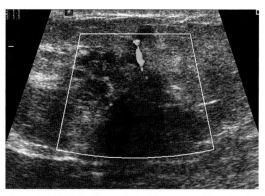

Fig. 17. Vascularity in an irregular mass with microlobulated and angular margins (BI-RADS category 5). Core-needle biopsy revealed invasive ductal carcinoma.

colleagues[18] reported that circumscribed, oval or gently lobulated, nonpalpable, hypoechoic masses had a risk for malignancy of less than 2%. Such lesions are classified as probably benign (category 3). Spiculations, angular margins, marked hypoechogenicity, shadowing, and presence of calcifications, duct extension, microlobulations, and a branching pattern are reported to be malignant features. They found that the addition of US to mammography increased sensitivity from 86% to 95% and specificity from 89% to 92%.

Rahbar and colleagues,[23] who evaluated 162 masses, reported that US features most predictive of a benign lesion were oval or round shape, circumscribed margins, presence of edge refraction, and width-to-anteroposterior (AP) dimension ratio. The features most predictive of breast cancers were spiculated or microlobulated margins, irregular shape, ill-defined margins, and a width-to-AP dimension ratio of 1.4 or less. They found that shape, margin, and width-to-AP dimension ratio are the most reliable criteria in differentiating benign from malignant breast masses. They reported that when these three criteria had been strictly applied to recommended biopsy, the overall cancer rate would have increased from 23% to 39%.

Skaane and colleagues[24] evaluated 336 masses (142 fibroadenomas and 194 invasive ductal carcinomas) with respect to shape, margin, echotexture, echogenicity, sound transmission, and surrounding tissue. They reported that irregular shape and margins, extensive hypoechogenicity, echogenic halo, shadowing, and distortion of the surrounding tissue were the findings with the highest predictive value of malignancy. Using strict sonographic criteria, they found a negative predictive value (NPV) of 100% in palpable and 96% in impalpable tumors.

In their recent study, Graf and colleagues[22] reported that the overall NPV for a circumscribed solid lesion with morphologic features characterized by US as BI-RADS category 3 was 99.8%. They evaluated 448 masses in 409 women; most of these masses (78%) were mammographically negative. Shape (oval or macrolobulated); circumscribed margins of the entire circumference of the lesion; width greater than height (long axis parallel to the skin surface); echogenicity (isoechoic or mildly hypoechoic); and no acoustic shadowing were the US criteria used to define a probably benign lesion (category 3).

These studies have shown that follow-up of solid lesions with benign features on sonography may be an alternative approach to biopsy, with a low false-negative rate. The malignancy rate should be less than 2% in probably benign assessment (category 3) in the BI-RADS. These lesions are not expected to change over the follow-up interval.[8] NPV for a category 3 mass detected on breast US was reported to be 92.3% to 95% in the studies of Constanini and colleagues[25] and Lee and colleagues.[26]

Mammographic findings besides US features should be taken into account in the assessment of BI-RADS categories. Sometimes, mammography may reveal malignant features (such as microcalcifications and spiculated margins). Follow-up studies are recommended 6, 12, and 24 months after the initial probably benign assessment (see Box 2). In mammographically occult masses, only a directed US examination is adequate. If the mass is visible on both mammography and US, follow-up mammography may be performed besides US. If the mass remains stable for 24 months, it may be accepted as benign (category 2).[19,27] A new or enlarging BI-RADS category 3 lesion needs histopathologic evaluation. Gordon and colleagues[28] evaluated 194 growing fibroadenomas and reported that these masses may be safely followed up after needle biopsy for all ages if the mean change in dimension in a 6-month interval is 20%.

Although three-dimensional US may provide a high-image quality, Cho and colleagues[29] reported that it does not increase diagnostic accuracy in the characterization of solid breast masses. Further evaluation in larger clinical trials is needed to reveal the efficacy of three-dimensional US in breast imaging.

The suspicious abnormality assessment (category 4)

Category 4 encompasses a wide range of findings, from complicated cysts to irregular, indistinct masses. Although in the official reports the standard category 4 language (suspicious abnormality–biopsy should be considered) is mandated by the Food and Drug Administration, the category may be subdivided into 4a, 4b, and 4c (see Box 2). This division will let the physician estimate the degree of suspicion. He/she may prefer to follow up a category 4a lesion, whereas he/she may rebiopsy or excise a category 4c lesion if the result of a fine- needle aspiration is benign.[8] Lazarus and colleagues[19] found the positive predictive values (PPVs) of categories 4a, 4b, and 4c to be 6%, 15%, and 53%, respectively. In their study, 52 lesions were evaluated by mammograms and sonograms, 32 were evaluated by mammograms alone, and 10 were evaluated by sonograms alone. Constani and colleagues[25] reported the PPV for category 4 to be 46.6%. Lee and colleagues[26] found that PPVs for categories 4a, 4b, and 4c were 26%, 89%, and 90%, respectively.

The highly suggestive of malignancy assessment (category 5)

A sonographically detected and categorized as BI-RADS 5 lesion should have a 95% or higher risk for malignancy. The PPVs for this category are reported to be 87.3% to 97%.[20,25,26] If percutaneous image-guided core-needle biopsy is performed for histopathologic diagnosis, the pathologic findings should be correlated with the imaging features to determine whether they are concordant. Discordant pathologic findings should be discussed with the pathologist and a repeat core-needle biopsy or surgical biopsy should be considered.

Few studies validate US lexicon. Lazarus and colleagues[19] reported that for sonographic descriptors, substantial interobserver agreement was obtained for lesion orientation, shape, and boundary (κ = 0.61, 0.66, and 0.69, respectively). Interobserver agreement was moderate for lesion margin and posterior acoustic features (κ = 0.40 for both) and fair agreement for lesion echo pattern (κ = 0.29). Lee and colleagues[26] reported good inter- and intraobserver agreement with the BI-RADS lexicon for US and concluded that the use of BI-RADS lexicon can provide a consistent description of US findings and an accurate assessment of breast lesions.

PALPABLE MASSES

The primary role of breast US in the evaluation of a palpable mass is to determine whether it is cystic or solid. If the patient is older than 30 years, mammography should be the initial imaging modality. US should be performed if the mass is not visible on mammography because of its location or breast density. The accuracy of US in adjunct to mammography is high in palpable lesions. Soo and colleagues[30] reported that when mammography and targeted US were negative for palpable masses, the NPV value for cancer was 99.8%. In the study of Dennis and colleagues,[31] none of the 600 lumps in 486 women with no focal sonographic mass or mammographic finding in the area of clinical concern were malignant.

Cystic Lesions

Palpable simple cysts may be aspirated if the patient has symptoms, such as pain or a very large lump. Cytologic evaluation is not needed when the cyst fluid is typical for a benign cyst (cloudy yellow or greenish black).[10] Because Ciatto and colleagues[32] found only 5 papillomas with frankly bloody cyst fluid in 6,782 cysts, they recommend the use of cytology only when the aspiration fluid is bloody. Some other studies have suggested

discarding nonbloody aspiration fluid.[33,34] Cysts may recur after initial aspiration. Although some studies report that recurrent cysts may have apocrine epithelium, carrying a greater risk for subsequent breast cancer than those with flattened epithelial cysts,[35] Berg and colleagues[10] indicated that excision of a recurrent cyst may not be necessary.

Symptomatic complicated cysts are placed in category 4a and should be aspirated.[7,8] Cytologic evaluation is necessary only for bloody fluid. If clinical finding suggest an abscess, aspiration fluid should be sent for culture and Gram staining.[10]

Solid Masses

Today, the standard approach is to biopsy a palpable solid lesion, even if it has sonographic features suggesting a probably benign lesion. How palpability will affect the management of solid masses with benign sonographic features with parallel orientation is being researched.

Graf and colleagues[36] evaluated 157 palpable masses in 152 patients, classified as probably benign at initial mammography and US. The masses were solid, with round, oval, macrolobulated, circumscribed margins, and parallel orientation. Forty-four patients were biopsied and proved to have benign masses (fibroadenomas) and 108 patients were followed up at 6-month intervals for 2 years, followed by 12-month intervals. In this study, none of the 157 masses turned out to be malignant, so the likelihood of malignancy was estimated to be less than 2%.

In the fourth edition of the BI-RADS atlas, category 4a is recommended for a finding needing intervention but with low suspicion for malignancy. A palpable, partially circumscribed solid mass with US features suggestive of a fibroadenoma may be categorized as category 4a and a 6-month or routine follow-up after a benign biopsy or cytology is appropriate.[7,8]

SUMMARY

Breast US is not only useful in identifying the cystic content of breast masses but also in characterization of the solid masses. BI-RADS US lexicon, like the mammography lexicon, provides a standard terminology and assessment for breast US reports. Nonpalpable simple cysts and complicated cysts with mobile internal echoes or fluid-debris level are benign lesions and may be dismissed (category 2). Circumscribed, hypoechoic, nonpalpable solid lesions with parallel orientation may be categorized as probably benign (category 3) and followed up safely. Nonpalpable complicated cysts with homogeneous low-level echoes and clustered microcysts are other category 3 lesions. Cystic lesions with solid components and solid masses with irregular shape, microlobulated, indistinct, angular, or spiculated margins, and posterior acoustic shadowing, should be biopsied (category 4 and 5). Needle biopsy results should be correlated with sonographic findings. Rebiopsy should be considered if the findings are discordant. Preliminary studies suggest that palpable masses with benign features may be managed like probably benign nonpalpable masses after full diagnostic workup.

REFERENCES

1. Mehta TS. Current uses of ultrasound in the evaluation of the breast. Radiol Clin North Am 2003;41(4): 841–56.
2. Yang W, Dempsey PJ. Diagnostic breast ultrasound: current status and future directions. Radiol Clin North Am 2007;45(5):845–61.
3. Bassett LW, Kimme-Smith C, Sutherland LK, et al. Automated and hand-held breast US: effect on patient management. Radiology 1987;165(1):103–8.
4. ACR practice guideline for the performance of a breast ultrasound examination. January 10, 2007. Available at: http://www.acr.org/SecondaryMainMenu Categories/quality_safety/guidelines/us/us_breast. aspx. Accessed September 16, 2008.
5. Berg WA. Supplemental screening sonography in dense breasts. Radiol Clin North Am 2004;42(5): 845–51.
6. Mendelson EB. Problem-solving ultrasound. Radiol Clin North Am 2004;42(5):909–18.
7. ACRIN 6666 protocol. November 30, 2007. Available at: http://acrin.org/6666_protocol.html. Accessed May 20, 2008.
8. Mendelson EB, Baum JK, Berg WA, et al. American College of Radiology BI-RADS: ultrasound. 1st edition. In: Breast imaging reporting and data system: BI-RADS atlas. 4th edition. Reston (VA): American College of Radiology; 2003.
9. Berg WA, Blume JD, Cormack JB, et al. Lesion detection and characterization in a breast US phantom: results of the ACRIN 6666 Investigators. Radiology 2006;239(3):693–702.
10. Berg WA, Campassi CI, Ioffe OB. Cystic lesions of the breast: sonographic-pathologic correlation. Radiology 2003;227(1):183–91.
11. Kolb TM, Lichy J, Newhouse JH. Occult cancer in women with dense breasts: detection with screening US-diagnostic yield and tumor characteristics. Radiology 1998;207(1):191–9.
12. Buchberger W, DeKoekkoek-Doll P, Springer P, et al. Incidental findings on sonography of the breast: clinical significance and diagnostic workup. AJR Am J Roentgenol 1999;173(4):921–7.
13. Venta LA, Kim JP, Pelloski CE, et al. Management of complex breast cysts. AJR Am J Roentgenol 1999; 173(5):1331–6.
14. Berg WA. Sonographically depicted breast clustered microcysts: is follow-up appropriate? AJR Am J Roentgenol 2005;185(4):952–9.
15. Rosen EL, Bentley RC, Baker JA, et al. Imaging-guided core needle biopsy of papillary lesions of the breast. AJR Am J Roentgenol 2002;179(5):1185–92.
16. Liberman L, Bracero N, Vuolo MA, et al. Percutaneous large-core biopsy of papillary breast lesions. AJR Am J Roentgenol 1999;172(2):331–7.
17. Hong AS, Rosen EL, Soo MS, et al. BI-RADS for sonography: positive and negative predictive values of sonographic features. AJR Am J Roentgenol 2005;184(4):1260–5.
18. Stavros AT, Thickman D, Rapp CL, et al. Solid breast nodules: use of sonography to distinguish between benign and malignant lesions. Radiology 1995; 196(1):123–34.
19. Lazarus E, Mainiero MB, Schepps B, et al. BI-RADS lexicon for US and mammography: interobserver variability and positive predictive value. Radiology 2006;239(2):385–91.
20. Giuseppetti GM, Baldassarre S, Marconi E. Color Doppler sonography. Eur J Radiol 1998;27(Suppl 2): S254–8.
21. Leung JW, Sickles EA. Multiple bilateral masses detected on screening mammography: assessment of need for recall imaging. AJR Am J Roentgenol 2000;175(1):23–9.
22. Graf O, Helbich TH, Hopf G, et al. Probably benign breast masses at US: is follow-up an acceptable alternative to biopsy? Radiology 2007;244(1):87–93.
23. Rahbar G, Sie AC, Hansen GC, et al. Benign versus malignant solid breast masses: US differentiation. Radiology 1999;213(3):889–94.
24. Skaane P, Engedal K. Analysis of sonographic features in the differentiation of fibroadenoma and invasive ductal carcinoma. AJR Am J Roentgenol 1998;170(1):109–14.
25. Costantini M, Belli P, Ierardi C, et al. Solid breast mass characterization: use of the sonographic BI-RADS classification. Radiol Med (Torino) 2007; 112(6):877–94.
26. Lee HJ, Kim EK, Kim MJ, et al. Observer variability of Breast Imaging Reporting and Data System (BI-RADS) for breast ultrasound. Eur J Radiol 2008;65(2):293–8.
27. Leung JW, Sickles EA. The probably benign assessment. Radiol Clin North Am 2007;45(5):773–89.
28. Gordon PB, Gagnon FA, Lanzkowsky L. Solid breast masses diagnosed as fibroadenoma at fine-needle aspiration biopsy: acceptable rates of growth at long-term follow-up. Radiology 2003;229(1):233–8.
29. Cho N, Moon WK, Cha JH, et al. Differentiating benign from malignant solid breast masses:

comparison of two-dimensional and three-dimensional US. Radiology 2006;240(1):26–32.

30. Soo MS, Rosen EL, Baker JA, et al. Negative predictive value of sonography with mammography in patients with palpable breast lesions. AJR Am J Roentgenol 2001;177(5):1167–70.

31. Dennis MA, Parker SH, Klaus AJ, et al. Breast biopsy avoidance: the value of normal mammograms and normal sonograms in the setting of a palpable lump. Radiology 2001;219(1):186–91.

32. Ciatto S, Cariaggi P, Bulgaresi P. The value of routine cytologic examination of breast cyst fluids. Acta Cytol 1987;31(3):301–4.

33. Hindle WH, Arias RD, Florentine B, et al. Lack of utility in clinical practice of cytologic examination of nonbloody cyst fluid from palpable breast cysts. Am J Obstet Gynecol 2000;182(6):1300–5.

34. Smith DN, Kaelin CM, Korbin CD, et al. Impalpable breast cysts: utility of cytologic examination of fluid obtained with radiologically guided aspiration. Radiology 1997;204(1):149–51.

35. Dixon JM, Lumsden AB, Miller WR. The relationship of cyst type to risk factors for breast cancer and the subsequent development of breast cancer in patients with breast cystic disease. Eur J Cancer Clin Oncol 1985;21(9):1047–50.

36. Graf O, Helbich TH, Fuchsjaeger MH, et al. Follow-up of palpable circumscribed noncalcified solid breast masses at mammography and US: can biopsy be averted? Radiology 2004;233(3):850–6.

Ultrasound-Guided Breast Biopsies and Aspirations

Aysenur Oktay, MD

KEYWORDS

• Breast • Ultrasound • Biopsy

The development and widespread use of imaging-guided interventional procedures have expanded the role of radiologists in the management of breast diseases. Imaging-guided percutaneous needle biopsy techniques have become an alternative to open surgical biopsies in the diagnosis of breast cancer.[1–5] The advantages of the imaging-guided biopsy technique over open biopsy include decreased cost, absence of surgical scarring, no need for general anesthesia, and speed of the procedure. Its use has decreased the number of unnecessary surgical biopsies for benign lesions and reduced the number of surgical procedures required in patients who have a diagnosis of cancer.[6–9] Real-time visualization, lack of ionizing radiation, and the use of nondedicated equipment are other advantages of ultrasound (US) guidance. US-guided procedures are generally better tolerated than other biopsy methods because patients are supine for the procedure and breast compression is not necessary.[10–14]

Needle biopsies using either fine needle aspiration or the core technique can be performed under US guidance for any lesion easily visible on US. The vacuum-assisted system can also be used with US in selected cases.[14,15] Most US apparent abnormalities selected for biopsy are the American College of Radiology's Breast Imaging Reporting Data System (BI-RADS) 4 (suspicious) or 5 (highly suggestive of malignancy) lesions. Other lesions on which biopsy can be performed are complex cysts with mural nodules and, in some cases, BI-RADS 3 (probably benign) masses. Most US-guided biopsy procedures are performed on masses.

TECHNIQUE
Preprocedure Preparation

The patient is advised to discontinue anticoagulant therapy and aspirin at least 1 week before biopsy. An informed consent should be obtained before performing the biopsy or cyst aspiration. At the time of biopsy, a prepared biopsy kit containing all of the necessary biopsy items would facilitate the procedure. The materials needed for biopsy include needles, gauze, scalpel blade, sterile drape, and lidocaine.

The patient is positioned supine or oblique, depending on the location of the lesion. To provide a sterile place during the procedure, the transducer is put in a sterile plastic sheath or sterile glove containing coupling gel. A small amount of sterile gel or antiseptic solution such as povidone-iodine at the skin surface can provide acoustic transmission. Local anesthesia is required for the core needle biopsy and localization procedures. The skin is cleaned with povidone-iodine and alcohol. Lidocaine hydrochloride 1% is used to anesthetize the skin and breast tissue around the lesion. A tiny skin nick is done to allow the biopsy needle to pass into the breast.[13,14] After the procedure, application of pressure to the biopsy site will decrease bruising.

High-resolution, real-time US machines are appropriate for performing US-guided biopsies in the breast. Using high-frequency linear array and small transducers (10–13 MHz) provides better resolution, and makes the operation easier.[15] Multiband transducers are optimal for breast imaging because they provide excellent near-field resolution while maintaining good depth penetration, which is necessary for deep lesions.[16] The focal

Department of Radiology, Medical School of Ege University, Izmir, Turkey
E-mail address: aysenur.oktay@ege.edu.tr

Ultrasound Clin 3 (2008) 289–294
doi:10.1016/j.cult.2008.08.004

zone should be placed at the level of the lesion. Two techniques are used for targeting the lesions, the use of needle guides and the "free-hand" technique. The most commonly used one is the free-hand technique, which allows the operator flexibility and an easier approach. In this technique, the transducer is held by the operator's nondominant hand and stabilizes the lesion in the appropriate position. The needle in the dominant hand is advanced parallel to the US beam and can be visualized in real time when advancing toward the lesion. The lesions can be targeted by oblique, horizontal, or vertical needle approaches. Needle visualization is better in the first two approaches (**Fig. 1**). If visualizing the needle is difficult, a sweeping motion is used to identify it. It is preferable that the biopsy needle be parallel to the chest wall throughout the procedure. A larger, coaxial needle can be used to take multiple samples, especially in dense breasts.[14] It is important to see the tip of the needle and the lesion before advancing or firing into the lesion. For core

biopsy, the needle tip is placed at the edge of the lesion. The position should be checked to ensure that the distal throw of the needle will not result in chest wall injury.[16] After firing the needle, it must be confirmed that the needle traversed the lesion on both longitudinal and transverse images.

CYST ASPIRATION

US can characterize simple breast cysts accurately. They usually do not require aspiration; however, if cysts are painful, aspiration can be performed for relief of symptoms. Complicated cysts showing low-level internal echoes or nonpalpable lesions that cannot be classified reliably as simple or complicated cysts can be aspirated under US guidance to confirm the diagnosis. For complex masses containing cystic and solid components, and for intracystic mural nodules, tissue diagnosis is recommended instead of aspiration.[15,17] The presence of a residual mass is also an indication for biopsy.

For cyst aspiration, a 21-gauge needle is used most often. If it is bloody, the aspirated fluid should be sent for cytologic examination. For nonbloody aspirates, no consensus has been reached on the necessity for cytologic examination.[17–19]

FINE NEEDLE ASPIRATION BIOPSY

Fine needle aspiration biopsy (FNAB) is widely used for symptomatic patients. It can be done under US guidance for nonpalpable solid lesions.[20–25] A fine-gauge needle with a 10- to 20-mL syringe is used to perform aspiration. Lesions are sampled with to-and-fro and rotational movements of the needle with applied suction. Cytologic smears are air dried for Giemsa stain or fixed immediately with absolute alcohol for Papanicolaou stain.[13]

FNAB of the breast depends on the operators' technique and the skill of the cytopathologists. On-site evaluation to establish the adequacy of the samples may increase the accuracy of the results. A meta-analysis of 31 articles reported a mean absolute sensitivity and specificity of 62.4% and 86.9%, respectively, for stereotactic FNAB, and 90.5% and 98.3%, respectively, for core biopsy.[20] In a multicenter randomized trial, Radiation Oncology Diagnosis Group V (RDOGV), stereotactically guided and US-guided FNAB of nonpalpable masses were studied.[21] The reported overall accuracy for US-guided FNAB was 77%, compared with 99.2% for core needle biopsy of masses. In addition, in situ and invasive carcinoma cannot be distinguished reliably with FNAB.

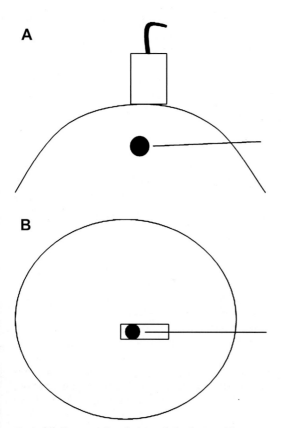

Fig. 1. (*A*) Cross-sectional view of the breast. The needle is approaching the lesion on a path parallel to the chest wall and perpendicular to the US beam. (*B*) Overhead view of the breast. The needle is aligned with the long axis of the transducer.

Therefore, in many centers, core needle biopsy is preferred over FNAB.[4,21,22]

ULTRASOUND-GUIDED LOCALIZATION OF NONPALPABLE BREAST LESIONS

Real-time US can be used for guidance in the localization of nonpalpable lesions with hook wires. Any lesion easily seen on US can be localized by this technique. Lesions in difficult locations for mammography localization can be targeted with US.[23,24] US guidance provides a shorter path to the lesion than mammographic guidance, with an oblique approach possible. The advantage of US guidance for needle localization is the ability to visualize the needle in real time. After the localization, mammograms should be taken for documentation. After excision, in addition to the specimen radiography, US should be performed.[25] Superficial lesions that are visible on US can be localized by simply marking the skin.

A metallic tumor marker can also be placed into the tumor if preoperative neoadjuvant chemotherapy is planned. The marker is used as a guide for subsequent preoperative needle placement, in case the tumor completely disappears after chemotherapy. Marker placement can also be performed after large core biopsy of subtle lesions, to facilitate localization when subsequent excision becomes necessary.[15,26]

ULTRASOUND-GUIDED CORE NEEDLE/VACUUM-ASSISTED BIOPSY

US-guided biopsy with a 14-gauge automated large core device was first described by Parker and colleagues[27] in 1993. Since then, US-guided percutaneous biopsy is widely used as an alternative to surgical biopsy in the diagnosis of nonpalpable lesions.[3–5,28] Fourteen-gauge needles have been found to be more accurate than smaller-diameter core biopsy needles (**Fig. 2**).[29] Fishman and colleagues[30] and Sauer and colleagues[31] reported that an accurate diagnosis can be obtained with a minimum of four core samples by using a 14-gauge needle with US guidance. A larger size (13-gauge) coaxial needle can be used to take multiple samples.[14] Handheld vacuum-assisted core biopsy devices are also used with either 11- or 8-gauge needles.[32] This technique allows rapid acquisition of multiple tissue specimens in an automated fashion. Vacuum-assisted devices allow the acquisition of larger amounts of tissue by using suction. False-negative results and histologic underestimation are less frequent for 11-gauge vacuum-assisted biopsy than for 14-gauge core needle biopsy.[14] During the

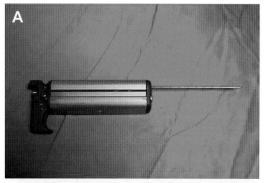

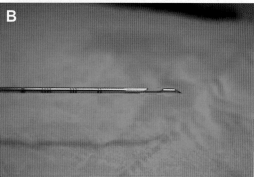

Fig. 2. (*A*) Device for automatic needle biopsy. (*B*) Cutting space of core biopsy needle.

procedure, it is important to document the biopsy needle before firing the device and while traversing the lesion after firing (**Fig. 3**). The needle position should be confirmed in the longitudinal and transverse planes (**Fig. 4**). After biopsy of subtle lesions, it may be useful to place a marker clip for subsequent localization.

The complications, although rare, after 14-gauge core needle biopsy include pneumothorax, ecchymosis, hematoma, implant rupture, and infection.[1,33] Seeding of the tumor cells along the needle track has been questioned; however, studies have not shown an increase in recurrence rates. Epithelial displacement, in which ductal carcinoma in situ may be confused with invasive carcinoma, is not an important issue for US-guided biopsies because most of these biopsies are performed for masses.[14,34] Not obtaining a diagnostic tissue sampling is another possible problem with core biopsy.

ULTRASOUND-GUIDED MARKER PLACEMENT

After core or vacuum-assisted biopsy, markers can be placed in breast masses using US guidance. This procedure can be performed for carcinomas in which neoadjuvant chemotherapy is planned. In noncalcified carcinomas having good

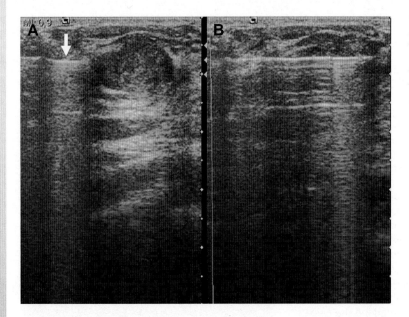

Fig. 3. (*A*) The needle tip (*white arrow*) is placed at the edge of the lesion before advancing into the lesion in prefire position. (*B*) Postfire image with the needle traversing the lesion.

response to chemotherapy, the tumor may disappear completely and cannot be shown by clinical or radiologic examination. In such cases, the markers will guide subsequent preoperative needle localization for surgical excision of the tumor bed. Marker placement can also be performed after large core biopsy of subtle lesions, to facilitate localization when subsequent excision becomes necessary, and after complex cyst aspiration when a suspicious hemorrhagic fluid is obtained and the cyst is completely evacuated.[15,26]

A coaxial needle is used for the procedure. The metallic marker is deployed while the needle tip is in the center of the mass. After withdrawing the

needle, mammograms are obtained to document the position of the marker.[15]

IMAGING–HISTOLOGIC CORRELATION

For successful biopsy results, good teamwork between radiologist and pathologist is important. Pathologic results must be correlated with the imaging findings.[3,4,28,32,35] The pathologist must have adequate information about the clinical and imaging findings of the lesion and the likelihood of malignancy when evaluating the specimens. BI-RADS is generally used to assess the likelihood of malignancy.[36]

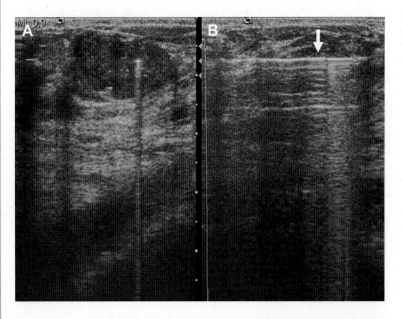

Fig. 4. The needle traversing the lesion is seen on both (*A*) transverse and (*B*) longitudinal images (*white arrow*).

To confirm results, imaging and pathologic findings are compared as in the "triple test" used in the FNAB protocol. Whether the pathology results adequately explain the imaging findings is ascertained. Careful imaging–histologic correlation will allow the detection of a substantial number of false-negative results immediately after needle biopsy, thereby avoiding delays in diagnosis.[14] In patients who have concordant imaging–pathology findings, a 6-month follow-up is recommended. The estimated false-negative rate in concordant benign lesions is less than 2%.[37] Concordant malignant cases are referred to surgery for definitive treatment. Preoperative diagnosis of malignancy usually results in a single therapeutic surgery. A discordant finding warrants repeat biopsy, usually in the form of a surgical biopsy. Imaging–pathology discordance rates for US-guided core biopsies using 14-gauge needles have ranged from 2.0% to 7.7%.[3,28,32,38,39] Sauer and colleagues[31] reported a 3.0% rate of discordance among 962 lesions subjected to 14-gauge core biopsy with US guidance. Rebiopsy of these lesions showed 27.6% malignancy. In Libermans's[39] study, the discordance rate was 3.3% among 580 cases, and 10.5% were cancers at rebiopsy of these lesions.

The limitations of core needle biopsy are sampling error and underestimation of disease. When the imaging–histologic results are discordant because of these limitations, excisional biopsy should be performed. In some benign and high-risk pathology results, underestimation of disease is a possibility. It is well established that after a core biopsy diagnosis of atypical ductal hyperplasia (ADH), open surgical biopsy is required. Underestimation rates for ADH on core needle biopsy range from 15% to 50%. Even with the use of an 11-gauge vacuum-assisted device, underestimation rates have been reported in 20% to 25% of diagnoses of ADH. The potential also exists to underestimate disease in the diagnosis of ductal carcinoma in situ on core biopsy. On the other hand, the need for open excisional biopsy is controversial in diagnoses of lobular neoplasia, radial scar, papillary lesions, and columnar cell lesions.[40–43]

The results of US-guided core needle biopsies should be monitored on a continuous basis. The results of subsequent surgical procedures, the number of cancer diagnoses, the number of inconclusive or inadequate samples, the number of complications, and follow-up findings should be monitored.[16]

SUMMARY

US is an efficient modality for guidance interventional procedures in the breast. It is inexpensive and well tolerated by patients, and the risks are rare. US-guided breast core biopsy is commonly used in many centers as an accurate alternative to surgical biopsy for suspicious lesions. A good imaging–histologic correlation is necessary to decrease false-negative results. Other interventional procedures like cyst aspiration and needle localization can also be performed easily under US guidance.

REFERENCES

1. Parker SH, Burbank F, Jackman RJ. Percutaneous large-core breast biopsy: a multi-institutional study. Radiology 1994;193:359–64.
2. Brenner RJ, Bassett LW, Fajardo LL, et al. Stereotactic core-needle breast biopsy: a multi-institutional prospective trial. Radiology 2001;218:866–72.
3. Smith DN, Rosenfield Darling ML, Meyer JE, et al. The utility of ultrasonographically guided large-core needle biopsy: results from 500 consecutive breast biopsies. J Ultrasound Med 2001;20:43–9.
4. Fajardo LL, Pisano ED, Caudry DJ, et al. Stereotactic and sonographic large-core biopsy of nonpalpable breast lesions: results of the Radiologic Diagnostic Oncology Group V study. Acad Radiol 2004;11: 293–308.
5. Crowe JP Jr, Rim A, Patrick RJ, et al. Does core needle breast biopsy accurately reflect breast pathology? Surgery 2003;134:523–6 [discussion: 526–8].
6. Liberman L, Goodstine SL, Dershaw DD, et al. One operation after percutaneous diagnosis of nonpalpable breast cancer: frequency and associated factors. Am J Roentgenol 2002;178:673–9.
7. Liberman L, Fachs MC, Dershaw DD, et al. Impact of stereotaxic core breast biopsy on cost of diagnosis. Radiology 1995;195:633–7.
8. Liberman L, LaTrenta LR, Dershaw DD. Impact of core biopsy on the surgical management of impalpable breast cancer: another look at margins. Am J Roentgenol 1997;169:1464–5.
9. Lind DS, Minter R, Steinbach B, et al. Stereotactic core biopsy reduces the reexcision rate and the cost of mammographically detected cancer. J Surg Res 1998;78:23–6.
10. Mainiero MB, Gareen IF, Bird CE, et al. Preferential use of sonographically guided biopsy to minimize patient discomfort and procedure time in a percutaneous image-guided breast biopsy program. J Ultrasound Med 2002;21:1221–6.
11. Rubin E, Mennemeyer ST, Desmond RA, et al. Reducing the cost of diagnosis of breast carcinoma: impact of ultrasound and imaging-guided biopsies on a clinical breast practice. Cancer 2001;91: 324–32.
12. Staren ED, O'Neill TP. Ultrasound-guided needle biopsy of the breast. Surgery 1999;126:629–34.

13. Fornage BD, Coan JD, David CL. Ultrasound-guided needle biopsy of the breast and other interventional procedures. Radiol Clin North Am 1992; 30:167–85.

14. Comstock CE. US guided interventional procedures. In: Feig SA. editor. Syllabus RSNA, breast imaging. Oak Brook (IL): RSNA, Inc.; 2005. p. 155–168.

15. Jackson VP, Reynolds HE. Other ultrasonographically guided interventional procedures. In: Bassett LW, Jackson VP, Fu KL, Fu YS, editors. Diagnosis of diseases of the breast. Philadelphia: Elsevier; 2005. p. 323–32.

16. Harvey JA, Moran RE, DeAngelis GA. Technique and pitfalls of ultrasound-guided core needle biopsy of the breast. Semin Ultrasound CT MR 2000;21:362–74.

17. Kinnard D. Results of cytological study of fluid aspirated from breast cysts. Am Surg 1975;41:505–6.

18. Ciatto S, Cariaggi P, Bularesi P. The value of routine cytologic examination of breast cyst fluids. Acta Cytol 1987;31:301–4.

19. Hindle WH, Arias RD, Florentine B, et al. Lack of utility in clinical practice of cytologic examination of nonbloody cyst fluid from palpable breast cysts. Am J Obstet Gynecol 2000;182:1300–5.

20. Britton PD. Fine needle aspiration or core biopsy. Breast 1999;8:1–4.

21. Pisano ED, Fajardo LL, Caudry DJ, et al. Fine-needle aspiration biopsy of nonpalpable breast lesions in a multicenter clinical trial: results from the Radiologic Diagnostic Oncology Group V. Radiology 2001;219: 785–92.

22. Clarke D, Sudhakaran N, Gateley CA. Replace fine needle aspiration cytology with automated core biopsy in the triple assessment of breast cancer. Ann R Coll Surg Engl 2001;83:110–2.

23. Edeiken BS, Fornage BD, Bedi DG, et al. US-guided implantation of metallic markers for permanent localization of the tumor bed in patients with breast cancer who undergo preoperative · chemotherapy. Radiology 1999;213:895–900.

24. Yang W, Dempsey PJ. Diagnostic breast ultrasound: current status and future directions. Radiol Clin North Am 2007;45:845–61.

25. Frenna T, Meyer J, Sonnenfeld M. Ultrasound of breast biopsy specimens. Radiology 1994;190:573.

26. Phillips SW, Gabriel H, Comstock CE, et al. Sonographically guided metallic clip placement after core needle biopsy of the breast. AJR Am J Roentgenol 2000;175:1353–5.

27. Parker SH, Jobe WE, Dennis MA, et al. US-guided automated large-core breast biopsy. Radiology 1993;187:507–11.

28. Crystal P, Koretz M, Shcharynsky S, et al. Accuracy of sonographically guided 14-gauge core-needle biopsy: results of 715 consecutive breast biopsies with at least two-year follow-up of benign lesions. J Clin Ultrasound 2005;33:47–52.

29. Nath ME, Robinson TM, Tobon H, et al. Automated large-core needle biopsy of surgically removed breast lesions: comparison of samples obtained with 14-, 16-, and 18-gauge needles. Radiology 1995;197:739–42.

30. Fishman JE, Milikowski C, Ramsinghani R, et al. US-guided core-needle biopsy of the breast: how many specimens are necessary? Radiology 2003;226: 779–82.

31. Sauer G, Deissler H, Strunz K, et al. Ultrasound-guided largecore needle biopsies of breast lesions: analysis of 962 cases to determine the number of samples for reliable tumour classification. Br J Cancer 2005;92:231–5.

32. Parker SH, Klaus AJ, McWey PJ, et al. Sonographically guided directional vacuum-assisted breast biopsy using a handheld device. AJR Am J Roentgenol 2001;177:405–8.

33. Meyer JE, Smith DN, Lester SC, et al. Large-core needle biopsy of nonpalpable breast lesions. JAMA 1999;281:1638–41.

34. Chen AM, Haffty BG, Lee CH. Local recurrence of breast cancer after breast conservation therapy in patients examined by means of stereotactic core-needle biopsy. Radiology 2002;225:707–12.

35. Philpotts LE, Hooley RJ, Lee CH. Comparison of automated versus vacuum-assisted biopsy methods for sonographically guided core biopsy of the breast. AJR Am J Roentgenol 2003;180:347–51.

36. American College of Radiology breast imaging reporting and data system. Breast imaging atlas. Reston (VA): American College of Radiology; 2003.

37. Memarsadeghi M, Pfarl G, Riedl C, et al. Value of 14-gauge ultrasound-guided large-core needle biopsy of breast lesions: own results in comparison with the literature. Rofo 2003;175:374–80.

38. Philpotts LE, Shaheen NA, Carter D, et al. Comparison of rebiopsy rates after stereotactic core needle biopsy of the breast with 11-gauge vacuum suction probe versus 14-gauge needle and automatic gun. AJR Am J Roentgenol 1999;172:683–7.

39. Liberman L, Drotman M, Morris EA, et al. Imaging-histologic discordance at percutaneous breast biopsy. Cancer 2000;89:2538–46.

40. Bassett LW, Mahoney MC, Apple SK. Interventional breast imaging: current procedures and assessing for concordance with pathology. Radiol Clin North Am 2007;45:881–94.

41. Hoyt AC, Bassett LW. After the imaging-guided needle biopsy. In: Feig SA. editor. Syllabus RSNA, breast imaging. 2005. p. 295–303.

42. Reynolds HE. Core needle biopsy of challenging benign breast conditions. AJR Am J Roentgenol 2000;174:1245–50.

43. Jacobs TW, Connolly JL, Schnitt SJ. Nonmalignant lesions in breast core needle biopsies: to excise or not to excise? Am J Surg Pathol 2002;26:1095–100.

Ultrasonography of the Postsurgical Breast Including Implants

Gul Esen, MD, Deniz Cebi Olgun, MD

KEYWORDS

- Breast • Breast neoplasms • US • Implants
- TRAM flap • Reduction mammoplasty
- Breast conserving surgery

The breast is one of the most common sites of surgical procedures performed for diagnostic and therapeutic or reconstructive purposes. Surgical interventions lead to many alterations in the breast tissue causing difficulty in the interpretation of clinical and radiologic findings. These changes resolve almost completely within the first year after benign biopsy, with minor architectural distortion and scarring remaining. They can be accentuated and prolonged considerably after cancer surgery, however, mostly as a result of the effects of radiation therapy.[1,2]

Although postsurgical changes can resemble malignant lesions in some patients, they also can mask signs of malignancy in others. It is important for radiologists to detect and appropriately recognize these alterations to diagnose recurrent tumor as early as possible, while there still is a chance for curative surgery. It also is important to avoid overdiagnosis in these patients so as not to lead to unnecessary biopsies of irradiated tissues where healing processes might be disturbed.

Ultrasonography (US) is a useful adjunct to mammography for the evaluation of operated breasts. It not only gives valuable information in the evaluation of palpable masses and suspicious mammographic opacities but also can increase diagnostic accuracy in the follow-up of these patients. Because it is a cross-sectional modality, it is less affected by the architectural distortion and edema caused by surgery and therapy. Augmented breasts also are easier to evaluate by US compared with mammography.

Evaluation of the treated breast is one of the most challenging aspects of breast imaging. This article reviews the sonographic findings in operated breasts with the main focus on the conservatively treated breast. Also reviewed are the findings associated with excisional biopsies, breast implants, augmentation, and reduction mammoplasties.

CONSERVATION THERAPY FOR BREAST CANCER

Prospective randomized trials have established that there is no significant difference in the survival outcome of patients treated with mastectomy versus breast conservation therapy.[3–8] The success of conservative treatment depends, however, on the appropriate selection and follow-up of eligible patients. It also depends on the trusted cooperation of a team of physicians; experienced radiologists are important members of this team.

During the preoperative period, the main responsibility of a breast radiologist is to determine the disease extent as accurately as possible. Tumor size is an important determinant in the choice between breast-conserving surgery and mastectomy. Although there is no absolute size measurement that makes breast conservation impossible, in patients who have tumors larger than 5 cm, mastectomy usually is preferred. The more important factors for determination of the type of surgery are the ratio of the size of the tumor to the size of the breast and presence of multicentric disease.[1,9,10] Studies have shown that US is more

Istanbul University, Cerrahpasa Medical School, Department of Radiology, 34300 Istanbul, Turkey
E-mail address: gulesen@istanbul.edu.tr (G. Esen).

Ultrasound Clin 3 (2008) 295–329
doi:10.1016/j.cult.2008.10.002

sensitive than mammography in demonstrating additional foci of tumor in patients who have breast cancer.[11–14] In the author's institution all patients who have breast cancer who have dense breast parenchyma (Breast Imaging Reporting and Data System [BI-RADS] 3 or 4) undergo US examination of bilateral breasts before type of surgery is determined. If multicentric foci or suspicious contralateral lesions are demonstrated, core-needle biopsy is performed. Although MR imaging is more sensitive in this context,[11–20] US is inexpensive, more rapid, practical, and almost as successful in experienced hands. If no additional lesions are seen on US, patients benefit from MR imaging, which has been shown to change management in 10% to 48% of patients.[11–13,17–22] This variability in results regarding the contribution of MR imaging to the preoperative assessment of tumor extent depends mainly on the differences in study designs and possibly also on the levels of expertise, especially for US examination. Additional tumor foci detected on MR imaging should be searched with second-look US. Demonstration of these lesions with US is important because of the chance for US-guided biopsy. It has been reported that as much as 23% to 55% of lesions (especially malignant ones) detected on MR imaging can be demonstrated with second-look US.[23,24] In the author's experience, however, the sensitivity of second-look US is much lower than this, probably because US always is performed before MR imaging and most of the lesions are detected on this primary US examination.

During the perioperative period, a breast radiologist has to localize any nonpalpable lesions and document accurate sampling and complete excision with specimen radiography. Specimen US also is possible for lesions that are visible only on US examination or that are localized under US guidance. Specimen US usually is performed for tumors that present as masses. For lesions, such as architectural distortions, or indistinct hipoechoic areas, specimen US examination may not be accurate.[10] Lesion localization and evaluation of the specimen also can be performed in an operating room with intraoperative US examination.[7,25–27]

Specimens should be evaluated while patients are in the operating room, and confirmation of excision and proximity to the margins should be reported. If a suspicious lesion is not seen in the specimen, or if a lesion is close to the margins, a surgeon is informed and re-excision is performed. The re-excision material also should be examined. On specimen radiography two orthogonal views are needed to determine whether or not the tumor extends to the margin of the specimen.

Evaluation of the margins is easier with US because it is possible to examine the specimen in different planes. It should be kept in mind, however, that clear margins on specimen radiography or specimen US are not enough to exclude margin involvement. Histologic evaluation is the gold standard, although sometimes histologic and radiologic evaluations can be complementary.[1,28]

Early postoperative evaluation of the breast generally is indicated only for tumors that present as microcalcifications. In these patients, mammography of the operated breast is obtained 2 to 4 weeks after the operation, before radiation therapy is initiated, to determine whether or not there are any residual calcifications.[10] Presence of residual calcifications does not necessarily mean residual tumor and absence of calcifications does not exclude residual disease. Therefore, demonstration of residual calcifications on postoperative mammograms may or may not lead to re-excision. However, their detection in this baseline mammogram may be helpful for the future follow-ups.[9,28] For noncalcified tumors that are excised with negative margins, early postoperative imaging usually is unnecessary, because architectural distortion, hematoma, and edema that develop in the breast make mammographic interpretation difficult.

In women who have positive margins on histologic examination, evaluation of the breast for residual disease may be necessary. MR imaging has been reported as the most accurate method in demonstrating the extent of residual disease in these patients, although it may lead to false-positive results resulting from early postoperative changes.[29–33] The superimposition of the residual fibroglandular tissue with architectural distortions, edema, and postoperative fluid collections usually impedes mammographic interpretation and inadequate compression of the painful edematous breasts makes interpretation more difficult. US may be more helpful in these patients and may show residual masses (**Fig. 1**). Because of the variable appearance and irregularity of the surgical cavity and postoperative hematoma, much experience is needed for US evaluation of the surgical bed. Occasionally, surgeons perform excisional biopsy of a suspicious palpable lesion without prior radiologic evaluation of the breast. On detection of malignancy, patients are sent to a radiology department before definitive treatment, even if the surgical margins are negative. They also benefit more from US examination, because of the reasons discussed previously, but mammography again is needed to exclude the possibility of residual malignant-type microcalcifications.

After radiotherapy is completed, a baseline mammogam is indicated in 3 to 6 months to

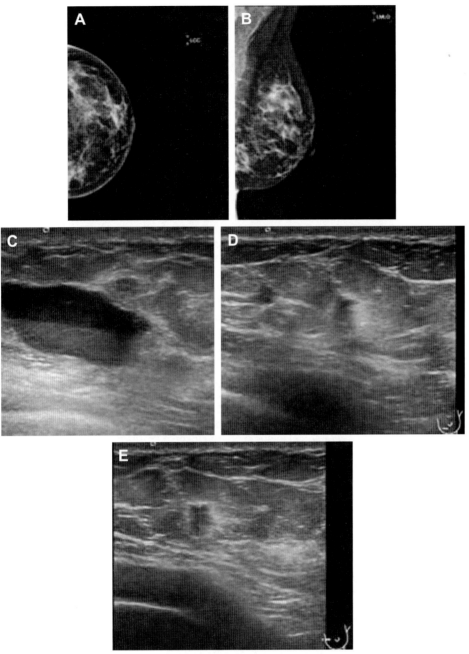

Fig. 1. Residual breast carcinoma. Excisional biopsy of a palpable mass with clinical features of a fibroadenoma detected in a 22-year-old woman proved to be invasive ductal carcinoma. Specimen margins were positive. Imaging was not performed preoperatively. (*A, B*) Mammograms taken 10 days after biopsy show an asymmetric opacity containing radiolucencies at the operation site. Mediolateral oblique mammogram also shows a small nodule with ill-defined margins above the opacity in front of the pectoralis muscle. (*C*) US demonstrates a collection corresponding to the asymmetric opacity seen on mammograms and a small residual tumor focus anteriorly. (*D, E*) Three other residual tumor foci are revealed on US imaging cranially to the operation site. Only one of them is seen on the mammograms.

demonstrate the new appearance of the breast.[9,10] This is the time when changes resulting from therapy are most accentuated. All findings, except for calcifications, which may appear years later, are expected to stay the same or decrease after this initial mammogram. Any increase may be associated with recurrence and should be investigated. The author finds it useful to evaluate the treated breast with mammography and US at the time of this first post-treatment assessment to document all findings in detail. This can be helpful in future follow-ups, in case suspicious findings are detected and need for comparison with previous evaluations arises. Although there is limited evidence in literature in the favor of routine US follow-up after breast conservation therapy,[34] the author uses mammography and US in the follow-up of these patients, especially for patients who have dense breast parenchyma.

There is no guideline for the timing of follow-up examinations. Some investigators recommend 6 months' follow-up of the treated breast for the first 2 or 3 years, although it has not been documented that this leads to early detection of recurrence or improves survival.[28] It probably is enough to image a treated breast initially within 6 months after completion of radiotherapy, image bilateral breasts at 1 year after treatment, and perform annual follow-up for both breasts thereafter.[28,34,35] The author performs mammography and US examination at the initial visit, continue with mammography, and add US examination whenever needed in the later follow-ups.

CHANGES RESULTING FROM BREAST CONSERVATION THERAPY

Breast surgery and radiation therapy cause some characteristic tissue changes. These are hematoma or seroma, fat necrosis, scar formation, edema, skin changes, lipophagic granuloma, and calcifications.[2,9,10,36] Hematoma and seroma usually occupy the surgical cavity but also may spread into the surrounding parenchyma, connective tissue, and adipose tissue. Traumatic injury of the

cell membrane causes tissue necrosis, which generally is called fat necrosis, although fat cells are not the only ones that are affected. This is followed by a healing process, where granulation tissue grows centripedally, beginning along the border of the cavity. Initially this tissue is hypervascular but later transforms into a poorly vascularized, densely packed fibrotic scar. Confluent foci of necrotic fat can liquefy centrally, producing oil cysts, which have a tendency to calcify.[36] Clinically, hematomas and seromas generally resolve completely or transform into scar tissue. Alternatively, fat necrosis presents as lipophagic granuloma or oil cysts, both of which can be difficult clinically to differentiate from malignancy.[37]

Breast imagers need to be familiar with the expected changes in the conservatively treated breast so that these are not mistaken for recurrence. Unnecessary biopsies can compromise the cosmetic result of conservation and should be avoided as much as possible. Sequential evaluation of radiologic findings, always comparing them with previous examinations, especially the oldest one, is important in the follow-up of these breasts.[9,10]

Fluid Collections

Fluid collections in the operation cavity, seromas and hematomas, are seen mammographically as round or oval masses that are fairly dense and well marginated. Sometimes there can be irregularity or small spiculations in the margins (**Fig. 2**). Some of these fluid collections also can appear as asymmetric soft tissue densities, where the borders might be obscured by the surrounding edema (see **Fig. 1**). These masses are present on the first postoperative mammogram and should not be

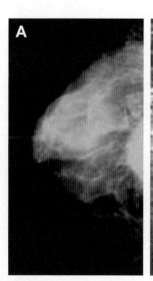 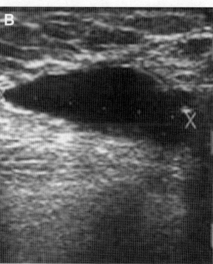

Fig. 2. Postoperative collection. (*A*) Craniocaudal mammogram demonstrates a mass with spiculated borders located at the surgical bed where a fibroadenoma was excised 1 month previously. (*B*) US reveals that the mass is a seroma.

mistaken for recurrences. Such an early recurrence, usually larger than the original mass, is unlikely, particularly if the resection margins are free of tumor.[1]

The fluid nature of these masses is easily demonstrated with sonography. The variety of different liquid contents makes the echogenicity of the lesions highly variable on US. Seromas usually appear as anechoic masses that show posterior acoustic enhancement whereas hematomas are hypoechoic or have echogenic components, which are distinguished from complex masses by fluctuating echoes on palpation.[36] Clots within a hematoma may be freely mobile or may be adherent to one wall resembling mural nodules (**Fig. 3**). Even so, knowing the clinical history, this should cause no difficulty in interpretation unless an excised tumor also was an intracystic mass or complete excision of the tumor was not documented. Fibrinous adhesions within seromas or hematomas can be resorbed over time or can persist as fibrous septations. Fluid collections conform to the size and shape of the surgical cavity and usually appear angular or elongated, which also is a clue as to the nature of these mass lesions.[37] These fluid collections rarely can become secondarily infected and then can evolve into abscesses. The sonographic findings of abscesses include increased echogenicity, thickened walls, and inreased peripheral vascularity. They can be uniocular or multilocular. They can be treated with US-guided aspirations or drained with the help of a catheter placed inside the abscess under US guidance if necessary.

Hematomas or seromas can develop as infrequent complications after primary closure of the surgical cavity or as the desired effect of not suturing the lumpectomy cavity closed. In cancer surgery, where a relatively large amount of tissue is excised, surgeons usually prefer to leave the cavity open with the hope that accumulating blood and serum minimizes the deformity of the overlying breast tissues and skin. Better cosmesis is achieved most of the time with this method, and these collections should not be aspirated. Sometimes, however, chronic collections progress through stages of fat necrosis to the fibrosis phase and retractile scar or cicatrix formation. This can produce severe deformity in some patients, especially after radiotherapy.[37] Hematomas and seromas usually are resorbed at the end of 1 year after benign biopsy. After cancer surgery and radiotherapy, however, it takes longer for them to disappear completely.[2,9,37] Usually the granulation tissue that surrounds the cavity grows thicker as the fluid collection gets thinner until it disappears completely and only the hypoechoic scar remains. Sometimes collections can persist as chronic hematomas or seromas or evolve into lipid cysts.[28,37]

Scar

Prominent scarring in the breast develops in more than 95% patients by the end of the second year after lumpectomy and radiation therapy. Benign biopsy changes often resolve more quickly and almost completely by the end of 1 year or 18 months.[38–40] The size of resection, volume of postsurgical fluid collection, and whether or not it was drained postsurgically may affect the rate of scar formation. Radiation therapy prolongs the resolution time of post-treatment changes to 2 years or more, and some findings may never disappear completely. On mammography, initially radiation mastitis obscures the scar, which then becomes increasingly conspicuous as the edema recedes. This should not be interpreted falsely as an enlarging scar suggesting local recurrence.[2,28,40]

Scars usually appear as architectural distortion, focal asymmetry, or spiculated opacity mammographically and have to be distinguished from recurrent tumors (**Fig. 4**). Clinical history, physical examination, and comparison with previous examinations are necessary for appropriate management. On physical examination, scarring uncomplicated by fat necrosis is perceived as induration rather than a mass.[9] On mammography, scars appear more suspicious and mass-like in one projection whereas they elongate in another. This changing appearance and the presence of radiolucencies within an opacity should suggest

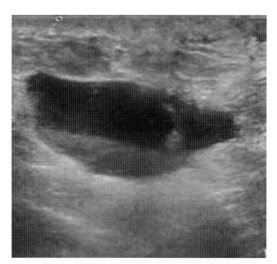

Fig. 3. Postoperative hematoma. A cystic mass is seen with layering echoes and an echogenic clot, which was demonstrated as mobile when the patient was turned on her side.

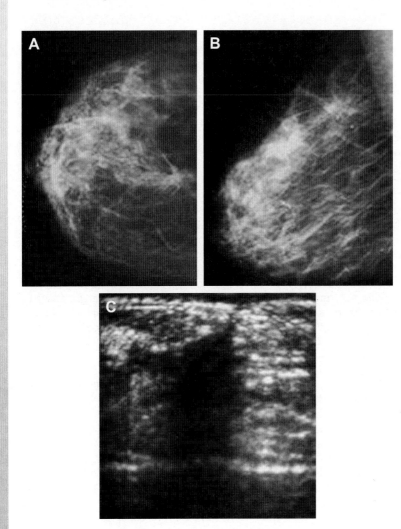

Fig. 4. Postoperative scar. (*A*, *B*) Screening mammograms demonstrate a spiculated mass with malignant features in the 12 o'clock position in the right breast. The patient recalls having a benign biopsy in her right breast some years before but does not remember the exact position. (*C*) US shows a lesion with dense posterior acoustic shadowing. The linear anterior border is the clue for the correct diagnosis. The lesion did not show any contrast enhancement on control MR imaging.

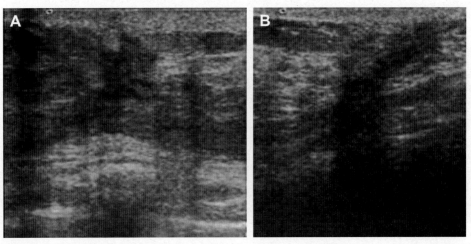

Fig. 5. US images of the surgical beds in two different patients with different types of surgical operations (*A*) Breast-conserving surgery where the surgical cavity was left open and appears 3-D and mass-like. (*B*) Benign biopsy where the surgical cavity was closed and appears linear and elongated.

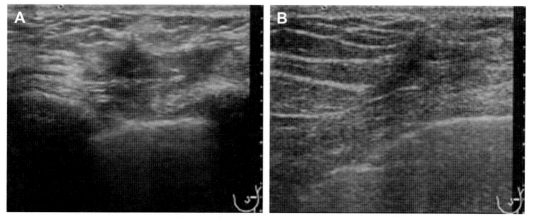

Fig. 6. Postoperative scar. The lesion looks ill defined and suspicious in one plane (*A*) but the linear extent is seen when scanned in the perpendicular plane (*B*).

scarring.[2,9] The radiolucencies represent fat entrapped by fibrous stranding and may be seen similarly in scarring, fat necrosis, and sclerosing lesions (radial scar) and also in some malignancies, such as invasive lobular cancers, which do not have a central tumor focus.[41,42] Scars usually are marked with wires taped over the incision on the skin before mammograms are obtained. The operation site within the breast, however, may not be directly beneath the incision site on the skin. This sometimes may cause confusion while evaluating mammograms.

US can demonstrate the surgical bed easily and more accurately, thus showing the location of a suspicious opacity in relation to the operation site. On US examination, a surgical cavity that has been closed looks like a linear hipoechoic area in the plane perpendicular to the plane of incision whereas a cavity that has been left open appears 3-D and mass-like (**Fig. 5**). In the plane parallel to the long axis of the scar, all cavities appear similarly suspicious because of hypoechogenicity and shadowing. The elongation and changing appearance of the lesion are the clues to correct diagnosis.[37]

The advantages of US over mammography are that it is multiplanar and cross-sectional thus eliminating false images caused by superimposition of tissues. It also is possible to evaluate compressibility of lesions, a feature helpful in the differential diagnosis of post-treatment changes. On US, scars appear as hipoechoic areas with indistinct or irregular borders that usually cast an acoustic shadow. They can look entirely different on two

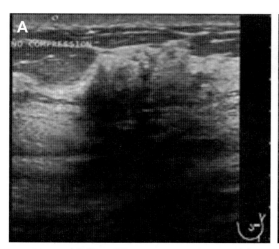
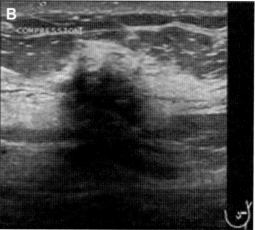

Fig. 7. Compressibility of the postoperative scar. (*A*) An ill-defined lesion with posterior shadowing is seen in a patient who has undergone breast-conserving therapy 3 years previously. (*B*) The lesion is smaller when it is compressed. It has been detected in the first evaluation 3 months after radiation therapy and has been stable since then.

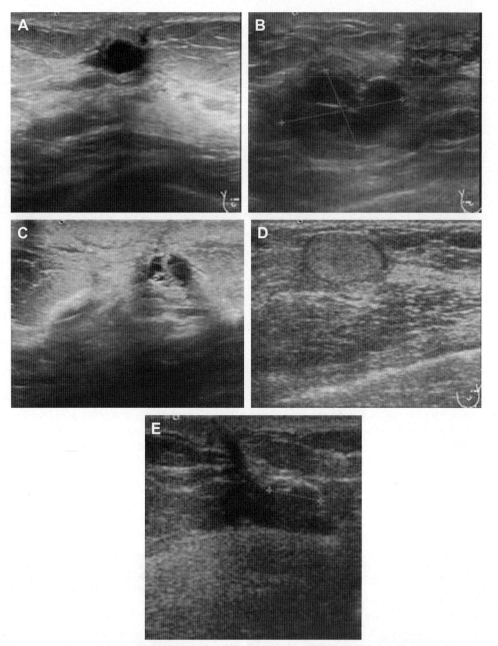

Fig. 8. Oil cysts have a spectrum of findings on US. They can appear pure cystic (*A*), multiloculated and septated (*B*), of mixed echogenicity (*C*), solid (*D*), or calcified (*E*).

projections and as the transducer is moved along the course of the scar, the linear extent of the defect and its continiuty with the skin incision can be appreciated (**Fig. 6**). When an ill-defined hypoechoic area is seen at the surgical bed, its compressibility should be assessed. Showing that the lesion is more than 10% to 15% compressible favors post-treatment changes, such as chronic hematoma, seroma, or lipid cyst, instead of a recurrent tumor (**Fig. 7**). With compression, the

hypoechogenicity and shadowing also should decrease. Prominent fibrosis and fat necrosis in the form of lipogranuloma, however, usually are uncompressible and this sign can be misleading.

Color or power Doppler US might be helpful in differential diagnosis but is not reliable. Post-treatment changes usually are avascular after approximately 6 months, whereas recurrent tumors often have demonstrable vacularity. Granulation tissue that develops in the walls of the cavity also has demonstrable blood flow in the first 6 months after surgery.[37] As is always the case, however, a positive Doppler study is more valuable than a negative Doppler study and absence of flow does not exclude malignancy.

Increasing size of the scar (after stability is achieved) is considered suspicious for malignancy.[9] This sign can be evaluated more reliably on mammograms where on each visit a standard image with the same exposure conditions, same angles, and same compression thickness can be obtained. In US examinations, the images usually are taken on whichever plane the lesion is best seen and a lesion that changes shape on different planes may not be able to be measured in the same way each time objectively. This is true especially in a setting where each examination is performed by different applicators.

Fat Necrosis

Fat necrosis can have variable and sometimes atypical appearances radiologically.[43–49] Lipid cysts have a characteristic and definitely benign (BI-RADS 2) appearance on mammography but they have a spectrum of findings on US (**Fig. 8**). Early in the course of development, before the water component has been resorbed, they are seen as completely anechoic cystic lesions with or without posterior acoustic enhancement. As the water component begins to resorb, they may show fat-fluid levels that shift when a patient is examined in different positions. They may appear far more suspicious, however, as hypoechoic lesions with acoustic shadowing or complex cystic masses with varying amounts of anechoic and hyperechoic components. They may have suspicious features, such as mural nodules and thick walls, or they may appear highly echoic and solid.[37,44,45,47,49] The sonographic appearance evolves in time and they may become more solid appearing or, on the contrary, more cystic. They mostly decrease in size but they also may stay stable. Fortunately, when interpreted together with mammograms, diagnosis is straightforward. Lipid cysts tend to calcify, showing typical eggshell-type calcification on mammography. These also can be appreciated on US with their highly echogenic walls and acoustic shadowing. High amounts of calcification can make interpretation difficult because of dense shadowing. In indeterminate cases elastography may assist diagnosis, demonstrating the benign and liquid nature of the lesion (**Fig. 9**).

Lipid cysts at the surgical bed are easily detected on mammograms most of the time in treated patients. Being familiar with the

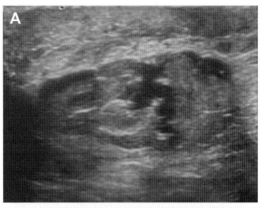

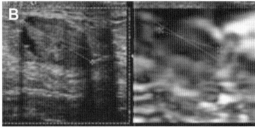

Fig. 9. Oil cyst. (*A*) US shows a complex cystic mass with mixed echogenicity. (*B*) On US elastography the lesion is consistent with a cyst (mixed colors with dimensions smaller than the B-mode image). Elastography can assist in differential diagnosis when mammograms are not available.

sonographic appearances of lipid cysts and fat necrosis and the evolution of these patterns, however, can be helpful in other patients where these lesions can be detected incidentally on US examinations and may not be appreciated as easily on mammograms or where they present as palpable nodules and are evaluated primarily with US examination.[47–49] Thus, unnecessary biopsies may be avoided.

Fat necrosis is a complex ischemic process that has traumatic and inflammatory elements and some sign of foreign body reaction. Factors that increase the likelihood of ischemia increase the risk for fat necrosis. Large fatty breasts, long excisions, extensive resection, and radiation all increase the risk for ischemia and fat necrosis.[37] Besides lipid cysts, fat necrosis can appear in the form of mastitis, foreign body granuloma (lipophagic granuloma), and fibrosis. All of these processes, except for lipid cysts, increase the echogenicity of fatty tissue in the beginning, similar to edema, but later on they usually progress to final stages of dense fibrosis. This resembles fibrosis of postoperative scarring but usually is more extensive and indistinguishable from recurrent tumor mammographically or sonograpically.

It is seen as an irregular hypoechoic area with dense shadowing that is present on all planes and not compressible.[40] Granulomas also can appear in other areas besides the surgical bed in the irradiated breast. Although fibrosis usually does not enhance on MR imaging, some forms of fat necrosis, especially lipogranulomas, may enhance even years after therapy (**Fig. 10**).[36,45] Findings of fat necrosis are reported as much more pronounced in patients who have been treated with intraoperative radiation therapy as opposed to conventional postoperative radiotherapy.[50,51] Frequently, core-needle biopsy is needed for the differential diagnosis of lipohagic granuloma and fibrosis from recurrent tumor. Fine-needle aspiration biopsy (FNAB) is not useful because these lesions are hypocellular and because radiation therapy may cause atypical changes in the cells, which is a problem in the cytologic evaluation.[1,36]

In one series, however, it was reported that differentiation of recurrence from scarring was possible with FNAB.[52] Again, a positive result is more valuable than a negative one in this setting.

Diffuse Changes

Conservative treatment for breast cancer also causes diffuse changes in the breast as a result of radiation therapy. The acute or early radiation-induced changes are dominated by edema. Mammograms usually show thickening of the skin, enlargement of the breast, and hazy increased density and increased trabecular markings more apparent in the subcutaneous fat.[3,37] These findings are similar in all pathologies that cause edema or mastitis in the breast. Sonographically, edema is characterized by increased echogenicity of the subcutaneous fat lobules and decreased echogenicity of the Cooper's ligaments. In severe cases of

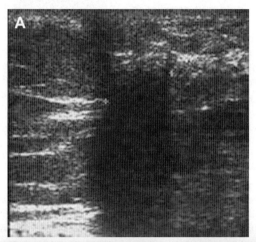

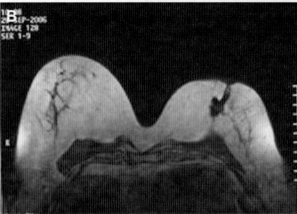
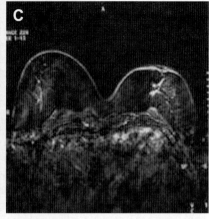

Fig. 10. Fat necrosis–lipogranuloma. (*A*) In a patient who had undergone breast-conserving therapy 5 years previously, US evaluation of a palpable mass near the operation site revealed an ill-defined hypoechoic lesion with dense acoustic shadowing. It was not compressible. Because she had no previous US examinations available for comparison, MR imaging was performed. (*B*) The lesion was nodular and very hypointense on T2-weighted image (*B*) and showed contrast enhancement (*C*). The histologic diagnosis on core-needle biopsy was lipogranuloma.

edema, anatomic distinction between tissues may become almost completely obscured. Small effusions may form within the subcutaneous tissue and the Cooper's ligaments (**Fig. 11**). Skin becomes diffusely thicker (>2 mm) and less echogenic, but this is most prominent in the lower quadrants (**Fig. 12**). Skin thickening is the most common finding after breast-conserving therapy, reported as present in up to 90% of patients, and usually returns to normal in 46% to 60% of patients by 2 to 3 years.[28,53,54] Because of edema, the breast also becomes thicker and in some patients edema may prevent adequate penetration of the tissues with the usual high frequency transducers. It may be necessary to use a 5-MHz linear transducer. The sonographic signs of edema begin to regress after 12 to 18 months in most patients, but may persist in some, especially in those patients who have axillary blockage resulting from axillary dissection. Chronic edema usually does not produce prominent changes in the breast and is discernable only when compared with the opposite breast. In some patients, edema can progress to fibrosis, which can make the breast progressively smaller.[9]

Besides evaluating and monitoring the changes caused by surgery and radiation therapy, another responsibility of radiologists is to localize the lumpectomy cavity for radiation therapy booster doses. Complications from radiation limit the dose that can be delivered to the whole breast, chest wall, and axilla, but higher radiation booster doses can be delivered to small areas of the breast that are at especially high risk for local recurrence. Most recurrences occur in the walls of the surgical cavity or in the immediately surrounding tissues. Therefore, booster doses are delivered to this area. The skin incision, however, does not always

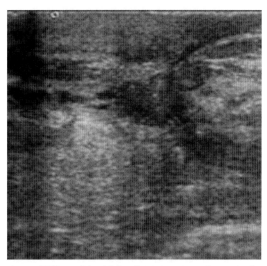

Fig. 12. Diffuse skin thickening more prominent at the incision site. Note decrease in the echogenicity of the skin.

correlate with the surgical cavity inside the breast. With US, patients are scanned in the same position they will be in for therapy, preferably on a radiation therapy table. The entire lumpectomy cavity can be mapped; its depth from the skin and the dimensions of any fluid collections can be determined.[37,55] More recently, an alternative approach to external whole-breast irradiation has become an option: brachytherapy. In this procedure radioactive seeds are delivered to the lumpectomy site through a balloon catheter. Although delivering high doses to lumpectomy cavity for maximum local control, the rest of the breast and other tissues are spared from the side effects of irradiation. These catheters can be placed during surgery or later under US guidance. US also can be used to determine eligibility. The seroma should be round if possible and at least 3 cm in diameter. Also important is the distance from the skin to the to the anterior wall of the cavity, which must be at least 7 mm to ensure equal and even radiation throughout the field.[55,56]

LOCAL TREATMENT FAILURE AFTER BREAST CONSERVATION THERAPY

Local treatment failure occurs at rates of 5% to 10% at 5 years and 10% to 15% at 10 years after completion of therapy.[57–59] In the first 5 to 7 years, recurrent tumor is most likely at or near the site of the original cancer, with mean time to recurrence 3 years. Rather than a real recurrence, it usually represents residual disease that was not recognized and resected at the time of surgery and that has not been controlled by the immune

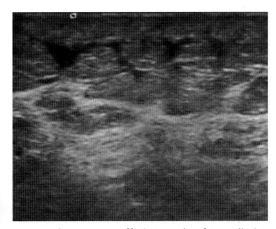

Fig. 11. Subcutaneous effusions early after radiation therapy.

system, radiation therapy, or chemotherapy. Local treatment failure after 5 to 7 years increasingly is found in other quadrants and mostly the result of new tumors that have grown in the meantime.[9,10,37] Because the stage of tumor recurrence is related to survival, early diagnosis is important. Recurrences that are still intraductal or smaller than 2 cm have better prognosis.[60] Risk factors for local treatment failure remain controversial but include young age at the time of diagnosis (especially younger than 30 years), an extensive intraductal component, vascular or lymphatic invasion, multiple tumors at presentation, positive margin of resection, high nuclear grade, larger tumor size, nonductal histologic type, and intraductal carcinoma of the comedo type.[61,62]

Sensitivity of mammography in the conservatively treated breast is considerably low compared with the untreated breast resulting from architectural distortion and increased density. Mammography reportedly has been unable to detect 19% to 50% of local recurrences after breast conservation therapy.[35,63–66] Alternatively, 29% to 42% of local recurrences, mostly in the form of ductal carcinoma in situ (DCIS), have been detected only with mammography.[35,64,67] Recurrences detected with mammography usually contain microcalcifications. Tumors of invasive lobular histology are

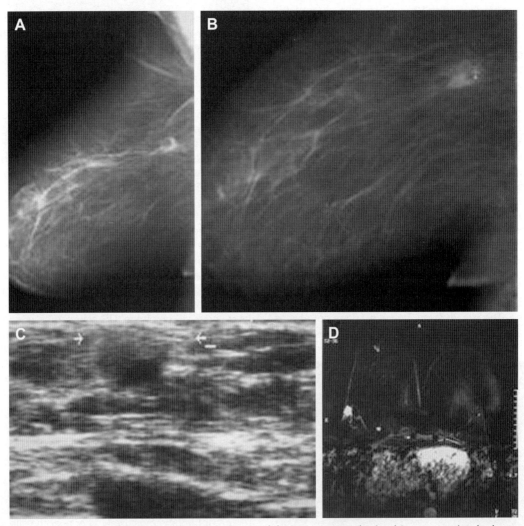

Fig. 13. Local recurrence after breast-conserving therapy. (A) Mammogram obtained 2 years previously shows an oil cyst with calcifications in the posterior wall. (B) New mammogram shows an interval ill-defined opacity surrounding the oil cyst. If the previous mammogram was not available it could have been misdiagnosed as scar or fat necrosis. (C) US shows a hypoechoic solid mass surrounding a cystic lesion in the subcutaneous tissue. (D) Subtraction MR imaging confirms the subcutaneous recurrence and demonstrates a second nodular lesion also diagnosed as an invasive tumor at mastectomy.

especially hard to detect with mammography. Overall, mammography can identify or confirm local recurrence in two thirds of patients.[35]

Recurrences rarely occur before 18 months after adequate treatment. In this follow-up period, the lumpectomy site should be imaged fully with spot compression and magnification views if needed. The author also performs US examination routinely in this period. Any changes detected in the breast on mammography and US should be documented so that comparison is possible if any suspicious findings are observed in future follow-ups. Mammographically, recurrences can appear as masses or new microcalcifications but usually findings are subtle. Sometimes just an enlargement in the scar (**Fig. 13**), thickening in the skin, or diffuse increase in density after stabilization of post-treatment changes can be a clue for recurrence.[9,10,28,35] In order to appreciate these subtle changes, the same exposure parameters should be used in each examination. It has been reported that mammographic features of local recurrences are similar to those of the primary tumor in 66% of cases. Therefore, it is important to review the preoperative mammograms during follow-up of conservatively treated patients.[68]

Local recurrences can develop in the breast parenchyma and in the skin, Cooper's ligaments, chest wall, and axilla. Recurrences in Cooper's ligaments usually are the result of unresected microscobic foci of invasive tumor. Skin recurrences usually arrive there through invasion of Cooper's ligaments or through invaded lymphatic channels that tend to drain superficially from the malignant nodule to the skin and then to the periareolar network of lymphatics. Chest wall invasion can result from direct invasion or from invaded lymphatic channels along the deep surface of the lesions that tend to drain medially to the internal mammary leymph nodes. Chest wall also can be involved

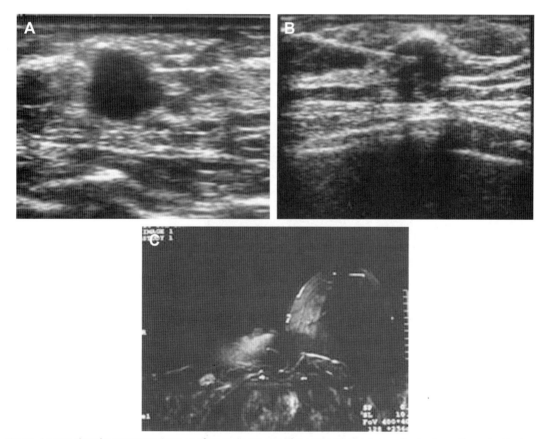

Fig. 14. Locoregional recurrence 9 years after mastectomy. The patient who was a doctor herself wanted to have US examination of the chest wall because of increasing tumor markers. (*A*) US shows an ill-defined vertically oriented nonpalpable solid mass in the chest wall (*B*) MR imaging shows that the lesion is located between the pectoralis major and minor muscles, consistent with Rotter's lymph node (*C*) US-guided FNAB followed by excisional biopsy confirmed the diagnosis. This was the author's first case with US diagnosis of a nonpalpable chest wall recurrence.

through perinodal invasion from internal mammary lymph nodes or from Rotter's lymph nodes that are located between the pectoralis major and pectoralis minor muscles (**Fig. 14**). Axilla also is a site for possible recurrence, usually within the lymph nodes but occasionally within the fat in patients who have perinodal inavasion. Axillary lymph node recurrences are more common in patients who have positive lymph nodes at the time of dissection but rarely can occur in patients who did not have axillary metastases.[37]

US is a useful adjunct to mammography in the detection of local failure in conservatively treated breasts. All the possible locations for recurrence can be evaluated with US. Shin and colleagues[34] have investigated the efficacy of US in detecting an occult malignancy after breast conservation therapy and found that it detected occult lesions that were not identified by clinical examination or mammography in 1.2% of the patients.

Sensitivity and specificity of US examination in this group were 70.6% and 98.3%, respectively, significantly higher than with mammography. Mendelson reports detecting recurrence in 6 out of 110 patients they followed with mammography and US. Four of these 6 tumors were positive on mammography and US whereas one palpable lesion was positive only on US. In the sixth patient, a new cluster of microcalcifications was detectable only by mammography. All of the false-positive lesions detected by US proved to be fat necrosis.[9] Alternatively, Balu-Maestro and colleagues[69] report that 95.5% of recurrences were identified mammographically and 90% by US. Only 45.5% of these lesions were detected by physical examination. US did not alter management in this series.

Recurrences inside the breast usually manifest as masses with irregular or indistinct, microlobulated borders, seperate from or in continuity with

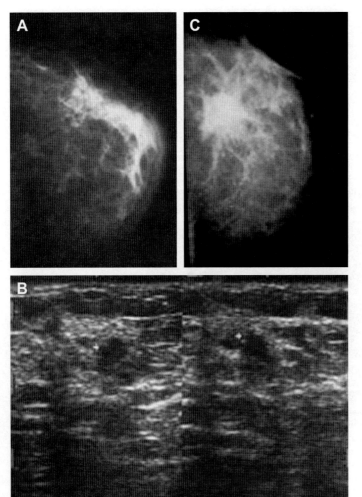

Fig. 15. Local recurrence after breast-conserving therapy. (*A*) Craniocaudal mammogram shows skin thickening and architectural distortion but no evidence of recurrence. (*B*) US examination performed on the same day reveals a 3-mm solid nodule near the surgical bed suspicious for local recurrence. US-guided biopsy was recommended but the oncologist ordered a 6-month follow-up instead. (*C*) The patient came back 1 year later for mammography. The lesion had grown in size and become mammographically evident.

the operation scar (**Fig. 15**). They sometimes may have acoustic shadowing or a hyperechoic halo surrounding them. Rarely, recurrent masses may present as multilobulated, well-defined lesions (**Fig. 16**). Recurrent tumors may or may not show typical features of malignancy on US. Unless they are definitely diagnosed as benign post-treatment changes, however, histologic diagnosis is needed in solid lesions especially if they are interval findings.

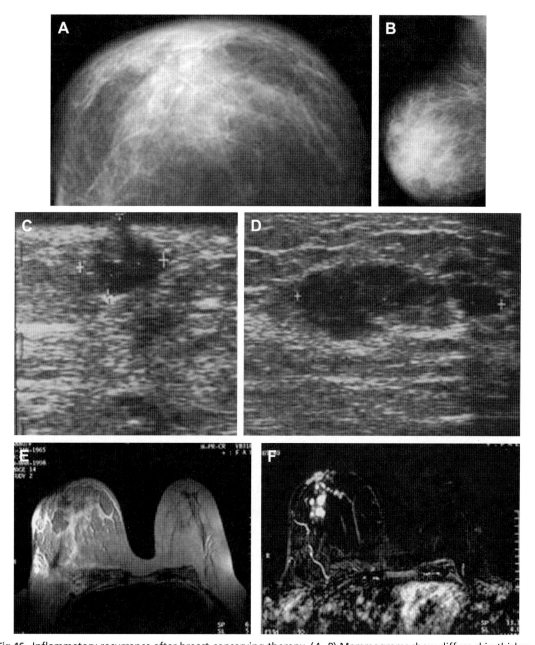

Fig. 16. Inflammatory recurrence after breast-conserving therapy. (*A, B*) Mammograms show diffuse skin thickening and increased opacity of the parenchyma, both of which were more prominent compared with previous examinations. Clinically, the breast had an inflamed appearance. (*C, D*) US images show an ill-defined subcutaneous heterogenous solid mass consistent with recurrence and a centrally located multilobulated hypoechoic lesion. (*E*) Diffuse edema in the breast is demonstrated on T2-weighted MR image. (*F*) Subtraction MR image shows multiple nodules consistent with recurrence corresponding to the multilobulated lesion detected on US. Although diffuse recurrence was suspected with mammography and US, the real extent of disease was demonstated more clearly with MR imaging in this case.

Compound imaging may be helpful in diagnosis because conspicuity of lesions and assessment of echotexture and margins are improved. Posterior shadowing may be increased, however, causing difficulty in interpretation.[70–73] In the author's experience, subtle recurrences, collections, and oil cysts usually are demonstrated more clearly on compound imaging whereas fibrotic scars and lipogranulomas appear much more suspicious (**Fig. 17**). In order to avoid unnecessary biopsy, compound imaging findings should be evaluated together with conventional images.

In diffuse forms of recurrence, skin thickening and edema may be the only detectable signs. Sometimes the whole or part of the parenchyma may appear hypoechoic with or without posterior acoustic shadowing. This may be difficult to appreciate in an irradiated breast; therefore, objective and progressive increase in skin thickening is important in the follow-up of these patients. Skin nodules appear as well-circumscribed solid lesions. Recurrences in the internal mammary lymph nodes may cause chest wall invasion and can be demonstrated with US if they are big enough. Lesions deep in the chest wall may be difficult to appreciate, however, because of radiation fibrosis and difficulty in penetration of tissues with high-frequency transducers. Recurrences in the axilla mostly are in the lymph nodes and share the same findings with metastatic lymph nodes (**Fig. 18**).[37] These are round shape, loss in the echogenic hilum, and asymmetric thickening of the cortex with or without subcapsular vascularization seen on power Doppler US studies.[74] Recurrences in the axillary fatty tissue are rare and manifest as solid masses with irregular borders and posterior acoustic shadowing (**Fig. 19**).

Although US is sensitive in the detection of recurrent tumors in the breast, its positive predictive value may be low. A high level of experience is needed for accurate interpretation of US findings that may be detected in treated breasts. Lipogranulomas and fat necrosis especially can simulate recurrent tumors and require biopsy for

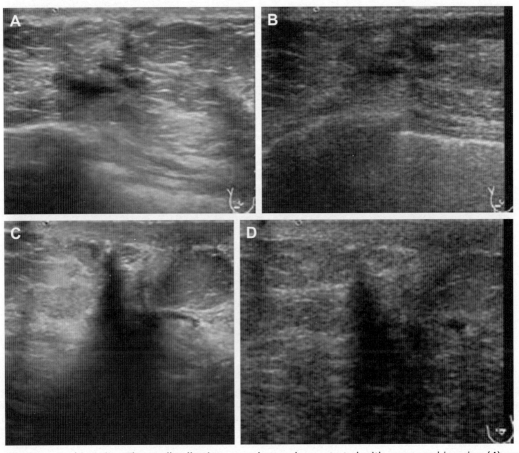

Fig. 17. Compound imaging. The small collections were better demonstrated with compound imaging (*A*) compared with conventional US image (*B*). Alternatively, the acoustic shadowing behind the scar also is more prominent and looks more suspicious with compound imaging (*C*) compared with conventional US image (*D*).

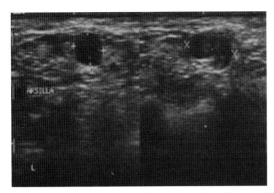

Fig. 18. Metastatic lymph node in the axilla with loss of hilum and round shape.

differentiation most of the time, even in experienced hands. Diagnosis of suspicious findings is best achieved by US-guided core-needle biopsy.[36] MR imaging is excellent in the differentiation of post-treatment changes from recurrent tumor because fibrotic tissue does not show contrast enhancement (**Fig. 20**). In the first 3 to 6 months after operation and the first 12 to 18 months after radiation therapy, there may be some false-positive enhancement, but after this period MR imaging usually is reliable.[36,75,76] In some patients, however, active scar can enhance for many years after surgery (see **Fig. 10**). Therefore, diagnosis of recurrence on MR imaging should be based not only on contrast enhancement but also on morphologic assessment.[76] MR imaging is not indicated for the routine follow-up (screening) of patients who have breast conservation because of low rated of local recurrences and significant increase in costs.[77,78]

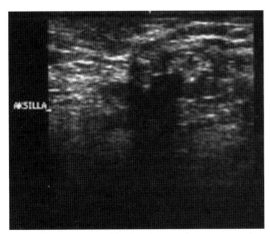

Fig. 19. Axillary recurrence in the fatty tissue. An ill-defined solid mass with posterior shadowing is demonstrated. Biopsy is needed to verify malignancy because fibrosis resulting from radiotherapy can look very similar.

Theoretically no vascularization should be detected in scar tissue on color or power Doppler US 6 months after the operation. Thus, differentiation from recurrent tumor, which is expected to be highly vascular, should be possible. It is not always as expected in practice, however.[9] Some investigators have found contrast-enhanced Doppler US more accurate in the evaluation of postoperative changes and recurrences.[75,79,80]

CHANGES RESULTING FROM MASTECTOMY

Today most mastectomies are simple or modified radical (simple mastectomy and axillary dissection) mastectomies. Radical mastectomies in which the pectoralis muscle is removed are abandoned mostly for cosmetic reasons. Mastectomy is performed for tumors that are too extensive to be treated with conserving therapy. These are lesions that are too large (>5 cm) or large compared with the size of the breast, are multifocal, are multicentric, or have direct invasion to the skin or the nipple. Patients whose tumors are detected by clinical examination tend to undergo mastectomy more often than those found by screening mammography or US.[81] Patients who have high-grade DCIS usually are treated with mastectomy. Mastectomy also may be preferred for patients who are not able to complete radiation therapy or for patients who are too anxious about the risk for recurrence.[9,10]

Mastectomy cavities are not left open to accumulate blood or serum; drains are placed to prevent any possible collections. If the drains are removed too early, collections can appear. When they do appear they tend to be elongated in a direction that is parallel to the long axis of the scar. Sonography using extended field of view is useful in demonstrating such collections. Similar collections also may be seen in the axilla after axillary dissection. The mastectomy incision is much longer compared with lumpectomy incision and extends to the axilla. Thus the scar also is longer. The postoperative scar of mastectomy usually causes no diagnostic problem because its linear extent is easily seen when scanned in its long axis, although sometimes it may appear as a mass-like lesion. Fat necrosis is not common because normally skin lies directly on the chest wall with no remaining breast tissue. Sometimes, however, variable amounts of tissue, mostly fatty tissue, might be left behind in which edema (if irradiated) or small oil cysts can be detected. Exuberant scarring, fibrosis, and fat necrosis sometimes is seen in the axilla, especially if the axillary region is irradiated. This may be difficult to differentiate from axillary recurrence.[4] In patients who

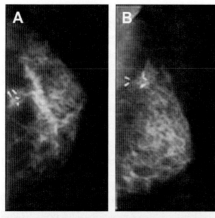

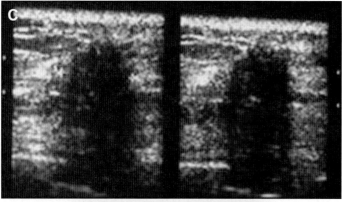

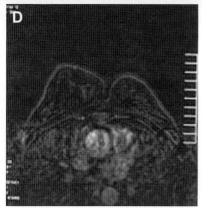

Fig. 20. Fat necrosis–lipogranuloma. (A, B) Mammograms taken 1 year after radiation therapy reveal an irregular opacity at the surgical bed where the surgical clips are seen. (C) US shows an irregular solid mass with shadowing also suspicious for recurrence. (D) Subtracted MR image shows no enhancement at the surgical bed, consistent with fibrosis. MR imaging is useful in these cases, eliminating the need for biopsy.

have sentinel node biopsy and no axillary dissection, there usually are no perceptible changes with US.

The frequency of local recurrence after mastectomy is lower compared with breast-conserving therapy. When it does occur, however, it is a sign of poor prognosis, with an increased risk for distant metastases and contralateral breast cancer.[82–85] Local failure after mastectomy occurs mostly in the skin or the chest wall.[1,37] The efficacy of routine mammography of the remaining tissue on the chest wall or the axilla has been reported by many investigators and

not found cost effective, most recurrences being evident on physical examination or manifested by chest wall pain or signs of distant metastases.[1,82,86] US is successful and reliable in the evaluation of the chest wall, especially when there is a finding of clinical concern. Skin nodules are readily apparent and need no radiologic evaluation. Other clinically suspicious lesions should be evaluated with US. They may correspond to oil cysts, chronic collections, or fat necrosis/mastitis in the subcutaneous tissues as a result of radiotherapy (Fig. 21). Recurrent tumors may be in the form of well-circumscribed

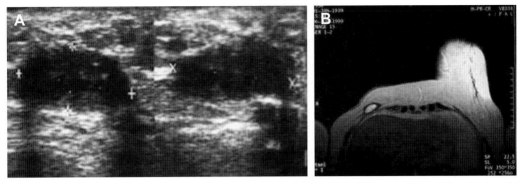

Fig. 21. Chronic collection after mastectomy. The patient was referred for US examination of the chest wall because of a palpable firm mass suspicious for local recurrence. (*A*) US shows a lobulated heterogeneous mass with internal septations and posterior enhancement. In spite of the US diagnosis of postoperative collection, MR imaging was requested because of clinically suspicious findings. (*B*) MR imaging clearly demonstrated a cystic lesion with thick walls consistent with a chronic seroma confined within the granulation tissue.

nodules or nodules with irregular borders and posterior acoustic shadowing; frequently there may be more than one lesion. US-guided FNAB is highly accurate in diagnosis.[87]

It generally is believed that all chest wall recurrences are palpable and there is no need to examine the mastectomy site if there is no finding in the physical examination. Rissanen and colleagues,[87]

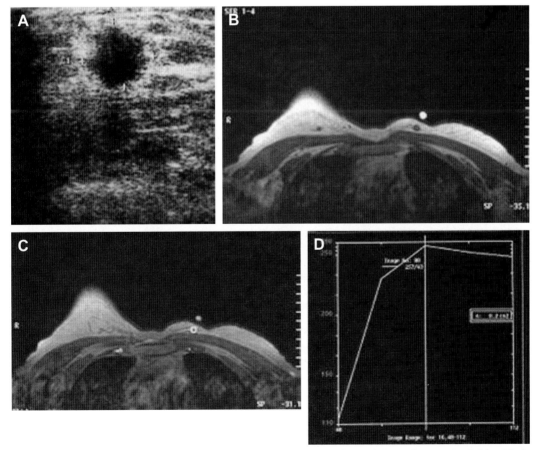

Fig. 22. Local recurrence after mastectomy. (*A*) A nonpalpable solid nodule wih irregular margins is identified on US examination of the chest wall. (*B*) Precontrast axial MR image shows a round hypointense nodule in the inner aspect of the chest wall, just underneath the skin marker placed over the sonographically detected lesion. (*C, D*) The nodule shows type 3 enhancement with washout. Excisional biopsy revealed invasive ductal carcinoma.

however, have reported a sensitivity of 91% for US detecting palpable and nonpalpable recurrences. The author's practice has encountered many cases of postmastectomy recurrences that were not detectable clinically and were found on US examination of the chest wall (**Fig. 22**). In a preliminary series of 27 cases, the author and colleagues compared accuracy of clinical examination, US, and MR imaging for detecting postmastectomy recurrences. The sensitivity and specificities respectively were 90% and 88.2%, respectively, for US and 70% and 35%, respectively, for clinical examination. MR imaging was found 100% accurate.[88] As a result, whenever US examination for the contralateral breast is needed in patients who have mastectomy, the author also examines the operation site (chest wall or transverse rectus abdominis myocutaneous [TRAM] flap and the axilla) in the clinic, although the need to do so has not been definitely established in the literature. The author and colleagues are in the process of collecting data; therefore, it is impossible to report if it is cost effective. US examination of the chest wall is fast, however, and usually not complicated by post-treatment changes, with few false-positive findings, so the author believes it is worthwhile in the follow-up of mastectomy patients. There also are supportive reports in the literature stating that early detection of recurrences after mastectomy is important in survival.[84,89]

CHANGES RESULTING FROM RECONSTRUCTIVE SURGERY

Several reconstructive surgical procedures can be performed after cancer surgery, especially after mastectomy. There are four types of mastectomies: (1) radical mastectomy, (2) modified radical mastectomy, (3) simple mastectomy, and (4) skin-sparing mastectomy. Radical mastectomy involves resection of the pectoralis muscle and all breast tissue, all overlying skin, including the nipple and axillary dissection. The only difference in modified radical mastectomy is that the pectoralis muscle is preserved. Simple mastectomy removes all breast tissue and overlying skin but does not include axillary dissection. In skin-sparing mastectomy, all breast tissue, the skin overlying the cancer site, and the nipple are removed but the rest of the skin is preserved. Except for skin-sparing mastectomy, all of these procedures involve extensive resection of the skin, after which reconstruction can be done only with myocutaneous flaps. Skin-sparing mastectomy, alternatively, allows for other options, including implants. The most commonly used reconstructions today are autologous myocutaneous flaps. There are two main types: latissimus dorsi flaps and TRAM flaps. Latissimus dorsi flaps are more appropriate in size for repair of partial mastectomy defects, whereas TRAM flaps are used after mastectomy.[37]

Normal mammographic and sonographic findings in myocutaneous flaps include predominance of fatty appearance, vascular pedicle, and surgical scar. The most common abnormal findings in autologous tissue transfers are fat necrosis and calcifications (**Fig. 23**), but recurrent tumor also can be detected. Local recurrences rarely appear in the transplanted autologous tissue; they are seen more commonly in the native breast skin that was spared at the time of mastectomy, the axilla, or the chest wall. At the time of local recurrence, distant metastases are present in more than 75% of cases.[37,90,91] US examination usually can successfully demonstrate palpable and nonpalpable lesions suspicious for malignancy and findings of fat necrosis (**Fig. 24**).

There are no guidelines regarding surveillance mammography or US examination for women who have undergone mastectomy and breast reconstruction. There are many reports of nonpalpable recurrences detected with mammography or US.[90–94] Edeiken and colleagues[92] report that 21 of the 39 (64%) recurrent cancers depicted at US were clinically occult. Mammography was obtained in only 25 of these recurrences and detected 14 (56%). US-guided FNAB helped establish a definitive diagnosis in 96% of the tumor specimens sampled. Alternatively, Lee and colleagues[93] state that routine mammography of TRAM flap reconstructions are not indicated because of low detection rates for nonpalpable recurrent breast cancer. MR imaging also is reported as highly accurate in showing recurrences and clarifying clinical suspicious findings (see **Fig. 24**).[95]

Color duplex sonography sometimes is called on preoperatively to help a surgeon decide whether or not to sacrifice the inferior or the superior epigastric artery when performing a TRAM flap reconstruction. To swing the flap free so that it can be implanted into the breast, one of them must be sacrificed. The relative contributions of these vessels to the blood supply of the rectus abdominis muscle vary from patient to patient. To improve the chances of success and minimize complications, the vessel with the least contribution is sacrificed. Blood flow can be estimated by measuring the sizes, blood flow velocities, and resistivity indices of the vessels on color duplex sonography.[37,96]

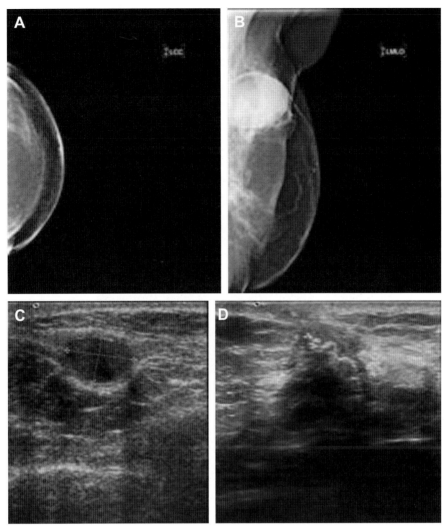

Fig. 23. Patient who had a plapable mass in the TRAM flap. (*A, B*) Mammograms show several oil cysts and calcifications of fat necrosis. (*C*) US evaluation of the palpable nodule reveals a well-defined hypoechoic lesion corresponding to an oil cyst on mammogram. (*D*) Triangular-shaped vascular pedicle.

CHANGES RESULTING FROM REDUCTION MAMMOPLASTY

Reduction mammoplasty is a plastic surgical procedure performed to address problems of self-image, to achieve breast symmetry, or to treat macromastia, which may lead to back pain, kyphosis, brachial plexus sypmptoms, or chronic intertrigo under the breasts. Breast asymmetry may be physiologic or a result of contralateral breast conservation therapy, mastectomy, and recontruction.[97]

Although there are many variations, the surgical procedure involves a circumareolar incision, an inframammary incision, and a vertical incision between the two, with removal of breast tissue, fat, and skin from a combination of these vertical and horizontal incisions. Breast tissue is removed predominantly from the lower breast, and the nipple-areolar complex is brought upwards.[9,98–100] All women undergoing reduction mammoplasty, especially those older than 35 years, should have a preoperative mammogram to detect any lesion that requires further investigation or removal at the time of the operation.

Preoperative mammogram is of no use after the procedure and the new appearance of the breast should be established with a baseline mammogram obtained 6 to 12 months after the operation. Mammographic features of reduction mammoplasty reflect the removal and redistribution of tissue and include linear strands, parenchymal bands, spiculated scars, calcifications, and skin

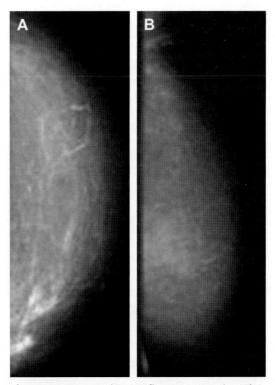

Fig. 24. Chest wall recurrence after mastectomy and TRAM flap reconstruction. The patient was referred for a skin nodule in the lower aspect of the flap. (*A, B*) Mammograms of the flap are unremarkable except for an indistinct opacity in the inner aspect on craniocaudal projection. (*C, D*) In addition to the skin nodule, US reveals two more irregular solid lesions located apparently in the flap and some hypoechoic areas with no definite borders. MR imaging was performed to determine the real extent of recurrent tumor. (*E, F*) MR images show recurrent tumor focus in the skin and a very irregular diffuse recurrence in the pectoralis mucle.

thickening (**Fig. 25**). Retroareolar fibrotic bands are characteristic. Usually there are asymmetric areas of soft tissue densities in both breasts. Findings are most pronounced in the lower aspect of the breast where the greatest amount of tissue has been excised.[98,101] Extensive fat necrosis may occur because of attenuated blood supply in these usually very fatty breasts. This may cause problems in the interpretation of mammographic and sonographic findings. Sonography especially tends to overestimate the BI-RADS categories of many findings in postreduction mammoplasty patients. Therefore, suspicious sonographic findings should be correlated carefully with mammograms before recommending biopsy.[37]

There is evidence that women have a somewhat lower breast cancer risk after reduction mammoplasty.[102] Their prognosis and mortality rates, however, are similar to general population.

ULTRASONOGRAPHIC EVALUATION OF BREAST IMPLANTS

Breast implants are used for augmentation or reconstruction purposes. Silicone gel prosthesis is the most well-known type of prosthesis; however, over the years, many variations have been developed to improve the cosmetic results and to reduce the percentage and severity of complications. Various types of implants have various normal sonographic appearances.

The most common implant type consists of a single-lumen, smooth-surfaced silicone elastomer membrane (shell) filled with silicone gel. The silicone elastomer shell is permeable, and microscopic amounts of silicone can pass through the shell outside to the breast parenchyma. This phenomenon is known as gel bleed. Silicone that passes outside the shell incites a foreign-body reaction that is believed responsible for the formation of a fibrous capsule around the implant. The addition of fluorsilicone to the elastomer membrane decreases its permeability and decreases problems with gel bleed and contracture.[103,104] Textured silicone gel implants have shells whose outer surfaces have been roughened. These implants have less severe fibrous capsular reaction and therefore have less capsular contraction.[105]

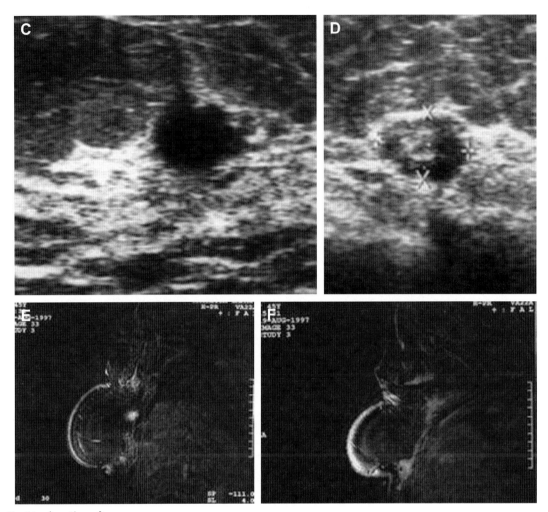

Fig. 24. (*continued*)

Single-lumen saline implants are the types implanted most frequently. Saline implants have advantages of being implantable through a smaller incision, and less prone to capsular contracture, and less dense on mammograms than the silicone gel implants. The disadvantages of saline implants are that the cosmetic result is inferior compared with silicone implants and they are more prone to rupture with minor trauma. Double lumen implants generally are constructed with an inner silicone-filled elastomer bag and outer saline-filled elastomer shell. The reverse configuration also exists and is used as a tissue expander after mastectomy (**Fig. 26**). The implantation site of implants also varies. Implants can be placed in subglandular or subpectoral locations. Implants can be placed from inframammary, periareolar, and axillary routes and they also can be placed endoscopically through paraumbilical incisions.[103,105]

Mammography is not considered the ideal tool for studying breast implants because of low sensitivity for the detection of implant complications and for the evaluation of other abnormalities in the breast.[106–110] Recent studies comparing sonography with MR imaging, mammography, and physical examination have found sonography superior to mammography for the detection of implant rupture but less sensitive than MR imaging.[111,112] Currently, MR imaging is considered the gold standard, with a sensitivity higher than 90%.[113–116] Patients who are evaluated solely for implant integrity, therefore, usually undergo MR imaging rather than sonography. Patients who have implants, however, like those who do not have implants, frequently have clinically or mammographically detected abnormalities for which targeted sonography is the procedure of choice. These abnormalities may be caused by

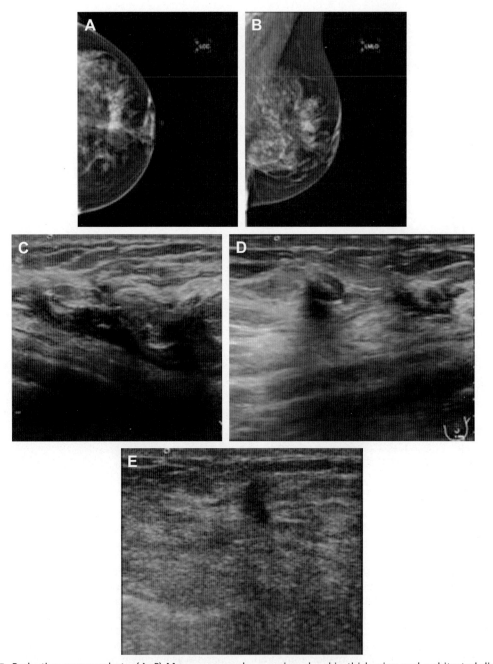

Fig. 25. Reduction mammoplasty. (*A, B*) Mammograms show periareolar skin thickening and architectral distortion and redistribution of fibroglandular tissue especially in the central and lower parts of the breast. (*C–E*) US demonstrates irregular hypoechoic lesions consistent with scar most of which are located in the lower quadrants. Sonographic interpretation may be impaired in patients with reduction mammoplasty because of these irregular hypoechoic lesions.

implant complications or by other breast pathologies.

Evaluation of implants may be the primary or the secondary goal of sonography. Overlying breast tissues and the implant can be evaluated with US. Although the diagnostic accuracy of US is controversial according to the literature, it has a high sensitivity if it is performed by a skilled radiologist.[117–122]

Evaluation of the peripheral edges of the implant usually is possible with 7.5- to 12-MHz probes. Evaluation of the center of the implant is more

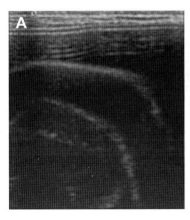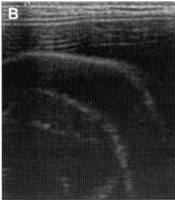

Fig. 26. (*A, B*) Double-lumen implant placed after mastectomy. The echogenic lines inside the implant represent the inner shell and should not be confused with intracapsular rupture. Note also the three echogenic lines anterior to the implant representing the outer shell and the capsule (*B*).

likely to require lower-frequency, more deeply focused 5-MHz linear or curved linear transducers, especially in patients who have capsular contracture or intracapsular rupture in which the elastomer shell has completely collapsed and fallen to the posterior aspect of the intracapsular space.[103,123] Some patients may have palpable folds or wrinkles in the implant shell that are palpable only in certain positions. They should be scanned in the position in which the abnormality is palpated and in the routine positions.

When evaluating implants, split-screen, mirror image scanning is suggested. Split-screen mirror image uses contralateral side as a cross-control at the same location. This approach is important in evaluating the alterations in internal echogenicity that occurs in patients who have intracapsular rupture of single-lumen silicone gel implants. Using very light compression during scanning of implants helps minimize reverberation echoes in the near field.[103]

NORMAL SONOGRAPHIC FINDINGS

The normal sonographic appearances of implants vary, depending on the type of implant and implantation site.

Echogenicity of Implant Contents

The contents of single-lumen silicone gel and single-lumen saline implants appear sonolucent (anechoic). Reverberation and ring-down artifacts can be present in the near field (**Fig. 27**). Reverberation artifacts commonly are encountered in the anterior aspects of intact implants and these echoes should not be confused with abnormalities. As a general rule, reverberation artifacts should be no thicker than the breast tissue anterior to the implant.[103,123,124] Recent technical developments, such as high frequency code harmonics, can reduce reverberation artifacts significantly.

Normally, silicone gel within the single-lumen implants is anechoic except for reverberation artifacts. In some patients who have neither intracapsular nor extracapsular rupture, however, heterogenous echoes may be scattered throughout the gel. These echoes may represent saline, povidone-iodine, antibiotics, or some other substance that was injected at the time of implantation, but in many cases their cause is unknown. These normal varient echoes are more heterogenous than the diffusely increased echogenicity that occurs within ruptured implants.[103]

Folds and Lobulations of the Elastomer Implant Membrane

The degree of wrinkling, folding, and lobulation in the implant membrane varies, and generally is

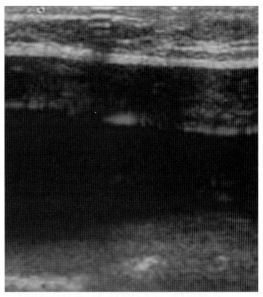

Fig. 27. Reverberation artifacts in the anterior aspect of the implant.

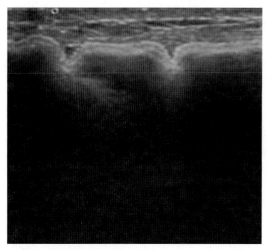

Fig. 28. Lobulations on the anterior surface of the implant. Note that the fibrous capsule and the outer shell are together and parallel.

more marked in saline than silicone gel implants. Wrinkles should be distinguished from the folds. In wrinkles, outer contour of the implant is lobulated, but the fibrous capsule is tightly opposed to the shell throughout the course of the lobulation, and the capsule and the elastomer shell remain parallel (**Fig. 28**). Radial folds are echogenic lines extending from the periphery of the implant to interior. In radial folds, elastomer shell invaginates and separates from the capsule, creating a potential space between the shell and the capsule. Radial folds are dynamic structures and are not fixed in position and size. Radial folds commonly are found in normal implants but seen more frequently and may be more prominent in the presence of capsular contracture.[2,123,124] If the folds occur on the anterior surface of the implant shell, they may be palpable.

The peri-implant fibrous capsule and shell complex of implants is represented by three echogenic lines: outer line representing surface of the capsule, middle echogenic line consisting of the fused echogenic lines of inner surface of the capsule and the outer surface of the shell, and the inner echogenic line representing the inner surface of the shell. The isoechoic or anechoic space between the outer and middle echogenic lines represents the thickness of the capsule or the thickness of the capsule together with the peri-implant effusion. The anechoic space between the middle and inner echogenic lines represents the thickness of the shell (see **Fig. 26 and 27**). Microscopic gel bleed or fat necrosis can lead to capsular calcifications that form along the inner surface of the fibrous capsule.[103]

Peri-implant Fluid Collections

Peri-implant effusions are normal findings. Normal effusions are small, not under pressure, and generally along the periphery of the implants or within the radial folds (**Fig. 29**). Any type of implant may induce a surrounding fluid collection but it is encountered more frequently in textured implants compared with smooth implants. This peri-implant fluid is anechoic or nearly anechoic. It can become echogenic over time for a variety of reasons. In some cases it can be difficult to distinguish between echogenic peri-implant effusion and mildly echogenic or extravasated silicone associated with implant rupture.[104]

Implantation Site

In subglandular or prepectoral implants, breast tissue and fibrous capsule lie superficial to the implant and pectoralis major muscle lies posterior to the implant. In retropectoral implants, pectoralis

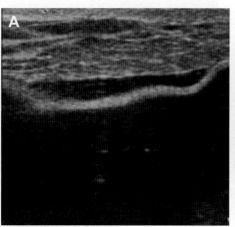
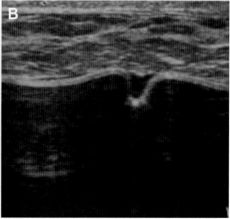

Fig. 29. (*A, B*) Peri-implant effusion.

major muscle lies superficially. Pectoralis major muscle covers only the superior part of the implant. Thus, when sonographically evaluating an implant site, the axillary segment must be evaluated, where the muscle is thickest. If the inferior part is scanned below the free edge of the pectoralis muscle, sonographic appearance is indistinguishable from that of a subglandular implant.[103]

OMPLICATIONS OF IMPLANTS

Complications of implants may occur immediately after surgery or months to years after implantation. Acute complications include bleeding and infection, asymmetry, loss of nipple sensation, pain, and tenderness. Long-term complications are encapsulation and capsular contracture, rupture (intracapsular or extracapsular), migration, herniation, hematoma/seroma, infection, capsular calcifications, and explantation or revision. Possible long-term complications include autoimmune disorder (human adjuvant disease) and carcinogenesis. In early complications (acute or subacute bleeding and local infection), US represents a useful diagnostic tool for diagnosis and for interventional procedures, such as drainage. Interventional US reduces the number of reoperations, allowing a fast problem solution and reduction of cost.[122]

Capsular Contracture

Even though capsular contracture is a clinical diagnosis, US findings may confirm clinical suspicion and give additional information about implant integrity. Demonstrable sonographic findings are abnormal spherical shape, abnormal thickening of the capsule (more than 1.5 mm), increased redundancy of the shell, and increased number of radial folds. The abnormal spherical shape can be identified when the anteroposterior dimension is greater than the transverse dimention and the posterior wall of the implant has a convex outward shape on the side of the capsular contracture.[103]

Implant Herniation

Implant herniation occurs most commonly in patients who have capsular contraction with very uneven thickening of the capsule. Herniation tends to occur through the thinnest segments of the capsule. Sonographically focal defect in the fibrous capsule and implant herniation through a rent in peri-implant fibrous capsule can be identified. In the herniated portion of an implant, there are only two thin echogenic lines instead of the three echogenic lines. Herniation can cause palpable abnormalities and, as is the case for radial folds, can be positional.[103]

Extracapsular Rupture

The most reliable sign of an extracapsular rupture is the presence of macroscopic amount of silicone gel outside of the implant shell and the peri-implant capsule. Extravasated silicone gel leads to formation of silicone granulomas, which may cause tender or nontender palpable lumps. Silicone granulomas represent free silicone globules, fibrosis and foreign body reaction. The most typical sonographic finding in silicone granuloma is a snowstorm appearance, which consists of a markedly and homogeneously hyperechoic nodule with a well-circumscribed, rounded anterior border; and dirty, incoherent posterior shadowing that obscures its posterior border. Besides the snowstorm appearance, silicone granulomas can present as cystic, complex cystic, semisolid nodules, or spiculated masses with acoustic shadowing. Complex cystic and snowstorm phases commonly coexist (**Fig. 30**).[120,125,126] Only the snowstorm appearance is diagnostic for extracapsular rupture sonographically. Demonstration of cystic or semisolid nodules can suggest the diagnosis is not specific.

Extravasated silicone gel can migrate away to the chest wall, the upper abdomen, or the axilla. Migrated silicone also presents with snowstorm appearance and its demonstration is evidence of extracapsular rupture.[127,128] In the presence of implant rupture, macroscopic amount of silicone also can be carried through lymphatic channels to the axillary lymph nodes. Lymph nodes appear hyperechoic; snowstorm shadowing begins in the hilum and progresses outward to the cortex with time. It is more difficult to define the structure as that of a lymph node.

Intracapsular Rupture

Intracapsular implant ruptures occur when silicone gel escapes through a rent in shell but remains confined within the surrounding fibrous capsule. Radial folds are common places for fatigue fractures to occur and, therefore, are common sites for intracapsular rupture to begin. The classically described sonographic findings in intracapsular rupture are the presence of abnormally echogenic extravasated silicone gel that lies outside the implant shell but remains confined within the intracapsular space and the stepladder sign (the sonograpic counterpart to the MR imaging linguini sign). The stepladder sign consists of horizontal echogenic straight or curvilinear lines, somewhat

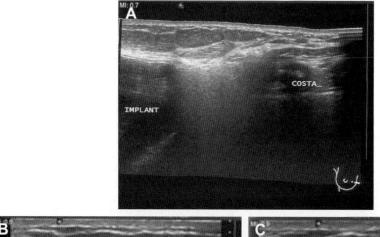

Fig. 30. Extracapsular rupture. (*A*) Snowstorm appearance represented by an echogenic area with shadowing. (*B*) The implant shell is freely floating inside the implant (stepladder sign). Note that there are only two echogenic lines at the anterior surface of the lumen instead of three because the shell is separated from the fibrous capsule. (*C*) Free silicone (silicone granuloma) inside the breast.

parallel, traversing the interior of the implant. This sign represents the collapsed elastomer shell floating within the implant (**Figs. 30** and **31**).[129] Another sign related to internal structure is presence of increased low level homogeneous echoes within the implant.[118] When US signs of intracapsular rupture is present, a thorough search for extracapsular rupture should be performed,

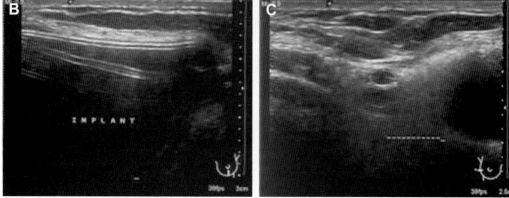

Fig. 31. Intra- and extracapsular rupture. (*A, B*) The echogenicity of the implant is increased and mixed because of extravasation of silicone outside the shell. The echoenic lines inside the implant represent the collapsed elastomer shell floating inside the implant (stepladder sign). There also were signs of extracapsular rupture not shown here.

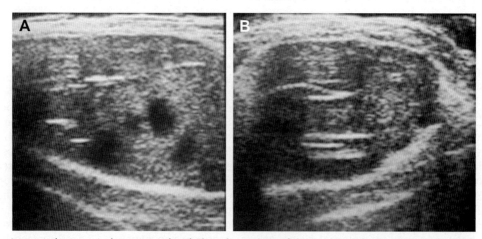

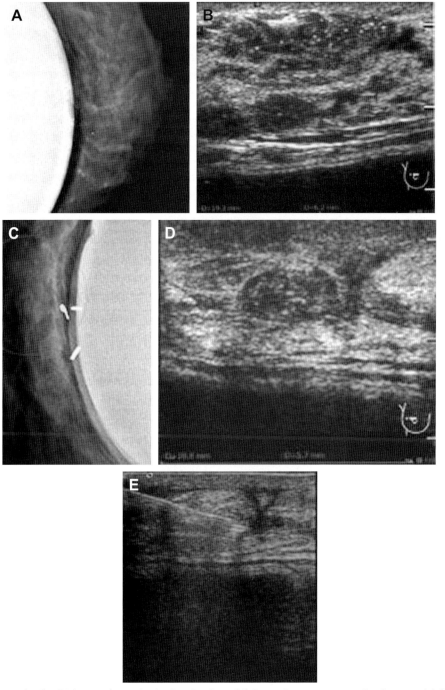

Fig. 32. Diagnosis of DCIS in a patient who had an implant. (*A*) Screening mammography shows multiple clusters of nonuniform low density microcalcifications. (*B*) US demonstrates the microcalcifications clearly. The patient refused mastectomy and underwent breast conserving therapy. (*C*) One year after the operation, control mammogram showed residual microcalcifications and surgical clips at the operation site. (*D*) The residual focus of microcalcifications also was identified on US. (*E*) The patient refused to have mastectomy again. The calcifications were excised after US-guided needle localization and residual high-grade DCIS was confirmed.

including careful scanning of the axilla to look for silicone granulomas.

There is a wide spectrum of findings in intracapsular rupture that varies with the size of the defect in the shell and the degree of collapse. In most patients who have intracapsular rupture, the shell defect is small, and the degree of collapse is less than complete. Traditionally, MR imaging has been reported as more accurate[112,130] in cases with less than complete collapse because the classic sonographic findings usually are associated with complete collapse of the implant.

Primary and Recurrent Tumors

Breast carcinoma may develop after breast augmentation. Breast augmentation alone does not increase the cancer risk in these patients, but women who have reconstructions after mastectomy have elevated breast cancer risk because of their personal history of breast malignancy. It has been shown that breast cancer diagnosis can be delayed in patients who have implants. Handel reported that in a study of 4082 breast cancer patients (3953 nonaugmented and 129 augmented), that augmented patients presented more frequently with palpable invasive tumors, axillary nodal metastases, and false-negative mammograms. Although the sensitivity of mammography was reduced in augmented women, tumors were diagnosed at a similar stage and their prognosis were similar to nonaugmented women.[131] Tuli and colleagues[132] also report that implants reduce mammographic sensitivity and interfere with mammographic detection, leading to delay in cancer diagnosis. In their experience, 8 out of 12 patients who had implants presented with palpable lumps whereas only 4 were diagnosed mammographically. Breast conservation was possible in only 50% of these patients.

US is a better alternative than mammography for the evaluation of breasts with implants. With subglandular and retropectoral implantations, all of the diagnostically relevant breast tissue lies anterior to the implants and is easily accessible to US evaluation. The appearance of tumors is the same as in breasts without implants (**Fig. 32**). A potential problem is that silicone granulomas may be palpable and present as hypoechoic masses with irregular margins, mimicking carcinoma. But the diagnosis still can be established and surgery avoided using US-guided needle biopsy. Usually FNAB is preferred in these patients to avoid rupture of the implant. It is reported to be highly accurate.[133] Only experienced examiners should attempt to biopsy a lesion in such a confined space.

SUMMARY

Superimposition of post-treatment changes with the fibroglandular tissue is the main reason for the decreased sensitivity and accuracy of mammography in treated breasts. Post-treatment changes in the breast can be visualized clearly and directly with US. Its main advantage over mammography is that it is tomographic, each image representing a thin slice of tissue, thus eliminating superimposition of structures. The technical developments in US have increased considerably its role in all aspects of breast imaging, including evaluation of the treated breasts. It no longer is only an adjunct to mammography for the evaluation of fluid collections but increases accuracy in the follow-up of operated breasts. It can serve as a problem-solving method in patients who have clinical or mammograpic abnormalities and as a guide for interventional procedures to avoid surgical biopsies. Its role as a screening adjunct to mammography in the follow-up of operated breasts has yet to be established but it increases sensitivity and accuracy, especially in dense breasts and breasts that are difficult to evaluate mammographically because of prominent post-treatment changes. As is the case for all US examinations, however, experience is important for correct interpretation of US findings, which can be misleading, especially in those patients who have prominent fibrosis and fat necrosis. Detailed documentation of all findings at the first examination after surgery is necessary to serve as a baseline for future follow-ups and to avoid unnecessary biopsies and anxiety. MR imaging also is a good problem solving method in operated breasts and should be included in the work-up whenever necessary.

REFERENCES

1. Mendelson EB, Tobin CE. Imaging the breast after rediation and surgery. In: Friedrich, Sickles, editors. Radiological diagnosis of breast lesions. Berlin: Springer Verlag; 2000.
2. Krishnamurty R, Whitman GJ Stelling C, Kushwaha AC. Mammographic findings after breast conserving therapy. Radiographics 1999;S53–62 Spec No.
3. Arriagada R, Le MG, Rochard F, et al. Conservative treatment versus mastectomy in early breast cancer: patterns of failure with 15 years of follow-up data. Institut Gustave-Roussy Breast Cancer Group. J Clin Oncol 1996;14:1558–64.
4. Bichert-Toft M, Rose C, Anderson JA, et al. Danish randomized trial comparing breast conservation therapy with mastectomy: six years of life-table

analysis. J Natl Cancer Inst Monographs 1992;11: 19–25.

5. Fisher B, Anderson S, Redmond CK, et al. Reanalysis and results after 12 years of follow-up in a randomized clinical trial comparing total mastectomy with lumpectomy with or without irradiation in the teatment of breast cancer. N Engl J Med 1995;33: 1456–61.

6. Jacobson JA, Dandorth DN, Cowan KH, et al. Ten-year results of a comparison of conservation with mastectomy in the treatment of stage I and II breast cancer. N Engl J Med 1995;332:907–11.

7. van Dongen JA, Voogd AC, Fentimen IS, et al. Long-term results of a randomized trial comparing breast conserving therapy with mastectomy: European organization for Research and Treatment of Cancer10801 trial. J Natl Cancer Inst 2000;92: 1143–50.

8. Veronesi U, Salvadori B, Luini A, et al. Conservative treatment of early breast cancer: long-term results of 1232 cases treated with quadrentectomy, axillary dissection, and radiotherapy. Ann Surg 1990;211: 250–9.

9. Mendelson EB. Evaluation of the postoperative breast. Radiol Clin North Am 1992;30(1):107–38.

10. Dershaw DD. Breast imaging and the conservatively treatment of breast cancer. Radiol Clin North Am 2002;40(3):501–516101.

11. Zhang Y, Fukatsu H, Naganawa S, et al. The role of contrast-enhanced MR mammography for determining candidates for breast conservation surgery. Breast Cancer 2002;9(3):231–9.

12. Berg WA, Gutierrez L, NessAiver MS, et al. Diagnostic accuracy of mammography, clinical examination, US and MR imaging in preoperative assessment of breast cancer. Radiology 2004; 233(3):830–49.

13. Schelfout K, Van Goethem M, Kersschot E, et al. Contrast-enhanced MR imaging of breast lesions and effect on treatment. Eur J Surg Oncol 2004; 30(5):501–7118.

14. Hata T, Takahashi H, Watanabe K, et al. Magnetic resonance imaging for preoperative evaluation of breast cancer: a comparative study with mammography and ultrasonography. J Am Coll Surg 2004; 198(2):190–7.

15. Boetes C, Mus RDM, Holland R, et al. Breast tumors: comparative accuracy of MR imaging relative to mammograhy and US to demonstrating extent. Radiology 1995;197:743–7.

16. Yang WT, Lam WWM, Cheung H, et al. Sonographic, magnetic resonance imaging and mammographic assessments of preoperative size of breast cancer. J Ultrasound Med 1997;16:791–7.

17. Hlawatsch A, Teifke A, Schimidt M, et al. Preoperative assessment of breast cancer: sonography versus MR imaging. AJR Am J Roentgenol 2002; 179:1493–501.

18. Bagley FH. The role of magnetic resonance imaging mammography in the surgical management of the index breast cancer. Arch Surg 2004;139(4): 380–3.

19. Schnall M. MR imaging evaluation of cancer extent: is there clinical relevance? Magn Reson Imaging Clin N Am 2006;14(3):379–81.

20. Liberman L, Morris EA, Dershaw DD, et al. MR imaging of the ipsilateral breast in women with percutaneously proven breast cancer. AJR Am Jroentgenol 2003;180:901–10.

21. Fisher U, Kopka L, Grabbe E. Breast carcinoma: effect of preoperative contrast-enhanced MRI on the therapeutic approach. Radiology 1999;213: 881–8.

22. Bedrosian I, Mick R, Orel SG, et al. Changes in the surgical management of patients with breast carcinoma based on preoperative magnetic resonance imaging. Cancer 2003;98:468–73.

23. La Trenta LR, Menell JH, Morris EA, et al. Breast lesions detected with MR imaging: utility and histopathologic importance of identification with US. Radiology 2003;227:856–61.

24. Shin JH, Choe YH, Ko K, et al. Targeted ultrasound for MR detected lesions in breast cancer patients. Korean J Radiol 2007;8(6):475–83.

25. Haid A, Knauer M, Dunzinger S, et al. Intra-operative sonography: valuable aid during breast-conserving surgery for occult breast cancer. Ann Surg Oncol 2007;14(11):3090–101.

26. Bennett IC, Greenslade J, Chiam H. Intraoperative ultrasound-guided excision of nonpalpable breast lesions. World J Surg 2005;29(3):369–74.

27. Kaufman CS, Jacobson L, Bachman B, et al. Intraoperative ultrasonography guidance is accurate and efficient according to results in 100 breast cancer patients. Am J Surg 2003;186(4):378–82.

28. Dershaw DD. The conservatively treated breast. In: Bassett LW, Jackson V, Fu K, editors. Diagnosis of diseases of the breast. 2nd edition. Philadelphia: Elsvier; 2005. p. 585–99.

29. Newstead GM. Clinical role of breast MR imaging. In: Karellas A, Giger ML, editors. RSNA 2004 Syllabus: advances in breast imaging: physics, technology, and clinical applications. Brook (IL): RSNA; 2004. p. 279–89.

30. Frei KA, Kinkel K, Bonel HM, et al. MR imaging of the breast in patients with positive margins after lmpectomy: influence of the time interval beween lumpectomy and MR imaging. AJR Am J Roentgenol 2000;175:1577–8.

31. Lee JM, Orel SG, Czerniecki BJ, et al. MRI before reexcision surgery in patients with breast cancer. AJRAm J Roentgenol 2004;182(2):473–80.

32. Orel SG, Renolds C, Schnall MD, et al. Breast carcinoma: MR imaging before re-excisional biopsy. Radiology 1997;205:429–36.

33. Hwang ES, Kinkel K, Esserman LJ, et al. Magnetic resonance imaging in patients diagnosed with ductal carcinoma in situ: value in the diagnosis of residual disease, occult invasion and multicentricity. Ann Surg Oncol 2003;10:381–8.

34. Shin JH, Han BK, Choe YH, et al. Ultrasonographic detection of occult cancer in patients after surgical therapy for breast cancer. J Ultrasound Med 2005; 24(5):643–9.

35. Ashkanani F, Sarkar T, Needham G, et al. What is clearly achieved by surveillence after breast conservation treatment for breast cancer? Ann J Surg 2001;182(3):207–10.

36. Heywang S, Dershaw DD, Schreer I, editors. Post-traumatic, post-surgical, and post-therapeutic changes. In: Diagnostic breast imaging. 2nd edition. New York: Thieme; 2001.

37. Sonographic evaluation of the iatrogenically altered breast. In: Stavros AT, editor. Breast Ultrasound. Philadelphia: Lippincott Williams & Wilkins; 2004. p. 778–832.

38. Mendelson EB. Imaging the post-surgical breast. CT, MR. Semin in Ultrasound 1989;10:154–70.

39. Singletary SE, McNeese M. Segmental mastectomy and irradiation in the treatment of breast cancer. Am J Clin Oncol 1988;11:679–83.

40. Madjar H, Mendelson EB. Scars—the treated breast. In: The practice of breast ultrasound: techniques, findings, differential diagnosis. New York: Thieme; 2008. p. 157–66.

41. Mendelson EB, Harris KM, Doshi N, et al. Infiltrating lobular carcinoma: mammographic patterns with pathologic correlation. AJR Am J Roentgenol 1989;153:265–71.

42. Miller CL, Feig SA, Fox JW. Mammographic changes after reduction mammoplasty. AJR Am J Roentgenol 1987;149:35–8.

43. Tan PH, Lai LM, Carrington EV, et al. Fat necrosis of the breast—a review. Breast 2006;15(3):313–8.

44. Baillie M, Mok PM. Fat necrosis in the breast: review of the mammographic and ultrasound features, and a strategy for management. Australas Radiol 2004;48(3):285–8.

45. Chala LF, Barros N, de Camargo Moraes P, et al. Fat necrosis of the breast: mammographic, sonographic, computed tomography, and magnetic resonance imaging findings. Curr Probl Diagn Radiol 2004;33(3):106–26.

46. Kinoshita T, Yashiro N, Yoshigi J, et al. Fat necrosis of breast: a potential pitfall in breast MRI. Clin Imaging 2002;26(4):250–3.

47. Bilgen IG, Ustun EE, Memis A. Fat necrosis of the breast: clinical, mammographic and sonographic features. Eur J Radiol 2001;39(2):92–9.

48. Soo MS, Kornguth PJ, Herzberg BS. Fat necrosis in the breast: sonographic features. Radiology 1998; 206(1):261–9.

49. Harvey JA, Moran RE, Maurer EJ, et al. Sonographic features of mammay oil cysts. J Ultrasound Med 1997;16(11):719–24.

50. Wasser K, Schoeber C, Kraus-Tiefenbacher U, et al. Early mammographic and sonographic findings after inraoperative radiotherapy (IORT) as a boost in patients with breast cancer. Eur Radiol 2007;17(7):1865–74.

51. Della Sala SW, Pellegrini M, Bernardi D, et al. Mammographic and ultrasonographic comparison between intraoperative radiotherapy (IORT) and conventional external radiotherapy (RT) in limited-stage breast cancer, conservatively treated. Eur J Radiol 2006;59(2):222–30.

52. Mitnick JS, Vazquez MF, Roses DF, et al. Recurrent breast cancer: streotaxic localization for fine-needle aspiration biopsy. Radiology 1992;182:103–6.

53. Dershaw DD, Shank B, Reisinger S. Mammographic findings after breast cancer treatment with local excision and definitive irradiation. Radiology 1987;164:455–561.

54. Roebuch EJ. The subcutaneous reaction: a useful mammographic sign. Clin Radiol 1984;35:311–5.

55. Mendelson EB. Problem solving ultrasound. Radiol Clin North Am 2004;42(5):909–18.

56. Zannis VJ, Walker LC, Barclay-White B, et al. Postoperative ultrasound-guided percutaneous placement of a new breast brachytherapy balloon catheter. Am J Surg 2003;186(4):383–5.

57. Osborne MP, Borgen PL. Role of mastectomy in breast cancer. Surg Clin North Am 1990;70: 1023–46.

58. Dewarz JA, Arriagada R, Benhamou S, et al. (for the IGR breast Cancer Group). Local relapse and contralateral tumor rates in patients with breast cancer treated with conservative surgery and radiotherapy (Institut Gustave-Roussy 1970–1982). Cancer 1995;76:2260–5.

59. Stotter AT, McNeese MD, Ames FC, et al. Predicting the rate and extent of locoregional failure after breast conservation therapy for early breast cancer. Cancer 1989;64:2217–25.

60. Kurtz JM, Spitalier JM, Almaric R, et al. Results of wide-excision for local recurrence after breast-conserving therapy. Cancer 1989;61:1969–72.

61. Harris JR, Recht A. Conservative surgery and radiotherapy. In: Harris JR, Hellman S, Henderson IC, editors. Breast diseases. 2nd edition.. Philadelphia: JB Lippincott; 1991. p. 338–419.

62. Arriagada R, Le MG, Guinebretiere JM, et al. Late local recurrences in a randomized trial comparing conservative treatment with total mastectomy in early breast cancer patients. Ann Oncol 2003; 14(11):1617–22.

63. Fowble B, Solin LJ, Schultz DJ, et al. Breast recurrence following conservative surgery and radiation. Patterns of failure, prognosis and pathologic findings from mastectomy specimens with implications for treatment. Int J Radiat Oncol Biol Phys 1990;19: 833–42.

64. Dershaw DD, McCormick B, Osborne MP. Detection of local recurrence after conservative therapy for breast carcinoma. Cancer 1992;70:493–6.

65. Locker AP, Hanley P, Wilson AR, et al. Mammography in the pre-operative assessment and post-operative surveillance of patients treated by excision and radiotherapy for primary breast cancer. Clin Radiol 1990;41:388–91.

66. Stomper PC, Recht A, Barenberg AL, et al. Mammographic detection of recuurent cancer in the irradiated breast. AJR Am J Roentgenol 1987;148: 39–43.

67. Orel SG, Fowble BL, Solin LJ, et al. Mammographic detection of recurrence after lumpectomy and radiation therapy for early-stage disease: prognostic significance of detection method. Radiology 1993; 188:189–94.

68. Gunhan-Bilgen I, Oktay A. Mammographic features of local recurrence after conservative surgery and radiation therapy: comparison with that of the primary tumor. Acta Radiol 2007;48(4):390–7.

69. Balu-Maestro C, Bruneton JN, Geoffray A, et al. Ultrasonographic posttreatment follow-up of breast cancer patients. J Ultrasound Med 1991;10:1–7.

70. Mesurolle B, Helou T, El-Khoury M, et al. Tissue harmonic imaging, frequency compound imaging, and conventional imaging: use and benefit in breast sonography. J Ultrasound Med 2007; 26(8):1041–51.

71. Weinstein SP, Conant EF, Sehgal C. Technical advances in breast ultrasound imaging. Semin Ultrasound CT MR 2006;27(4):273–83.

72. Huber S, Wagner M, Medl M, et al. Real-time spatial compound imaging in breast ultrasound. Ultrasound Med Biol 2002;28(2):155–63.

73. Cha JH, Moon WK, Cho N, et al. Differentiation of benign from malignant solid breast masses: conventional US versus spatial compound imaging. Radiology 2005;237(3):841–6.

74. Esen G, Gurses B, Yılmaz MH, et al. Gray-scale and power Doppler US in the preoperative evaluation of axillary metastases in breast cancer patients with no palpable lymph nodes. Eur Radiol 2005;15: 1215–23.

75. Aichinger U, Schulz-Wendtland R, Kramer S, et al. Scars or recurrrence—comparison of MRI and color-coded ultrasound with echo signal amplifiers. Rofo 2002;174(11):1395–401.

76. Morris EA. Diagnostic breast MR maging: current status and future directions. Radiol Clin North Am 2007;45(5):863–80.

77. Gorechlad JW, McCabe EB, Higgins JH, et al. Screening for recurrences in patients treated with breast conserving surgery: is there a role for MRI? Ann Surg Oncol 2008;1(6):1703–9.

78. Khatcheressian J, Swainey C. Breast cancer follow-up in the adjuva setting. Curr Oncol Rep. 2008; 10(1):38–46.

79. Baz E, Madjar H, Reuss C, et al. The role of enhanced Doppler ultrasound in differentiation of benign vs. malignant scar lesion after breast surgery for malignancy. Ultrasound Obstet Gynecol 2000; 15(5):377–82.

80. Winehouse J, Douek M, Holz K, et al. Contrast-enhanced colour Doppler ultrasonography in suspected breast cancer recurrence. Br J Surg 1999; 86(9):1198–201.

81. Freedman GM, Anderson PR, Goldstein LJ, et al. Routine mammography is associated with earlier stage disease and greater eligibility for breast conservation in breast carcinoma patients age 40 years and older. Cancer 2003;98(5):918–25.

82. Tarja J, Rissanen MD, Hanna P, et al. Breast cancer recurrence after mastectomy: diagnosis with Mammography and US. Radiology 1993;188:463–7.

83. Zimmerman KW, Montague ED, Fletcher GH. Frequency, anatomical distribution and management of local recurrences after definitive therapy for breast cancer. Cancer 1996;19:67–74.

84. DeVita VT, Hellmann S, Rosenberg S. Local recurrence after mastectomy. In: Cancer: Principles and practice of oncology. 5th edition. Lippincott-Raven Publishers; 1997. p. 1582–3.

85. Horiguch J, Koibuchi Y, Yoshida T, et al. Significance of local recurrence as a prognostic factor in the treatment of breast cancer. Anticancer Res 2006;26(1B):569–73.

86. Fajardo LL, Roberts CC, Hunt KR. Mammographic surveillence of breast cancer patients: should the mastectomy site be imaged? AJR Am J Roentgenol 1993;161:953–5.

87. Rissanen TJ, Apaja-Sarkkinen MA, Makarainen HP, et al. Ultrasound-guided fine needle aspiration biopsy in the diagnosis of breast cancer recurrence after mastectomy. Acta Radiol 1997;38(2):232–9.

88. Yilmaz MH, Esen G, Ayarcan Y, et al. The role of US and MR imaging in detecting local chest wall tumorrecurrences after mastectomy. Diagn Interv Radiol 2007;13(1):13–8.

89. Willner J, Kiricuta IC, Kolbl O. Locoregional recurrence of breast cancer following mastectomy: always a fatal event? Results of univariate and multivariate analysis. Int J Radiat Oncol Biol Phys 1997;37(4):853–63.

90. Kim SM, Park JM. Mammographic and ultrasonographic features after autogenous myocutaneous flap reconstruction mammoplasty. J Ultrasound Med 2004;23(2):275–82.

91. Barnsley GP, Grunfeld E, Coyle D, et al. Surveillance mammography following the treatment of primary breast cancer with breast reconstruction: a systematic review. Plast Reconstr Surg 2007; 120(5):1125–32.

92. Edeiken BS, Fornage BD, Bedi DG, et al. Recurrence in myocutaneous flap reconstruction after mastectomy for primary breast cancer: US diagnosis. Radiology 2003;227(2):542–8.

93. Lee JM, Georgian-Smith D, Gazelle GS, et al. Detecting nonpalpable recurrent breast cancer: the role of routine mammographic screening of transverse rectus abdominis myocutaneous flapreconstructions. Radiology 2008;248(2):398–405.

94. Helvie MA, Bailey JE, Roubidoux MA, et al. Mammographic screening of TRAM flap breast reconstructions for detection of nonpalpable recurrent cancer. Radiology 2002;224(1):211–6.

95. Devon RK, Rosen MA, Mies C, et al. Breast reconstruction with a transverse rectus abdominis myocutaneous flap: spectrum of normal and abnormal MR imaging findings. Radiographics 2004;24(5):1287–99.

96. Temple CL, Strom EA, Youssef A, et al. Choice of recipient vessels in delayed TRAM flap reconstruction after radiotherapy. Plast Reconstr Surg 2005; 115(1):105–13.

97. Greco RJ, Dascombe WH, Williams SL, et al. Two-staged breast reconstruction in patients with symptomatic macromastia requiring mastectomy. Ann Plast Surg 1994;32:572–9.

98. Jackson V. Reduction mammoplasty. In: Bassett LW, Jackson V, Fu K, editors. Diagnosis of diseases of the Breast. 2nd edition. Philadelphia: Elsevier; 2005. p. 617–22.

99. Hidalgo DA, Franklyn EL, Palumbo S, et al. Current trends in breast reduction. Plast Reconstr Surg 1999;104:806–15.

100. Strombeck JO. Reduction mammoplasty. In: Strombeck JO, Rosato FE, editors. Surgery of the breast: diagnosis and treatment of breast diseases. New York: Georg Thieme; 1986. p. 277–311.

101. Brown FE, Sargent SK, Cohen SR, et al. Mammographic changes following reduction mammoplasty. Plast Reconstr Surg 1987;80:691–8.

102. Brown MH, Weinberg M, Chong N, et al. A cohort study of breast cancer risk in breast reduction patients. Plast Reconstr Surg 1999;103:1674–81.

103. Stavros AT. Nontargeted indications: mammary implants. In Stavros AT (editor). Breast ultrasound. Philadelphia, Lippincott Williams & Wilkins 2004, pp. 199–274.

104. Nemecek JAR, Young VL. How safe are silicone gel implants? Southampt Med J 1993;86:932–44.

105. Reynolds HE. Evaluation of the augmented breast. Radiol Clin North Am 1995;33(6):1131–45.

106. O'Toole M, Caskey CI. Imaging spectrum of breast implant complications: mammography, ultrasound, and magnetic resonance imaging. Semin Ultrasound CT MR. 2000;21:351–61.

107. AzavedoE Bone B. Imaging breast with silicone implants. Eur Radiol. 1999;9:349–55.

108. Eklund GW, Busby RC, Miller SH, et al. Improved imaging of the augmented breast. AJR Am J Roentgenol 1988;151:469–73.

109. Ganott MA, Haris KM, Ilkhanipour ZS, et al. Augmentation mammoplasty: normal and abnormal findings with mammography and US. Radiographics. 1992;12:281–95.

110. Destouret JM, Monsees BS, Oser RF, et al. Screening mammography in 350 women with breast implants: prevalence and findings of implant complications. Am J Roentgenol. 1992; 159:973–8.

111. Gorczyca DP, DeBruhl ND, Ahn CY, et al. Silicone breast implant ruptures in an animal model: comparison of mammography, MR imaging, US, and CT. Radiology 1994;190:227–32.

112. Everson LI, Parantainen H, Detlies T, et al. Diagnosis of breast implant rupture: imaging findings and relative efficacies of imaging techniques. AJR 1994;163:57–60.

113. Berg WA, Caskey CI, Hamper UM, et al. Single and double lumen silicone breast implants integrity: prospective evaluation of MR and US criteria. Radiolgy 1995;197:45–52.

114. Gorczyca DP. MR imaging of breast implants. Magn Reson Imaging Clin N Am. 1994;2:659–72.

115. Monticciolo DL, Nelson RC, Dixon WT, et al. MR detection of leakage from silicone breast implants: value of a silicone-selective pulse sequence. Am J Roentgenol. 1994;163:51–6.

116. Gorczyca DP. Magnetic resonance imaging of the failing implants. In: Gorczyca DP, Brenner RJ, editors. The augmented breast: radiologic and clinical perspectives. Stuttgart: Thime; 1997. p. 121–43.

117. Medot M, Landis GH, McGregor CE, et al. Effects of capsular contracture on ultrasonic screening for silicone gel breast implant rupture. Ann Plast Surg. 1997;39:337–41.

118. Caskey CI, Berg WA, Anderson ND, et al. Breast implant rupture: diagnosis with US. Radiology 1994;190:819–23.

119. Levine RA, Collins TL. Definitive diagnosis of breast implant rupture by ultrasonography. Plast Reconstr Surg. 1991;87:1126–8.

120. Rosculet KA, Ikeda DM, Forrest ME, et al. Rupture gel-filled silicone breast implants: sonographic findings in 19 cases. Am J Roentgenol. 1992;159: 711–6.

121. Harris KM, Ganot MA, Shestak KC, et al. Silicone implant rupture: detection with US. Radiology 1993;187:761–8.

122. Cilotti A, Marini C, Iacconi C, et al. Ultrasonographic appearance of breast implant complications. Ann Plast Surg 2006;56:243–7.

123. DeBruhl ND, Gorczyca DP, Basett LW. Imaging after breast implants. In: Friedrich M, Sickles EA, editors. Radiological diagnosis of breast lesions. Berlin: Springer Verlag; 2000.
124. DeBruhl ND, Michael D, Gorczyca DP, et al. The augmented breast. In: Bassett LW, Jackson V, Fu K, editors. Diagnosis of diseases of the breast. 2nd editon. Philadelphia: Elsevier; 2005. p. 600–16.
125. Herzog P. Silicone granulomas: detection by ultrasonography. Plast Reconstr Surg. 1989;84:856–7.
126. Meigel W, Winzer M, Berg A, et al. Siliconoma. Z Hautkr 1989;64(9):815–6.
127. Liebman AJ, Kossoff MB, Kruse BD. Intraductal extension of silicone from a rupture breast implant. Plast Reconstr Surg. 1992;89:546–7.
128. Capozzi A, DuBou R, Pennisi VR. Distant migration of silicone gel from a ruptured breast implant. Plast Reconstr Surg. 1980;62:302–3.
129. DeBruhl ND, Gorczyca DP, Ahn CY, et al. Silicone breast implants: US evaluation. Radiology 1993; 189:95–8.
130. Ikeda DM, Borofsky HB, Herfkens RJ, et al. Silicone breast implant rupture: pitfalls of magnetic resonance imaging and relative efficacies of magnetic resonance, mammography and ultrasound. Plast Reconstr Surg 1999;104:2054–62.
131. Handel N. The effect of silicone implants on diagnosis, prognosis and treatment of breast cancer. Plast Reconstr Surg 2007;120/7(suppl 1):815–93.
132. Tuli R, Flynn RA, Brill KL, et al. Diagnosis, treatment and management of breast cancer in previously augmented women. Breast J 2006;12(4):343–8.
133. Fornage BD, Sneige N, Singletary SE. Masses in breasts with implants: diagnosis with US-guided fine-needle aspiration biopsy. Radiology 1994; 191(2):339–42.

Ectopic Pregnancy

Safiye Gurel, MD

KEYWORDS
- Ectopic • Pregnancy • Ultrasonography

Ectopic pregnancy (EP) is any pregnancy occurring outside the endometrial cavity of uterus and was first described by the Arab physician El-Zahrawi (Albucasis) in the tenth century who is acknowledged as the chief surgeon of the middle ages and up to the Renaissance.[1] EP can be studied in several subsets in terms of localization of implantation as extrauterine (tubal, ovarian, abdominal) and intrauterine (cornual, interstitial, cervical), presence of accompanying normal intrauterine pregnancy (heterotopic pregnancy), and clinical presentation as acute or chronic EP.

EP is one of the major causes of maternal-fetal morbidity and mortality and loss of pregnancy. It remains the leading cause of maternal death in the first trimester, the second leading cause of maternal mortality overall, and has an associated mortality that is 4 times greater than that of childbirth and 38 times greater than that of a legal induced abortion.[2,3] All causes of EP are associated with abnormalities of tubal structure or transport. It is much higher in the population treated with assisted reproductive techniques, with a prior history of EP, tubal surgery, tubal obstruction resulting from pelvic inflammatory disease (PID) or endometriosis, and use of intrauterine contraceptive device.[4,5] Cigarette smoking is another etiologic factor, in direct proportion to the total dose, possibly as a result of impaired tubal function.[6,7] Other risk factors such as vaginal douching, early onset of sexual activity, and multiple partners probably increase the risk of EP indirectly by increasing the risk of infection.[8] Contraceptive use is known to decrease the total incidence of EP. On the other hand, when a contraception method—mostly with intrauterine devices, progestin-based contraceptives, and tubal ligation—failure occurs, the risk of EP is relatively higher than among women not using contraception.[9,10]

Recent studies show that the incidence of EP is increasing worldwide, particularly in industrialized countries such as Northern Europe (from 11 to 19 per 1000 pregnancies between 1976 and 1993), United Kingdom (11,000 cases per year), and United States (from 0.5% to 1% to 2% in the past 30 years).[2,11,12] This remarkable increase in the prevalence of EP during the past 2 decades might be a result of several factors such as more sensitive ultrasound (US) examinations using advanced technology, more infertility treatment, increased incidence of PID and endometriosis, and widespread use of laparascopy.[5] Parallel to the increase in the prevalence of EP, a steady decrease in its morbidity and mortality is observed mostly because of earlier and prompt diagnosis with advanced technology of transvaginal US (TVUS).

CLINICAL PRESENTATION

The clinical finding of EP has a wide spectrum ranging between a completely asymptomatic status and peritoneal irritation resulting from rupture and consequent bleeding into the peritoneal cavity and hypovolemic shock.[13] The classic clinical triad of "pain, abnormal vaginal bleeding, palpable adnexal mass" is present in only 45% of patients with EP and this triad has a positive predictive value of only 14%.[14] Today, the ability to diagnose and evaluate pregnancy at very early gestational ages has altered the traditional presenting symptoms of EP. Up to 9% of patients report no pain, and 36% of them lack adnexal mass.[1,11,13] In spite of absence of pathognomonic symptoms and physical findings, a history of delayed or irregular menstrual period, prior history of assisted reproductive surgery, patient age, smoking, use of contraceptive methods, or prior tubal surgery can provide useful hints for suggesting EP in the differential diagnosis.

DIAGNOSIS

The mainstay parameters to use confidently in diagnosing an EP, after quite much discussion

Department of Radiology, Izzet Baysal University School of Medicine, Golkoy, 14280, Bolu, Turkey
E-mail address: safiyegurel@hotmail.com

Ultrasound Clin 3 (2008) 331–343
doi:10.1016/j.cult.2008.07.003

and debate, is a combination of TVUS findings and serial serum β-hCG levels.[15–18]

β-hCG, used in most laboratories today, becomes positive at approximately 23 menstrual days, in other words 9 days after conception, which is before a sac can be seen with TVUS.[19] In normally developing intrauterine pregnancies, serum levels of β-hCG approximately double in value every 48 hours during the first 10 weeks after the last menstrual period. The serum level of β-hCG peaks at approximately 10 menstrual weeks, and then begins to decline. During the first 10 weeks, a 66% rise over 2 days is generally considered acceptable evidence of a viable intrauterine pregnancy. However, rates of increase over 48 hours as high as 228% and as low as 53% have been documented in viable pregnancies.[16] In ectopic pregnancies, values may plateau or increase at a slower than normal rate. In one recent study, almost 30% of women with ectopic pregnancies had patterns of β-hCG change that mimicked either intrauterine pregnancy or complete miscarriage.[20] Thus, serial β-hCG is most useful when combined with TVUS. At a β-hCG level of 1000 mIU/mL (Second International Standard, IS) or 2000 mIU/mL (International Reference Preparation, IRP), an intrauterine pregnancy should be clearly visible if present, and this serum β-hCG level is defined as the "discriminatory zone."[21–23] In case of β-hCG level lower than the discriminatory zone and absence of an intrauterine pregnancy, an ectopic pregnancy, a miscarriage, or a very early intrauterine pregnancy should be considered. Decreasing β-hCG values before 10 weeks' gestation usually indicate pregnancy loss, but do not identify the site of the pregnancy. Women with ruptured or nonruptured ectopic pregnancies have been reported to display a wide range of β-hCG values; therefore, women who are symptomatic require further evaluation regardless of β-hCG level.[24–26] A negative β-hCG value does not reliably rule out EP, as chronic ectopic pregnancy is reported to be present with its low titers or a negative β-hCG value.[27,28]

TVUS, defined as the "ultimate diagnostic tool," has brought a revolution in the early diagnosis of EP.[29] Sensitivity, specificity, and positive and negative predictive values of TVUS in diagnosing EP are found to be over 90% in different studies while diagnostic reliability of transabdominal sonography has been shown to be 70%.[29,30] However, both transabdominal and transvaginal scanning play a complementary role in diagnosis of EP. Transabdominal views are important to screen for hemoperitoneum and to visualize ectopic pregnancies beyond the range of the transvaginal probe.[31,32] Transvaginal scanning is important for detailed visualization of endometrial contents and evaluation of adnexa. If the patient has an empty bladder, it is easy and reasonable to begin with a transvaginal scan; however, if the adnexa are beyond the field of view of the endovaginal probe and not well evaluated, a transabdominal scan with a full bladder is necessary. Another important point while examining with US is to scan above and below the ovaries and between the uterus and ovaries, as most ectopic pregnancies are located within the tubes. Although very rare, abdominal pregnancy should be sought with US as a whole abdominal examination in the presence of positive serum β-hCG values and absence of intrauterine pregnancy.

Gestational sacs grow at a rate of 0.8 mm/day; therefore, a follow-up sonography in 2 to 3 days will demonstrate growth in normal pregnancy. Ectopic pregnancies do grow as in normal pregnancies, may hemorrhage, and become (5% to 18%) more apparent on follow-up US. If an exact diagnosis is not established at the time of initial scanning, and if the patient is stable, follow-up sonography, accompanied with or without serum β-hcG level is necessary.[15,33]

SONOGRAPHIC DIAGNOSIS OF ECTOPIC PREGNANCY
Endometrial Findings

Several endometrial patterns and cut-off values for endometrial thicknesses have been studied in the prediction of EP;[34–37] however, no specific and sensitive endometrial pattern or thickness has been determined. In EP, the endometrial cavity can exhibit various appearances such as trilaminar, homogeneously hyperechoic, heterogeneously hyperechoic, containing decidual cyst or pseudogestational sac, and thickness such as normal, thickened or thin. However, EP can be associated with thinner endometrium compared with normal intrauterine pregnancy and first trimester loss possibly in correlation with serum progesterone and β-hCG levels.[34,38]

Decidual cyst is a small fluid collection without an echogenic rim, which might represent an early breakdown of the decidua. They are typically located at the junction of the endometrium and myometrium (**Fig. 1**).[39] It is neither specific nor sensitive for EP as it can be seen in intrauterine pregnancy and in nonpregnant patients as well.[4,40] Multiplicity of decidual cyst, although not a truly distinguishing feature, and absence of an echogenic rim might help in differentiating it from an intradecidual sign.

Pseudosac or pseudogestational sac or pseudosac is a fluid collection within the endometrial

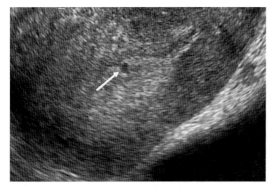

Fig. 1. Decidual cyst. An anechoic fluid collection without a perceptible echogenic wall (*arrow*) is seen eccentrically within the endometrial cavity on sagittal transvaginal image. (*From* Gurel S, Sarikaya B, Gurel K, et al. Role of sonography in the diagnosis of ectopic pregnancy. J Clin Ultrasoun 2007;35(9):509–16; with permission. **Fig. 1** is used.)

cavity (**Fig. 2**). It represents blood and debris in the endometrial cavity, which can be seen in both intrauterine and ectopic pregnancy. It is found to be present in 20% of EP.[41] It might be seen as a simple or complex and at times moving fluid. It is centrally located within the endometrial cavity and surrounded by only one echogenic layer corresponding to the endometrial decidual reaction. Central localization of pseudogestational sac helps in differentiation from decidual cyst, while central localization and one echogenic rim helps in differentiation from double decidual sac sign seen in early intrauterine pregnancy.[42]

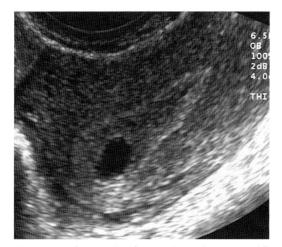

Fig. 2. Pseudogestational sac. A cystic area with a weekly echogenic rim, different from the surrounding two prominent echogenic rims double decidual sac sign, located centrally within the endometrial cavity is demonstrated on sagittal transvaginal image. (*From* Gurel S, Sarikaya B, Gurel K, et al. Role of sonography in the diagnosis of ectopic pregnancy. J Clin Ultrasoun 2007;35(9):509–16; with permission. **Fig. 2** is used.)

Adnexal Findings

Tubal pregnancy is the most common location of EP, constituting 99% of extraovarian EP, with 75% in the ampullary portion, 10% in the isthmic portion, 5% in the fimbrial end, 2% to 4% in the interstitial end.[1,43] The combination of positive β-hCG, absence of intrauterine pregnancy and presence, of an adnexal mass other than a simple intraovarian cyst should be regarded as an EP until proven otherwise. Sonographic adnexal findings of EP can appear in four different ways as given below in decreasing order of specificity:

(1) An extrauterine live embryo with positive heart motion
(2) An extrauterine gestational sac containing a yolk sac with or without an embryo
(3) A tubal ring without an embryo or yolk sac
(4) A complex or solid adnexal mass separate from the ovary

The pathognomonic finding of EP, a live embryo with positive heart motion, is present in only 8% to 26% of ectopic pregnancies on TVUS (**Fig. 3**A, B).[32] The second most specific sign "an extrauterine gestational sac containing a yolk sac with or without an embryo" carries the risk of being confused with a hemorrhagic cyst containing debris mimicking a yolk sac or embryo (**Fig. 4**).[44] The tubal ring is an oval, round, or, if ruptured, irregular mass with hyperechoic rim of trophoblastic tissue and has a specificity of 40% to 68% for EP (**Fig. 5**). A complex or solid adnexal mass separate from the ovary is slightly less specific but more common than a tubal ring.[45–51]

Adnexal findings, other than a live embryo, need to be differentiated from a hemorrhagic corpus luteum cyst arising from the ovary. A sonographic clue for this differentiation is echogenicity of the wall of the corpus luteum, which is more hypoechoic when compared to the wall of the tubal ring and endometrium (**Fig. 6**A–C).[52,53] Follow-up sonographic examinations help to detect the changes in a hemorrhagic corpus luteum as the blood products within it evolve. When it is unclear if the mass is ovarian or extraovarian, a maneuver performed while scanning with gentle pressure on the endovaginal probe and anterior abdominal wall can be used to demonstrate that a corpus luteum moves with the ovary, while tubal EP moves separately from the ovary.

Pelvic Fluid

In normal pregnancies usually a small amount of free fluid, accepted as physiological, is seen in the pelvis. In both intrauterine and ectopic

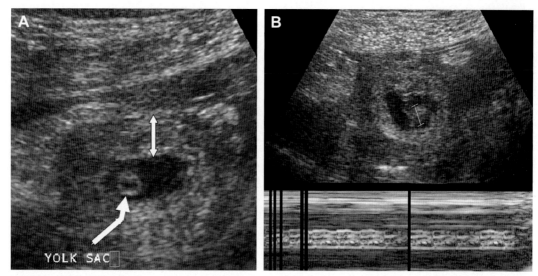

Fig. 3. Tubal ectopic pregnancy. A tubal ring (echogenic trophoblastic tissue) (*arrow*) containing a yolk sac (*angled arrow*) is seen on transabdominal axial image. (*A*) Fetal pole (*cursor*) is also present and a live embryo is identified on M-Mode scanning (*B*).

pregnancies, free fluid accumulates in the cul-de-sac, which is the most dependent location in the pelvis. In EP, free pelvic fluid is seen either because of a response to the distention of the fallopian tube or bleeding from the damaged tube or the EP itself.[54] It can have a simple (anechoic) or complex appearance with floating echoes, or a layering appearance. Complex fluid suggests hemoperitoneum and, sometimes, even blood clot can be seen, surrounding the uterus giving its contours an ill-defined appearance. Complex pelvic fluid when present in a patient with a positive β-hcG level has a positive predictive value of 86% to 93% in the diagnosis of EP and may be the only endovaginal sonographic finding (**Fig. 7**).[44,55,56]

It should be kept in mind that a moderate amount of echogenic fluid might be present owing to retrograde passage of blood in an intrauterine pregnancy when the patient is bleeding or a hemorrhagic corpus luteum cyst ruptures. Although quantification of pelvic fluid is not necessary, it is important to scan up by the hepatorenal space (Morrison's pouch) to assess for the degree of hemoperitoneum. In general, when pelvic complex fluid is seen extending beyond the cul-de-sac, EP should be considered in the differential diagnosis.[57,58]

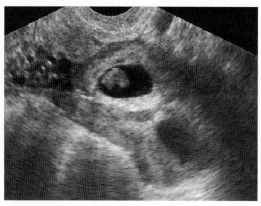

Fig. 4. A tubal ectopic pregnancy with a well-formed gestational sac containing a nonliving embryo.

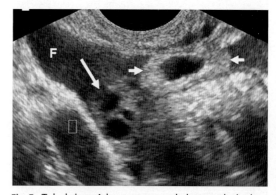

Fig. 5. Tubal ring. A homogeneously hyperechoic ring-like structure, representing trophoblastic tissue, (*short arrows*) with a central cystic component is illustrated on a transvaginal coronal image in a case of ampullary EP. The tubal ring is adjacent to the ovary (*long arrow*) and accompanying periovarian free fluid (F) with low-level echoes is present.

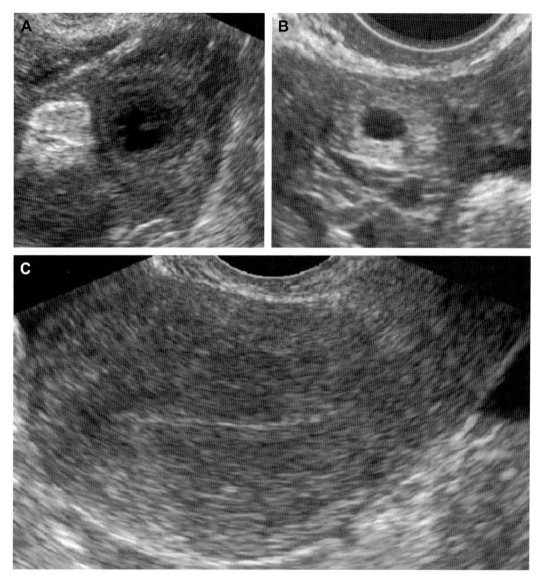

Fig. 6. Echogenicity of the wall of corpus luteum (*A*) is seen as more hypoechoic compared to the wall of the tubal ring (*B*) and endometrium (*C*) on coronal and sagittal transvaginal images respectively.

Doppler Findings

The process of implantation shows local hemodynamic changes characterized as high-velocity and low-impedance flow, whether it occurs within or other than the endometrial cavity. Regarding the asymmetry between two adnexa, the increased blood flow around the conceptus of a tubal EP is defined as "ring of fire."[59,60] The limitation for this finding is that the blood flow pattern of corpus luteum, "luteal flow," may have a similar appearance and to avoid an overestimation, it should be remembered that corpus luteum cysts are much more common than EP (**Fig. 8**A, D). Peripheral hypervascularity is a nonspecific finding and may also be seen surrounding a normal maturing follicle or corpus luteal cyst or hemorrhagic cyst. As a result of all studies and reports up to now, there is no pathognomonic or specific Doppler finding for EP because of the overlap with a corpus luteum cyst, at least in resistive indices.[61] The only discriminating feature between these two entities is the location. A corpus luteum cyst is always located in the ovary, whereas an EP is 90% unilateral to the corpus luteum.[53] Recently, a finding called "the leash sign," a combination of gray-scale and Doppler sonographic findings was reported by Ramanan and Gajaraj.[62] This sign mostly depends on the abnormal implantation

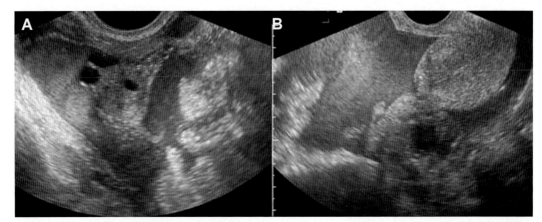

Fig. 7. Free fluid. A ruptured tubal ectopic pregnancy presenting with massive—periovarian (*A*), cul-de-sac, and pelvic (*B*)—echogenic (hemorrhagic) free fluid.

and tubal trophoblast invasion causing marked blood flow changes in the adjacent supplying vessels.[63,64] The sign has 3 parts: (1) gray-scale identification of an adnexal abnormality (eg, a swollen tube or a ring-like structure suggestive of an EP); (2) a linear artery supplying the tube at one point; (3) a low-resistance placental type of flow on spectral Doppler interrogation of the above artery. With fulfillment of the above criteria, a sensitivity of 100% and a specificity of 98% have been

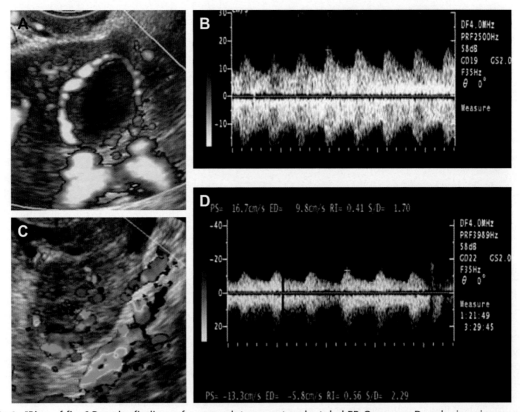

Fig. 8. "Ring of fire." Doppler findings of a corpus luteum cyst and a tubal EP. On power Doppler imaging corpus luteum cyst is encircled with a rim of color (*A*) and displaying a low-resistance (resistive index: 0.41) high blood flow pattern (*B*). On color Doppler imaging, tubal EP demonstrates an intense color rim (*C*) with a low resistance spectral pattern (*D*) similar to corpus luteum cyst. (*From* Gurel S, Sarikaya B, Gurel K, et al. Role of sonography in the diagnosis of ectopic pregnancy. J Clin Ultrasoun 2007;35(9):509–16; with permission. **Fig. 9**A is used.)

reported in the diagnosis of an early EP in a limited number of cases. However, an overlap was shown to be present in an ovary with a mature cystic teratoma, therefore, this sign still needs to be verified both with larger series and various ovarian pathologies.

Color Doppler is most helpful when an EP is not seen, but highly suspected. At that time, Doppler imaging can be used to find a mass representing an EP.

RARE TYPES OF ECTOPIC PREGNANCY
Ovarian

Ovarian pregnancy is very rare, constituting 3% of all ectopic pregnancies.[65] It has an estimated frequency ranging from 1 in 2100 to 1 in 7000 pregnancies and there is a high frequency of rupture and hemorrhage if the diagnosis is delayed.[66,67] The exact diagnosis is by demonstration of a yolk sac or embryo either on the surface or within the parenchyma of the ovary (**Fig. 9**). On TVUS, ovarian EP is usually seen as a well-defined echogenic ring which is indistinguishable from a corpus luteum cyst and the diagnosis is usually confirmed histopathologically.[67,68] Therefore, a complex cyst is the least specific finding for the diagnosis of an ovarian EP, as corpus luteum cyst is much more

common than an ovarian EP, which is less than 1% of all EP.

Abdominal

Abdominal pregnancy is implantation of blastocyst anywhere within the peritoneum or retroperitoneum. It is very rare, with a varying reported incidence between 1 in 3372 and 1 in 7931 pregnancies.[69] Reported sites for abdominal pregnancy are pouch of Douglas, posterior uterine wall, uterine fundus, liver, spleen, omentum, diaphragm, and retroperitoneum.[69–71] Symptoms might be quite intriguing when compared with classical tubal pregnancy. The most common symptom is severe abdominal pain in which delay in menstruation or vaginal bleeding can be absent. In the presence of a negative TVUS, a positive serum β-hCG, and symptomatology, sonographic examination should be directed to encompass the whole abdomen, in populations with or without risk factors for EP (**Fig. 10**).

Interstitial

Interstitial pregnancy constitutes 2% to 4% of all EP. It occurs in the interstitial (intramyometrial) portion of the fallopian tube. Interstitial EP, as a term, is sometimes used interchangeably with cornual EP. However, it would be more

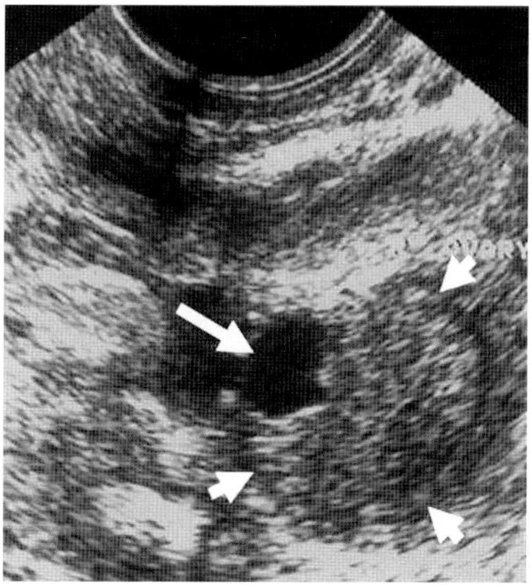

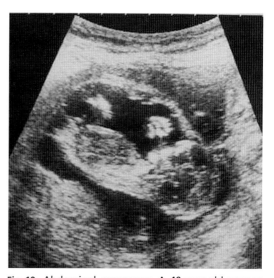

Fig. 9. Ovarian ectopic pregnancy. A true ovarian pregnancy located eccentrically within the ovarian parenchyma is demonstrated on transvaginal axial image. The gestational sac (*long arrow*) without a fetal pole or yolk sac is confirmed histopathologically. (*From* Gurel S, Sarikaya B, Gurel K, et al. Role of sonography in the diagnosis of ectopic pregnancy. J Clin Ultrasoun 2007;35(9):509–16; with permission. **Fig. 11** is used.)

Fig. 10. Abdominal pregnancy. A 40-year-old woman presented with irregular and minimal amount of vaginal bleeding and weight gain. An intra-abdominal extrauterine, live 14 weeks' gestation fetus overlooked with transvaginal sonography, is detected on transabdominal sonography. (*From* Gurel S, Sarikaya B, Gurel K, et al. Role of sonography in the diagnosis of ectopic pregnancy. J Clin Ultrasoun 2007;35(9):509–16; with permission. **Fig. 4** is used.)

appropriate to use cornual pregnancy for an intra-uterine pregnancy implanted in one horn of a sep-tated or bicornuate uterus. In these patients, pregnancy can continue for a longer period of time and present with myometrial rupture usually at the end of first trimester or in the beginning of the second trimester. Ruptured myometrium leads to life-threatening hemorrhage. Maternal mortality is in the range of 2.0% to 2.5%, which is approximately twice that of other tubal pregnancies.[72,73]

An eccentrically located gestational sac within the uterine wall (40% sensitivity and 62% specificity) that is surrounded by a thin myometrium (40% sensitivity and 74% specificity) can be seen on US. The surrounding myometrium can be either thin (<5 mm) or absent laterally.[48,74] Another finding, the "interstitial line sign"(80% sensitivity and 99% specificity) is described as an echogenic line reflecting the two opposing layers of endome-trium seen, not surrounding but just, adjacent to the gestational sac, owing to an interposing myometrium between the gestational sac and in-terstitial line.[75] Braxton-Hicks contractions, cornual pregnancy, and uterine fibroids might cause misdiagnosis of interstitial EP. Follow-up TVUS is helpful in detecting the transient nature of Braxton-Hicks contractions, whereas three-dimensional US is reported to help in demonstrat-ing uterine anomalies or fibroids with an eccentric gestational sac.[76–79]

Cervical

Cervical EP constitutes less than 1% of all EP.[80] Implantation occurs within the cervical mucosa, below the level of the internal os. It presents as painless bleeding in the first trimester. Preopera-tive diagnosis of cervical EP is important because, owing to the lack of cervical contractile tissue, therapeutic dilatation and curettage (D/C) frequently leads to excessive bleeding, ultimately

requiring hysterectomy. The differential diagnosis consists of spontaneous abortion. The most reliable sonographic finding of cervical EP is identification of a gestational sac with peritropho-blastic flow or a live embryo within the cervix. Follow-up scanning allows for differentiation as well, because in cases of ectopic pregnancy, the sac does not change in position, whereas in spon-taneous abortion the sac shape and position changes.[19] Some secondary sonographic find-ings, which are not entirely reliable but can be helpful in the differential diagnosis of cervical EP, are summarized in **Table 1**.[81]

Uterine Scar

A uterine scar pregnancy is a gestation separated from the endometrial cavity and completely sur-rounded by the myometrium and the fibrous tissue of the scar. The suggested mechanism is the entrance of the blastocyst into the myometrium through a microscopic dehiscent tract. This tract can develop from trauma from previous surgeries such as D/C, myomectomy, metroplasty and Cae-sarean section (C-section). They are most com-mon in the site of a previous C-section scar.[82,83] Vial and colleagues[84] suggested two different de-grees of implantation. One is implantation of the amniotic sac on a scar with a progression of the pregnancy toward the cervico-isthmic space and uterine cavity; the other is a deeper implantation in a C-section scar defect. These typically result in rupture and bleeding during the first trimester.

Although C-section scar EP is known to be the rarest form of EP, its true incidence is not known yet, and it is expected to be higher than the reported cases in the current literature because of the increasing rate of C-section deliveries all over the world. The women with placental pathol-ogy, ectopic pregnancy, multiple C-section

Table 1
Ancillary sonographic findings of cervical EP and spontaneous abortion

Cervical EP	Spontaneous Abortion
No evidence of intrauterine pregnancy	Residual placental tissue or fluid in the endometrial cavity
Minimal uterine enlargement	Uterine enlargement beyond the nongravid uterus state
Closed internal os	Open internal os
Eccentrically located gestational sac within the endocervical canal	Centrally located gestational sac within the endocervical canal
Hourglass-shaped uterus with a ballooned cervical canal (because of the resistance in the external os)	

Abbreviation: EP, ectopic pregnancy.

surgeries, and Caesarean breech delivery are at higher risk for C-section scar pregnancy.[85]

In C-section scar EP, the gestational sac can be seen in the lower part of the uterine cavity or at the level of the uterine isthmus. The differential diagnosis is spontaneous abortion in progress in the former and cervico-isthmic pregnancy in the latter form.

TVUS combined with color flow Doppler (CFD) is a reliable tool for early diagnosis of C-section scar EP.[86–88] Sonographic imaging criteria are as follows:

(1) Empty uterine cavity and cervical canal;
(2) A gestational sac in the anterior uterine wall at the isthmus (presumed site of the previous lower segment C-section scar);
(3) Absence of healthy myometrium between the bladder sac, allowing differentiation between from cervico-isthmic implantation
(4) A negative "sliding organs" sign, which is described as the inability to displace the gestational sac from its position at the level of the internal os with gentle pressure applied by the endovaginal probe
(5) Evidence of functional throphoblastic circulation on Doppler examination, defined by the presence of an area of increased peritrophoblastic vascularity on color Doppler examination

In the cervical phase of a proceeding spontaneous abortion, an avascular gestational sac, reflecting that the sac has been detached from its implantation site, is seen in the cervical canal and easily displaced while applying pressure with transvaginal probe (positive "sliding organ" sign).[88,89]

Heterotopic

Heterotopic pregnancy is defined as the simultaneous presence of an intrauterine and ectopic gestation. Spontaneous heterotopic pregnancy is rare and occurs in from 1 in 10,000 to 1 in 50,000 pregnancies,[90] but its incidence increases with age and multiparity. On the other hand, the incidence is as high as 1% in women undergoing assisted reproductive techniques. Particularly in this population, visualization of an intrauterine pregnancy is not reliable and adequate to rule out EP in a symptomatic patient and a careful search should be performed to look for an ectopic pregnancy.[91]

Chronic

Chronic ectopic pregnancy is an independent entity apart from acutely ruptured ectopic pregnancy. There is still no agreement about the

definition of this condition and its etiology is unknown. The incidence of chronic ectopic pregnancy varies from 6.5% to 84.0% of ectopic pregnancies, which might be a result of lack of consensus about its definition.[27,92] In most cases, it is assumed that it is a result of tubal abortion or ruptured EP in which the hemodynamic insult was subclinical and self-limited.

It may present with a long period of amenorrhea, abdominal pain, and a low or negative titer of β-hCG.[92,93] Chronic ectopic pregnancy is usually diagnosed intraoperatively or histopathologically because of the paucity of clinical and laboratory findings. Operative findings consist of an adnexal mass with a significant amount of adhesions incorporating uterus, bowel, or the contralateral adnexa. Histopathologically, it presents a delayed involutional process, because of intraluminal retention of extensive blood clot with inflammation and necrotic hyalinized or degenerated ghost chorionic villi.[94,95] There is not much data concerning the abdominal or transvaginal sonographic findings of chronic EP. Reported transabdominal US findings are

(1) An extrauterine complex mass occupying the adnexa uni- or bilaterally and cul-de-sac with a considerably varying ratio of cystic-solid components. Variations in the echo patterns might represent hematoceles consisting of liquid blood, fresh clot, organized hematoma and adhesions[96]
(2) Fluid in the cul-de-sac[97]
(3) Normal in 9% of chronic EP[96]

TVUS findings are similar to transabdominal US findings including an extrauterine complex mass occupying one or both adnexa or cul-de-sac accompanied with an empty uterus and simple or particulate fluid in the cul-de-sac/pelvis.[27]

Doppler findings are quite sparse in the literature demonstrating no blood flow within or in the periphery of the complex mass or extensive vascularization, aberrant vessels, arteriovenous shunting without an internal blood flow.[27,95]

The sonographic pattern of chronic EP is similar to pelvic inflammatory disease, endometrioma, leiomyoma, complex ovarian cyst and ovarian neoplasm and although definitive diagnosis is mostly operative and histopathological, a combination of absence of intrauterine gestation, low titers or absence of serum β-hcG, and an extrauterine mass can be helpful in the diagnosis of chronic EP. On the other hand, in the absence of β-hCG, differential diagnosis consists of a wide spectrum of adnexal and other pelvic pathologies.

Persistent

Persistent EP can be defined as the presence of residual trophoblastic tissue after surgical management of tubal pregnancy. It is commonly seen following conservative management with salpingostomy or fimbrial expression.[98,99] Women with a small ectopic pregnancy, less than 8 mm in diameter, detected by preoperative US are at high risk of developing or remaining residual trophoblastic tissue. It should be suspected in all patients with elevated or "plateauing" serum β-hCG levels 1 week after management of an ectopic pregnancy. Its management is based on symptomatology and follow-up serum β-hCG levels.[100]

In conclusion, when combined with serum β-hCG level, ultrasonography is the only and most effective radiologic modality in diagnosis of EP. Although transvaginal approach has brought high-resolution imaging of uterus and adnexa, complementary use of transabdominal ultrasonography should be performed whenever possible. Three-dimensional imaging US, which is quite new in routine practice, compared to three-dimensional imaging in CT and MR imaging, is continuing to evolve and it might bring new facilities in overcoming some limitations of today's sonographic display formats.

REFERENCES

1. Cotlar AM. Extrauterine pregnancy: a historical review. Curr Surg 2000;57(5):484–92.
2. Centers for Disease Control. Current trends in ectopic pregnancy: United States, 1990–92. MMWR Morb Mortal Wkly Rep 1995;44(3):46–8.
3. Grimes DA. The morbidity and mortality of pregnancy: still risky business. Am J Obstet Gynecol 1994;170(5Pt 2):1489–94.
4. Frates MC, Laing FC. Sonographic evaluation of ectopic pregnancy: an update. AJR Am J Roentgenol 1995;165(2):251–9.
5. Atri M, Leduc C, Gillet P, et al. Role of endovaginal sonography in the diagnosis and management of ectopic pregnancy. Radiographics 1996;16(4):755–74.
6. Coste J, Bouyer J, Ughetto S, et al. Ectopic pregnancy is again on the increase. recent trends in the incidence of ectopic pregnancies in France (1992–2002). Hum Reprod 2004;19(9):2014–8.
7. Saraiya M, Berg CJ, Kendrick JS. Cigarette smoking as a risk factor for ectopic pregnancy. Am J Obstet Gynecol 1998;178(3):493–8.
8. Pisarska MD, Carson SA, Buster JE. Ectopic pregnancy. Lancet 1998;351(9109):1115–21.
9. Furlong LA. Ectopic pregnancy risk when contraception fails. a review. J Reprod Med 2002;47(11):881–5.
10. Mol BW, Ankum WM, Bossuyt PM, et al. Contraception and the risk of ectopic pregnancy: a meta-analysis. Contraception 1995;52(6):337–41.
11. Tay JI, Moore J, Walker JJ. Ectopic pregnancy. BMJ 2000;320(7239):916–9.
12. Storeide O, Veholmen M, Eide M, et al. The incidence of ectopic pregnancy in Hordaland County, Norway 1976-1993. Acta Obstet Gynecol Scand 1997;76(4):345–9.
13. Lehner R, Kucera E, Jirecek S, et al. Ectopic pregnancy. Arch Gynecol Obstet 2000;263(3):87–92.
14. Schwartz RO, Di Pietro DL. Beta-hCG as a diagnostic aid for suspected ectopic pregnancy. Obstet Gynecol 1980;56(2):197–203.
15. Gracia C, Barnhart K. Diagnosing ectopic pregnancy: decision analysis comparing six strategies. Obstet Gynecol 2001;97(3):464–70.
16. Barnhart KT, Sammel MD, Rinaudo PF, et al. Symptomatic patients with an early viable intrauterine pregnancy; hCG curves redefined. Obstet Gynecol 2004;104(1):50–5.
17. Condous G, Okaro E, Khalid A, et al. The accuracy of transvaginal ultrasonography for the diagnosis of ectopic pregnancy prior to surgery. Hum Reprod 2005;20(5):1404–9.
18. Kirk A, Papageorghiou AT, Condous G. The diagnostic effectiveness of an initial transvaginal scan in detecting ectopic pregnancy. Human Reprod 2007;22(11):2824–8.
19. Dialani V, Levine D. Ectopic pregnancy: a review. Ultrasound Q 2004;20(3):105–17.
20. Dart RG, Mitterando J, Dart LM. Rate of change of serial β-human chorionic gonadotropin values as a predictor of ectopic pregnancy in patients with indeterminate transvaginal ultrasound findings. Ann Emerg Med 1999;34(6):703–10.
21. Mehta TS, Levine D, Beckwith B. Treatment of ectopic pregnancy: is a human chorionic gonadotropin level of 2,000 mIU/mLa reasonable threshold? Radiology 1997;205(2):569–73.
22. Dart RG. Role of pelvic ultrasonography in evaluation of symptomatic first-trimester pregnancy. Ann Emerg Med 1999;33(3):10–20.
23. Condous G, Kirk E, Lu C, et al. Diagnostic accuracy of varying discriminatory zones for the prediction of ectopic pregnancy in women with a pregnancy of unknown location. Ultrasound Obstet Gynecol 2005;26(7):770–5.
24. Korhonen J, Stenman UH, Ylöstalo P. Serum human chorionic gonadotropin dynamics during spontaneous resolution of ectopic pregnancy. Fertil Steril 1994;61(4):632–6.
25. Silva C, Sammel MD, Zhou L, et al. Human chorionic gonadotropin profile for women with ectopic pregnancy. Obstet Gynecol 2006;107(3):605–10.

26. Kriebs JM, Fahey JO. Ectopic pregnancy. J Midwifery Womens Health 2006;51(6):431–9.
27. Turan C, Ugur M, Dogan M, et al. Transvaginal sonographic findings of chronic ectopic pregnancy. Eur J Obstet Gynecol Reprod Biol 1996;67(2):115–9.
28. Brennan DF, Kwatra S, Kelly M, et al. Chronic ectopic pregnancy—two cases of acute rupture despite negative beta hCG. J Emerg Med 2000;19(3):249–54.
29. Shalev E, Yarom I, Bustan M, et al. Transvaginal sonography as the ultimate diagnostic tool for the management of ectopic pregnancy: experience with 840 cases. Fertil Steril 1998;69(1):62–5.
30. Cacciatore B, Stenman UH, Ylöstalo P. Diagnosis of ectopic pregnancy by vaginal ultrasonography in combination with a discriminatory serum hcG level of 1000 IU/L. Br J Obstet Gynaecol 1990;97(10):904–8.
31. Zinn HL, Cohen HL, Zinn DL. Ultrasonographic diagnosis of ectopic pregnancy: importance of transabdominal imaging. J Ultrasound Med 1997;16(9):603–7.
32. Nyberg DA, Mack LA, Jeffrey RB Jr, et al. Endovaginal sonographic evaluation of ectopic pregnancy: a prospective study. AJR Am J Roentgenol 1987;149(6):1181–6.
33. Cacciatore B, Stenman UH, Ylöstalo P. Early screening for ectopic pregnancy in high-risk symptom-free women. Lancet 1994;343(8896):517–8.
34. Hammoud AO, Hammoud I, Bujold E, et al. The role of sonographic endometrial patterns and endometrial thickness in the differential diagnosis of ectopic pregnancy. Am J Obstet Gynecol 2005;192(5):1370–5.
35. Lavie O, Boldes R, Neuman M, et al. Ultrasonographic 'endometrial three-layer' pattern: a unique finding in ectopic pregnancy. J Clin Ultrasound 1996;24(4):179–83.
36. Wachsberg RH, Karimi S. Sonographic endometrial three-layer pattern in symptomatic first-trimester pregnancy: not diagnostic of ectopic pregnancy. J Clin Ultrasound 1998;26(4):199–201.
37. Spandorfer SD, Barnhart KT. Endometrial stripe thickness as a predictor of ectopic pregnancy. Fertil Steril 1996;66(3):474–7.
38. Mehta TS, Levine D, McArdle CR. Lack of sensitivity of endometrial thickness in predicting the presence of an ectopic pregnancy. J Ultrasound Med 1999;18:117–22.
39. Ackerman TE, Levi CS, Lyons EA, et al. Decidual cyst: endovaginal sonographic signs of ectopic pregnancy. Radiology 1993;189(3):727–31.
40. Yeh HC. Some misconceptions and pitfalls in ultrasonography. Ultrasound Q 2001;17(3):129–55.
41. Marks WM, Filly RA, Callen PW, et al. The decidual cast of ectopic pregnancy: a confusing ultrasonographic appearance. Radiology 1979;133:451–4.
42. Bradley WG, Fiske CE, Filly RA. The double sac sign of early intrauterine pregnancy: use in exclusion of ectopic pregnancy. Radiology 1982;143(1):223–6.
43. Bren JL. A 21 year survey of 654 ectopic pregnancies. Am j Obstet Gynecol 1970;106(7):1004–19.
44. Russel SA, Filly RA, Damato N. Sonographic diagnosis of ectopic pregnancy with endovaginal probes: what really has changed? J Ultrasound Med 1993;12(3):145–51.
45. Cacciatore B. Can the status of tubal pregnancy be predicted with transvaginal sonography? A prospective comparison of sonographic, surgical, and serum hCG findings. Radiology 1990;177(2):481–4.
46. Thorsen MK, Lawson TL, Aiman EJ, et al. Diagnosis of ectopic pregnancy: endovaginal vs transabdominal sonography. AJR Am J Roentgenol 1990;155(2):307–10.
47. Brown DL, Doubilet PM. Transvaginal sonography for diagnosing ectopic pregnancy: positivity criteria and performance characteristics. J Ultrasound Med 1994;13(4):259–66.
48. Fleischer AC, Pennell RG, McKee MS, et al. Ectopic pregnancy: features at transvaginal sonography. Radiology 1990;174(2):375–8.
49. DiMarchi JM, Kosasa TS, Hale RW. What is the significance of the human chorionic gonadotropin value in ectopic pregnancy? Obstet Gynecol 1989;74(6):851–5.
50. Stiller RJ, Haynes de Regt R, Blair E. Transvaginal ultrasonography in patients at risk for ectopic pregnancy. Am J Obstet Gynecol 1989;161(4):930–3.
51. Filly RA. Ectopic pregnancy: the role of sonography. Radiology 1987;162(3):661–8.
52. Frates MC, Visweswaran A, Laing FC. Comparison of tubal ring and corpus luteum echogenicities: a useful differentiating characteristic. J Ultrasound Med 2001;20(1):27–31.
53. Stein MW, Ricci ZJ, Novak L, et al. Sonographic comparison of the tubal ring of ectopic pregnancy with the corpus luteum. J Ultrasound Med. 2004;23(1):57–62.
54. Dart R, McKeab SA, Dart L. Isolated fluid in the cul-de-sac: how well does it predict ectopic pregnancy? Am J Emerg Med 2002;20(1):1–4.
55. Nyberg DA, Hughes MP, Mack LA, et al. Extrauterine findings of ectopic pregnancy of transvaginal US: importance of echogenic fluid. Radiology 1991;178(3):823–6.
56. Sickler GK, Chen PC, Dubinsky TJ, et al. Free echogenic pelvic fluid: correlation with hemoperitoneum. J Ultrasound Med 1998;17(7):431–5.

57. Gurel S, Sarikaya B, Gurel K, et al. Role of sonography in the diagnosis of ectopic pregnancy. J Clin Ultrasoun 2007;35(9):509–16.

58. Levine D. Ectopic pregnancy. Radiology 2007;245(2):385–97.

59. Pellerito JS, Taylor KJ, Quedens-Case C, et al. Ectopic pregnancy: evaluation with endovaginal color flow imaging. Radiology 1992;183(2):407–11.

60. Taylor KJ, Meyer WR. New techniques in the diagnosis of ectopic pregnancy. Obstet Gynecol Clin North Am 1991;18(1):39–54.

61. Atri M. Ectopic pregnancy versus corpus luteum cyst revisited: best Doppler predictors. J Ultrasound Med 2003;22(11):1181–4.

62. Ramanan RV, Gajaraj J. Ectopic pregnancy—the leash sign. A new sign on transvaginal Doppler ultrasound. Acta Radiol 2006;47(5):529–35.

63. Kirchler HC, Kolle D, Schwegel P. Changes in tubal blood flow in evaluating ectopic pregnancy. Ultrasound Obstet Gynecol 1992;2(4):283–8.

64. Szabo I, Csabay L, Belics Z, et al. Assessment of uterine circulation in ectopic pregnancy by transvaginal color Doppler. Eur J Obstet Gynecol Reprod Biol 2003;106(2):203–8.

65. Bouyer J, Coste J, Fernandez H, et al. Sites of ectopic pregnancy: a 10-year population-based study of 1800 cases. Hum Reprod 2002;17(12):3224–30.

66. Hage PS, Arnouk IF, Zarou DM, et al. Laparoscopic management of ovarian ectopic pregnancy. J Am Assoc Gynecol Laparosc 1994;1(3):283–5.

67. Hallatt JG. Primary ovarian pregnancy: a report of twenty-five cases. Am J Obstet Gynecol 1982;143(1):55–60.

68. Comstock C, Huston K, Lee W. The ultrasonographic appearances of ovarian ectopic pregnancies. Obstet Gynecol 2005;105(1):42–5.

69. Martin JN Jr, Sessums JK, Martin RW, et al. Abdominal pregnancy: current concepts of management. Obstet Gynecol 1988;71(4):549–57.

70. Lee JW, Sohn KM, Jung HS. Retroperitoneal ectopic pregnancy. AJR Am J Roentgenol 2005;184(5):1600–1.

71. Onan MA, Turp AB, Saltik A, et al. Primary omental pregnancy: case report. Hum Reprod 2005;20(3):807–9.

72. Lau S, Tulandi T. Conservative medical and surgical management of interstitial ectopic pregnancy. Fertil Steril 1997;72(2):207–15.

73. Malinowski A, Bates SK. Semantics and pitfalls in the diagnosis of cornual/interstitial pregnancy. Fertil Steril 2006;86(6):1764.e11–4.

74. Graham M, Cooperberg PL. Ultrasound diagnosis of interstitial pregnancy: findings and pitfalls. J Clin Ultrasound 1979;7(6):433–7.

75. Ackerman TE, Levi CS, Dashefsky SM, et al. Interstitial line: sonographic finding in interstitial (cornual) ectopic pregnancy. Radiology 1993;189(1):83–7.

76. Lawrence A, Jurkovic D. Three-dimensional ultrasound diagnosis of interstitial pregnancy. Ultrasound Obstet Gynecol 1999;14(4):292–3.

77. Lee GS, Hur SY, Kown I, et al. Diagnosis if early intramural ectopic pregnancy. J Clin Ultrasound 2004;33(4):190–2.

78. Izquierdo LA, Nicholas MC. Three-dimensional transvaginal sonography of interstitial pregnancy. J Clin Ultrasound 2003;31(9):484–7.

79. Maymon R, Herman A, Ariely S, et al. Three-dimensional vaginal sonography in obstetrics and gynaecology. Hum Reprod Update 2000;6(5):475–84.

80. Ushakov FB, Elchalal U, Aceman PJ, et al. Cervical pregnancy: past and future. Obstet Gynecol Surv 1997;52(1):45–59.

81. Vas W, Suresh PL, Tang-Barton P, et al. Ultrasonographic differentiation of a cervical abortion from a cervical pregnancy. J Clin Ultrasound 1984;12(9):553–7.

82. Miller DA, Chollet JA, Goodwin TM. Clinical risk factors for placenta praevia-placenta accreata. Am J Obstet Gynecol 1997;177(1):210–4.

83. Fait G, Goyert G, Sundareson A, et al. Intramural pregnancy with fetal survival: case history and discussion of etiologic factors. Obstet Gynecol 1987;70(3 Pt 2):472–4.

84. Vial Y, Petignat P, Hohlfeld P. Pregnancy in a caesarean scar. Ultrasound Obstet Gynecol 2000;16(6):592–3.

85. Maymon R, Halperin R, Mendlovic S, et al. Ectopic pregnancies in Caesarean section scars: the 8-year experience of one medical centre. Human Reprod 2002;19(2):278–84.

86. Godin PA, Bassil S, Donnez J. An ectopic pregnancy developing in a previous caesarean section scar. Fertil Steril 1997;67(2):398–400.

87. Flystra DL. Ectopic pregnancy within a caesarean scar: a review. Obstet Gynecol Surv 2002;57(8):537–43.

88. Jurkovic D, Hillaby K, Woelfer B, et al. First trimester diagnosis and management of pregnancies implanted into the lower uterine segment caesarean section scar. Ultrasound Obstet Gynecol 2003;21(3):220–7.

89. Tan G, Chong YS, Biswas A. Caesarean scar pregnancy: a diagnosis to consider carefully in patients with risk factors. Ann Acad Med Singapore 2005;34(2):216–9.

90. Condous G, Okaro E, Bourne T. The conservative management of early pregnancy complications: a review of the literature. Ultrasound Obstet Gynecol 2003;22(4):420–30.

91. Moore C, Promes SB. Ultrasound in pregnancy. Emerg Med Clin N Am 2004;22(3):697–722.

92. Cole T, Corlett RC Jr. Chronic ectopic pregnancy. Obstet Gynecol 1982;59(1):63–8.
93. Ugur M, Turan C, Vicdan K, et al. Chronic ectopic pregnancy: a clinical analysis of 62 cases. Aust N Z J Obstet Gynaecol 1996;36(2):186–9.
94. Case records of the Massachusetts general hospital (case 11). N Engl J Med 1976;294(11):600–5.
95. Abramov Y, Nadjari A, Shushan A. Doppler findings in chronic ectopic pregnancy: case report. Ultrasound Obstet Gynecol 1997;9(5):344–6.
96. Rogers WF, Shaub M, Wilson R. Chronic ectopic pregnancy: ultrasonic diagnosis. J Clin Ultrasound 1977;5(4):257–9.
97. Bedi DG, Fagan CJ, Nocera RM. Chronic ectopic pregnancy. J Ultrasound Med 1984;3(8):347–52.
98. DiMarchi JM, Kosasa TS, Kobara TY, et al. Persistent ectopic pregnancy. Obstet Gynecol 1987;70(4):555–8.
99. Seifer DB, Gutmann JN, Doyle MB, et al. Persistent ectopic pregnancy following laparoscopic linear salpingostomy. Obstet Gynecol 1990;76(6):1121–5.
100. Nathorst-Böös J, Rafik Hamad R. Risk factors for persistent trophoblastic activity after surgery for ectopic pregnancy. Acta Obstet Gynecol Scand 2004;83(5):471–5.

Ultrasound Assessment of Premenopausal Bleeding

Raj M. Paspulati, MD[a], Ahmet T. Turgut, MD[b,c], Shweta Bhatt, MD[d],
Elif Ergun, MD[b], Vikram S. Dogra, MD[d],*

KEYWORDS

- Pregnancy • Abortion • Arteriovenous malformation
- Bleeding • Ultrasound • First trimester

First trimester pregnancy accounts for the majority of patients with premenopausal bleeding. In the first trimester of pregnancy, 25% of women experience vaginal bleeding. Nearly 50% of these women have an abnormal outcome, while the other 50% continue to term.[1] The differentiation between these two groups depends upon the identification of a normal intrauterine gestation in this early stage of pregnancy; thus, the radiologist must be familiar with the normal appearance of intrauterine gestation at various stages of first trimester pregnancy. It is important to recognize the sonographic appearance of abnormal intrauterine gestation and intrauterine changes of an ectopic pregnancy. Before the embryonic stage of pregnancy, a combination of serum quantitative beta human chorionic gonadotropin (hCG) and transvaginal ultrasonography (TVUS) is an accurate method of identifying a normal intrauterine gestation. The concept of the discriminatory zone, which is the serum beta hCG level at which an intrauterine gestation should be seen by TVUS, is an important landmark in identifying a normal intrauterine pregnancy.[2,3] This discriminatory zone varies between 1,000 IU/mL to 2,000 IU/mL and is commonly cited to be at 1,500 IU/mL.[2,4] The normal intrauterine gestational sac (GS), before the appearance of the yolk sac (YS), has a double decidual sac appearance because of the separation of the decidua capsularis overlying the GS from the deciduas parietalis by the endometrial cavity.[5,6] Identification of a YS within the GS is a definitive sign of intrauterine gestation.[7,8] An ectopic pregnancy is strongly considered when an extra ovarian adnexal mass is observed without an intrauterine GS and serum beta hCG is above the discriminatory level. Demonstration of an extrauterine GS with a YS or embryo is a definitive sign of an ectopic pregnancy. Hydatidiform mole is a more common manifestation of gestational trophoblastic disease (GTD), which is a spectrum of pregnancy-related proliferative trophoblastic abnormalities. A high or rapidly rising serum beta hCG and a complex intrauterine mass with cystic foci is indicative of a molar pregnancy. Arteriovenous malformation (AVM) is a rare but important cause of first trimester bleeding, and distinguishing this entity from retained products of gestation is vital, as its management is entirely different.[9,10] Important causes of first trimester bleeding are spontaneous abortion, ectopic pregnancy, gestational trophoblastic disease, and AVM.

This article provides an overview of ultrasound (US) scanning techniques, the normal sonographic landmarks of intrauterine gestation, and sonographic features of an abnormal intrauterine gestation in spontaneous abortion, ectopic pregnancy, GTD, and AVM of the uterus, accounting for premenopausal bleeding.

[a] Department of Radiology, University Hospitals, Case Medical Center, Case Western Reserve University 11100 Euclid Avenue, Cleveland, OH 44106, USA
[b] Department of Radiology, Ankara Training and Research Hospital, TR-06590, Ankara, Turkey
[c] 25. Cadde, 362. Sokak, Hüner Sitesi No: 18/30, TR-06530, Ankara, Turkey
[d] Department of Imaging Sciences, University of Rochester School of Medicine, 601 Elmwood Avenue, Box 648, Rochester, NY 14642, USA
* Corresponding author.
E-mail address: vikram_dogra@urmc.rochester.edu (V.S. Dogra).

Ultrasound Clin 3 (2008) 345–368
doi:10.1016/j.cult.2008.07.005
1556-858X/08/$ – see front matter © 2008 Elsevier Inc. All rights reserved.

Parameter	Transabdominal US	Transvaginal US
Gestational sac	–	Present at 5 weeks
Yolk sac	Always present with a MSD of >16 mm	Always present with a MSD of >8 mm
Embryo	Always present with a MSD of >25 mm	Always present with a MSD of >16 mm
Embryonic cardiac activity	CRL of >5 mm	CRL of >5 mm

Table 1
Normal sonographic milestones of first trimester pregnancy

Abbreviations: CRL, crown rump length; GS, gestational sac; MSD, mean sac diameter.

ULTRASOUND SCANNING TECHNIQUES

In women presenting with first trimester bleeding, transabdominal ultrasound (TAUS) with a 3.5-MHz transducer is initially performed with a full bladder to displace the bowel and provide an acoustic window. This provides a general overview of the uterus and adnexa. After the bladder is emptied, TVUS is performed using a 5-MHz to 10-MHz transducer. Higher frequency US and the closer position of the transducer to the imaging structures provides high-resolution images of the uterus and adnexa, which is essential to detect early intrauterine gestation and abnormalities associated with first trimester bleeding. Color flow Doppler and pulsed Doppler US should be used if necessary, but one should keep in mind the concept of "as low as reasonably achievable" to avoid potential harmful effects on the developing embryo.[11]

NORMAL SONOGRAPHIC LANDMARKS OF INTRAUTERINE GESTATION

Normal sonographic milestones of first trimester pregnancy are shown in **Table 1**. Approximately 1 week after fertilization, the blastocyst is implanted in the endometrium and is too small to be visualized by TVUS. Focal thickening of the endometrium with an increased trophoblastic flow on color flow Doppler at the implanted site is reported to be the earliest sign of an intrauterine gestation, but is a nonspecific and unreliable sign.[12] An eccentric anechoic focus within the thickened endometrium, described as an "intradecidual sign," is the earliest evidence of an implanted blastocyst (**Fig. 1**).[13]

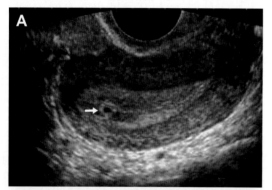

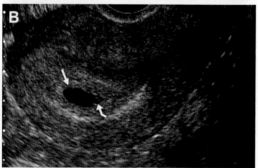

Fig. 1. Intradecidual sign. (*A*) Sagittal TVUS of the uterus demonstrates an eccentric anechoic focus (*arrow*) in the endometrial lining representing early blastocyst. (*B*) Follow up TVUS after two weeks shows a well-defined gestational sac (*arrow*) with a yolk sac (*curved arrow*) confirming an intrauterine gestation.

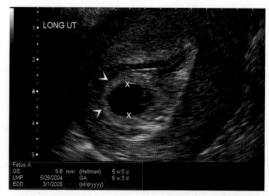

Fig. 2. Sagittal TVUS of the uterus shows a normal gestational sac (*within the calipers*) with a thick echogenic rim representing chorionic villi and decidual reaction (*arrowheads*).

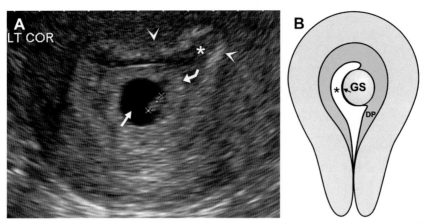

Fig. 3. Double decidual sac sign. (*A*) Coronal TVUS of the uterus reveals an intrauterine gestational sac (*arrow*), decidua capsularis (*curved arrow*), decidua parietalis (*arrowhead*), and effaced endometrial cavity (*asterix*). (*B*) The corresponding line diagram.

Gestational Sac

GS is the sonographic term for the fluid-filled chorionic cavity of the implanted blastocyst. It is seen as early as the first 4 weeks of gestational age as a 2-mm to 3-mm eccentric sonolucent focus with a surrounding echogenic rim formed by the combined trophoblastic and decidual reaction. This surrounding rim of a normal GS is more echogenic than the myometrium and is 2-mm to 3-mm thick (**Fig. 2**).[1] The double decidual sac sign (DDS) of a true intrauterine GS is caused by eccentric GS in the endometrium surrounded by the ipsilateral decidua basalis and decidua capsularis, which is separated from the decidua parietalis by the collapsed endometrial cavity (**Fig. 3**). This appearance distinguishes a true intrauterine GS before the appearance of a YS from a pseudogestational sac of ectopic pregnancy, which is caused by fluid in the endometrial cavity surrounded by thick decidual reaction.[5,6]

Yolk Sac

The secondary YS is the first extraembryonic structure to be seen by TVUS within the GS (chorionic cavity). It is visualized at 5 weeks and is the first reliable sign of intrauterine gestation. It is a well-defined, thin walled cystic structure that gradually increases in size from 5 to 11 weeks of gestation and reaches a maximum size of 5 mm to 6 mm; it is generally not seen after 12 weeks. In a normal intrauterine gestation, a YS should be seen when the mean sac diameter (MSD) is 8 mm (**Fig. 4**). The YS is located between the amnion and chorion and is connected to the embryo by a stalk-like vitelline or omphalomesenteric duct.[7,8,14]

Embryo

The earliest evidence of an embryo is seen as a focal thickening at the periphery of adjoining

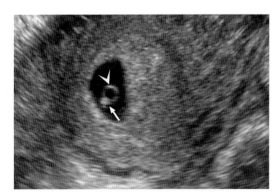

Fig. 4. TVUS of the uterus at 5-weeks menstrual age demonstrates an intrauterine gestational sac with a yolk sac (*arrowhead*) and an echogenic focus (*arrow*) adjacent to the yolk sac representing an early embryo.

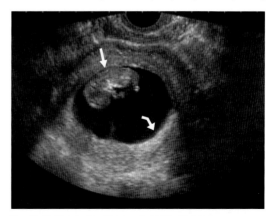

Fig. 5. Embryonic stage of intrauterine pregnancy. TVUS image of the uterus at 7 weeks of menstrual age demonstrates a well-developed embryo (*arrow*) within a gestational sac (*curved arrow*).

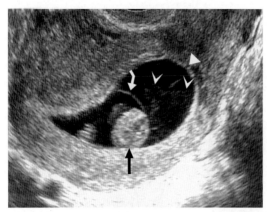

Fig. 6. Sagittal TVUS of the uterus demonstrates intra-uterine pregnancy with an embryo (*arrow*), thin amniotic membrane (*curved arrow*) adjacent to the embryo, and a peripheral thick chorionic membrane (*solid arrowhead*). The chorionic and amniotic membranes are not yet fused with low level echoes (*arrowheads*) between the unfused chorion and amnion.

the YS (see **Fig. 4**). With the currently available high-frequency transducers, embryonic cardiac activity is often appreciated adjacent to the YS, even before an embryo is well visualized.[15–17] An embryo should always be seen by TVUS when the MSD of the GS is 16 mm and by TAUS when the MSD is 25 mm (**Fig. 5**).[7,14] Cardiac activity should always be seen and documented in all embryos with a crown rump length (CRL) of 5 mm.[18,19] Cardiac activity increases gradually from 100 beats per minute (bpm) at 5 to 6 weeks gestation to about 140 bpms at 8 to 9 weeks of gestation and should be documented by M-mode.[20]

Box 1
Causes of spontaneous abortion
Genetic causes
Trisomy
Aneuploidy/polyploidy, translocations
Environmental causes
Uterus
Congenital uterine anomalies
Leiomyoma
Intrauterine adhesions or synechiae (Asherman's syndrome)
Endocrine
Progesterone deficiency (inadequate luteal phase)
Thyroid disease
Diabetes mellitus (uncontrolled)
Luteinizing hormone hypersecretion
Immunologic
Antiphospholipid syndrome, systemic lupus erythematosus (SLE)
Infections
Toxoplasma gondii,
Listeria monocytogens,
Chlamydia trachomatis,
Ureaplasma urealyticum,
Mycoplasma hominis,
Herpes simplex,
Treponema pallidum,
Borrelia burgdorferi,
Neisseria gonorrhoea

Table 2
TVUS features of abnormal outcome in first trimester bleeding

Ultrasound Findings	Comments
Serum beta hCG above discriminatory level (1,000 mIU/mL) without IUGS	Ectopic gestation has to be excluded
MSD of > 8 mm without a yolk sac	Follow-up with serum beta hCG and TVUS
MSD of >16 mm without an embryo	Anembryonic pregnancy
Embryo with CRL of 5 mm and >	Embryonic demise without cardiac activity
Embryo with bradycardia (<100 bpm)	Poor outcome and needs close TVUS follow-up
Small GS with a <5 mm difference between MSD and CRL	Poor out come with embryonic demise or oligohydramnios
Subchorionic hematoma	Correlation of the size of subchorionic hematoma with pregnancy outcome is not well established and needs TVUS follow-up

Abbreviations: bpm, beats per minute; IUGS, intrauterine gestational sac.

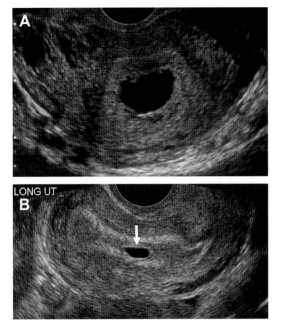

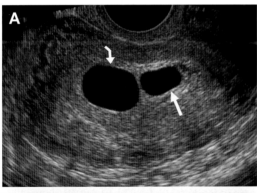

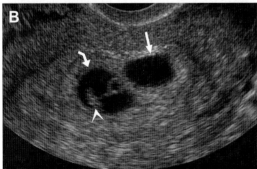

Fig. 7. Abnormal gestational sac in the pre embryonic stage. (*A*) A transverse TVUS image demonstrates a large, irregular intrauterine gestational sac without an embryo. (*B*) A sagittal TVUS image shows a low implantation of intrauterine gestational sac (*arrow*).

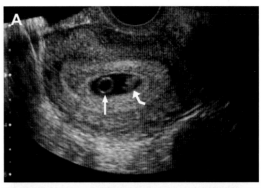

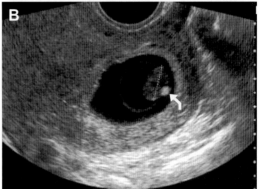

Fig. 9. Yolk sac signs of abnormal gestation. (*A*) TVUS at 6-weeks menstrual age demonstrates an intrauterine gestational sac with an embryo (*curved arrow*) and an abnormally large yolk sac (*arrow*). (*B*) TVUS of another patient at 7 weeks shows an intrauterine gestational sac with embryo and an echogenic yolk sac (*curved arrow*). Both patients eventually had complete abortion.

Fig. 8. Anembryonic gestation. (*A*) TVUS demonstrates at 4-weeks menstrual age demonstrates two intrauterine gestational sacs (*arrows*). (*B*) Follow up TVUS after 2 weeks demonstrates a yolk sac and embryo (*arrowhead*) in one gestational sac (*curved arrow*) and anembryonic second gestational sac (*arrow*).

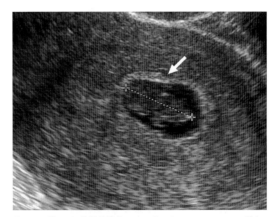

Fig. 10. Coronal TVUS image demonstrates a small intrauterine gestational sac (*arrow*) with an embryo (*cursors*). The difference between mean sac diameter and CRL is less than 5 mm. Follow-up US revealed embryonic demise.

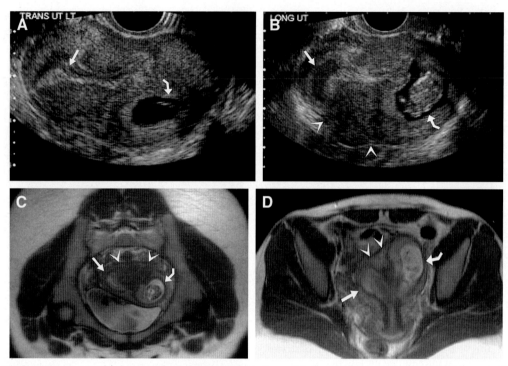

Fig. 11. Septate uterus with intrauterine gestation presenting with first trimester bleeding. TVUS images (*A, B*) demonstrate two separate endometrial cavities with gestational sac and embryo (*curved arrow*) in one endometrial cavity and decidual reaction with fluid in another endometrial cavity (*arrow*). Corresponding coronal (*C*) and axial (*D*) T2-weighted images of the pelvis confirm the septate uterus with intrauterine gestation in one endometrial cavity (*curved arrow*). The intervening septum (*arrowheads*) is demonstrated in both TVUS and MR images.

Chorio-Amniotic Membranes

The amniotic sac is formed at about 4 weeks of gestation and is visible by TVUS at 5 to 6 weeks as a separate cystic structure, separated from the YS by the embryonic disc. This appearance has been described as "the double bleb sign."[21] The amniotic sac gradually enlarges and completely surrounds the embryo and the YS is located outside the amniotic sac. The amniotic membrane is less than 0.5-mm thick and is best seen when the US beam is perpendicular to the membrane.[21] The amniotic sac gradually increases in size and fuses with the outer chorionic membrane between 14 and 16 weeks of gestation. Before 6.5 weeks of gestation, the amniotic membrane is closely aligned to the embryo and is not readily seen by TVUS. Separation of the amniotic and chorionic membranes is a normal feature before 14 weeks of gestation and is abnormal after 17 weeks.[22,23] The contents of the amniotic sac are anechoic; low-level echoes and linear strands can normally be seen within the chorionic cavity outside the amniotic membrane. This is because

of high proteinaceous contents, coagulum, and mesodermal strands (**Fig. 6**).[21]

SPONTANEOUS ABORTION

Spontaneous abortion is defined as termination of pregnancy during the first 20 weeks of gestation. It is more common in the first 16 weeks of gestation and the incidence decreases as gestational age increases. Genetic abnormalities are the most common cause of spontaneous abortion; autosomal trisomy is the most frequently identified abnormality.[24] Environmental factors account for the remaining small percentage of spontaneous abortions. The causes of spontaneous abortion are displayed in **Box 1**. Spontaneous abortion is classified clinically as threatened, missed, incomplete, and complete abortion.

Threatened abortion is the most common presentation and occurs in 25% of all pregnancies. After confirmation of the pregnancy by a urine pregnancy test and determination of the serum beta hCG levels, the management of these patients depends upon the viability of the gestation. TVUS is

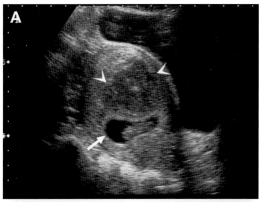

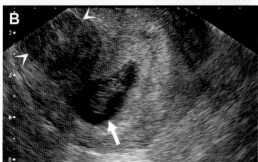

Fig. 12. Fibroid uterus with first trimester bleeding. Transabdominal (*A*) and TVUS (*B*) sagittal images demonstrate a fibroid in the ventral myometrial wall (*arrowheads*) deforming the intrauterine gestational sac with embryo (*arrow*). The pregnancy continued to term without complications.

necessary to confirm an intrauterine gestation and to assess the viability and probable outcome.

Sonography in Spontaneous Abortion

Knowledge of the normal sonographic milestones of first trimester pregnancy is essential to identify abnormal sonographic features and probable outcomes in these patients. The sonographic findings depend upon the stage of gestation and have to be correlated with serum beta hCG levels. TVUS features of an abnormal gestation are displayed in **Table 2**.

SONOGRAPHIC FEATURES OF ABNORMAL INTRAUTERINE GESTATION
Pre-Embryonic Stage

Correlation of ultrasonographic findings with serum beta hCG is essential in this early stage of gestation. A GS should be identified in the uterus when serum beta hCG has reached the discriminatory level, which ranges from 1,000 IU to 1,500 IU.[2,3,25] The appearance of the GS, YS, and the choriodecidual reaction determines the probable outcome for these patients.

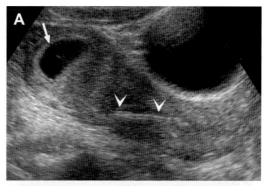

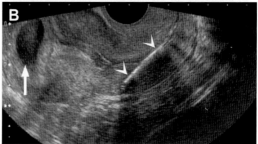

Fig. 13. Intrauterine pregnancy in a misplaced IUCD presenting with first trimester bleeding. Transabdominal (*A*) and TVUS (*B*) sagittal images demonstrate a low IUCD (*arrowheads*) with its tip extending into the posterior myometrial wall and an early intrauterine gestational sac (*arrow*). Follow-up TVUS after removal of the IUCD confirmed dichorionic diamniotic twin intrauterine gestation.

Gestational sac criteria

The GS size, shape, and location are important predictors of pregnancy outcome. A GS with an MSD of 8 mm to 10 mm without a YS, and a GS with an MSD of 16 mm to 20 mm without an embryo, is an indicator of abnormal gestation (**Fig. 7**A).[7,26] This empty GS without a YS or embryo is because of early embryonic demise and resorption of the embryo. An abnormal karyotype, such as autosomal trisomy or triploidy, is the cause for this early pregnancy failure. This anembryonic gestation is also called "blighted ovum" and "empty amnion sign" (see **Fig. 7**A; **Fig. 8**).[27,28] A GS small for the gestational age should be followed by US at 1- to 2-week intervals. A small GS with a growth rate of less than 1 mm per day is an indicator for a poor outcome.[29] A distorted GS, low lying GS, the absence of the double decidual sac sign, and thin (<2 mm) decidual reaction are other minor criteria of an abnormal gestation (**Fig. 7**B).[7,26]

Yolk sac criteria

Identification of a YS within the GS is the most reliable sign of intrauterine gestation in the pre-embryonic stage.[7,8] Absence of a YS in the

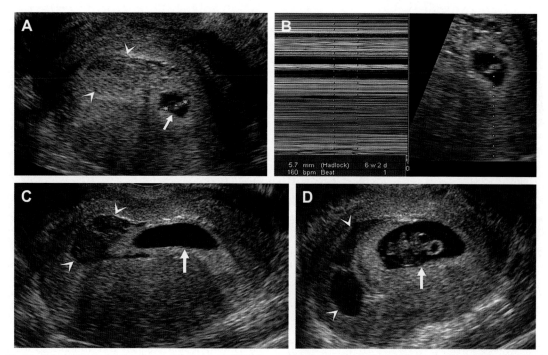

Fig. 14. Subchorionic hemorrhage. (*A*) Coronal TVUS image demonstrates an intrauterine gestational sac (*arrow*) with embryo (*cursors*) and an echogenic acute subchorionic hemorrhage (*arrowheads*). (*B*) Cardiac activity with a heart rate of 160 bpm is recorded. Follow-up TVUS after 2 weeks (*C*) demonstrates decrease in the echotexture of the hematoma (*arrowheads*) and after 4 weeks (*D*) demonstrates normal progression of the gestational sac and embryo (*arrow*) with a stable more anechoic subchorionic hematoma (*arrowheads*).

presence of an embryo is an indicator of poor outcome.[14,30] An abnormally large YS (>6 mm) or small, echogenic, and calcified YSs are associated with embryonic death (**Fig. 9**).[31–33] The YS is associated with nutritive, metabolic, and hemopoetic functions of the early embryo. The abnormal shape, size, and appearance of YS is a sequela of early embryonic demise rather than its cause.[34] An echogenic YS has also been associated with aneuploidy.[35] However, the significance of YS in predicting the pregnancy outcome is uncertain and follow up US is recommended.[36,37]

Embryonic Stage

Once an embryo is identified in the GS, documentation of embryonic cardiac activity is the primary criterion for assessment of pregnancy viability. Though cardiac activity can be identified in embryos as small as 2 mm, the accepted standard CRL at which cardiac activity should be identified is 5 mm.[26] An embryo with a CRL of 5 mm or greater without cardiac activity is a definite sign of nonviable gestation.[18] Embryos with CRL less than 5 mm without cardiac activity should undergo follow-up US.[19] Embryonic bradycardia and small sac size are poor prognostic signs in a viable embryo with cardiac activity. Embryonic bradycardia

is defined as a heart rate less than 100 bpm before 6.3 weeks and less than 120 bpm between 6.3 weeks and 7.0 weeks of gestation.[38,39] The relationship of the GS size to the embryo is an important prognostic feature. A difference of less than 5 mm between the mean GS diameter and CRL of embryo is associated with high incidence of abortion. This is called "small sac syndrome" or oligohydramnios (**Fig. 10**).[14,40] A follow up US is recommended in embryonic bradycardia and if there is a discrepancy between the CRL and mean GS diameter.

Anatomic Factors in Spontaneous Abortion

Anatomic uterine defects are associated with about 15% of recurrent spontaneous abortions.[41] These uterine abnormalities are because of congenital mullerian duct fusion anomalies, such as septate or bicornuate uterus, and acquired causes, such as uterine leiomyomas, intrauterine adhesions, and polyps. Recurrent abortions in a septate and bicornuate uterus are because of reduced intrauterine volume or from inadequate vascularity (**Fig. 11**).[42,43] The outcome of pregnancy in the presence of uterine leiomyomas depends upon their size, number, location, and relationship to the placenta. Large submucosal, and multiple and

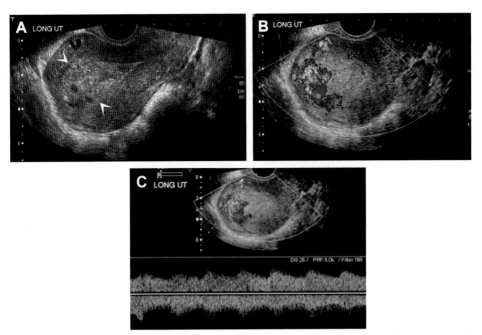

Fig.15. Retained products of conception. (*A*) Sagittal TVUS image in a patient with first trimester vaginal bleeding demonstrates heterogeneous intrauterine contents (*arrowheads*) without a definite gestational sac. Color flow Doppler (*B*) shows increased vascularity of the complex endometrial contents and pulsed Doppler (*C*) reveals low resistance arterial flow.

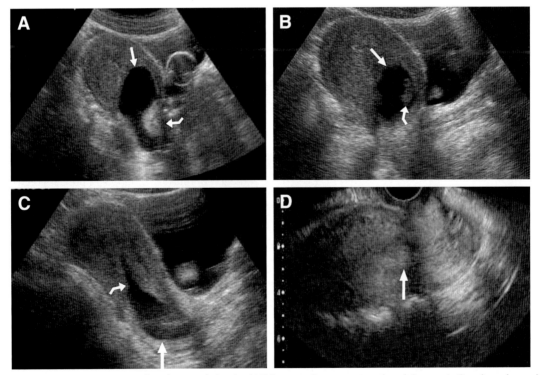

Fig. 16. Abortion in progress. (*A, B*) Transabdominal US images demonstrate a low-lying gestational sac (*arrow*) with trophoblastic tissue (*curved arrow* in *A*) and embryo (*curved arrow* in *B*). (*C*) Subsequent transabdominal scan shows extension of the products of conception through the internal os (*curved arrow*) into the cervix (*arrow*). (*D*) Final transabdominal US image shows a collapsed endocervical canal (*arrow*) after complete expulsion of the products of conception.

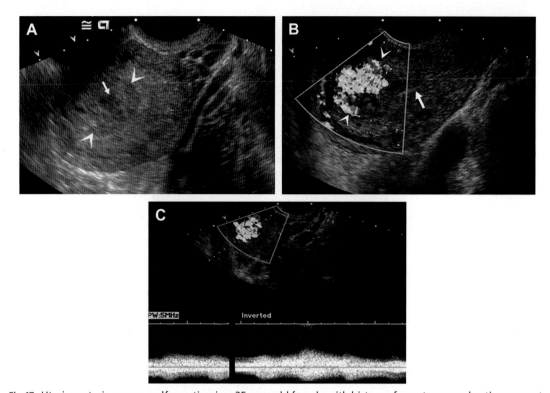

Fig. 17. Uterine arteriovenous malformation in a 35-year-old female with history of spontaneous abortion presenting with vaginal bleeding. She was referred to exclude retained products of conception. (*A*) TVUS shows a complex myometrial mass (*arrowheads*) with anechoic spaces (*arrow*). (*B*) Corresponding color flow Doppler demonstrates the mosaic pattern of flow within the mass (*arrowheads*). Arrow points to the collapsed endometrial cavity. (*C*) Pulsed Doppler demonstrates arterialized venous flow diagnostic of arteriovenous malformation.

retroplacental leiomyomas are associated with spontaneous abortion (**Fig. 12**).[44–46] Pregnancy associated with an intrauterine contraceptive device (IUCD) in situ is another acquired cause of vaginal bleeding and spontaneous abortion. US is useful to identify the IUCD and its relationship to the GS. The IUCD is extra-amniotic and generally away from the implantation site. Removal of an IUCD in the first trimester increases the chances of continuing a pregnancy to term (**Fig. 13**).[47–49]

Subchorionic Hemorrhage

Approximately 18% to 20% of women presenting with first trimester bleeding have sonographic evidence of subchorionic hematoma. They appear as extrachorionic crescentic anechoic or complex collection, with acute hematomas being more echoic (**Fig. 14**). The size of the hematoma can be measured by either volume or by the percentage of chorionic sac circumference elevated by the hematoma. There are variable reports regarding the outcome of pregnancy in patients with subchorionic hematoma.[50–55] The outcome depends upon the size of the hematoma, gestational age, and maternal age. The outcome is generally poor with

large hematomas in women over age 35 presenting before 8 weeks of gestation.[50–52,55]

Retained Products of Conception

Patients presenting with persistent bleeding following spontaneous abortion undergo TVUS for detection of retained products of conception. Retained products of conception are associated with an increased risk of bleeding and infection, and delayed complications, such as disseminated

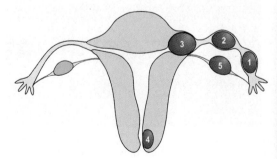

Fig. 18. Line diagram illustrates the various locations of ectopic pregnancy: (**1**) ampulla (**2**) isthmus (**3**) interstitial (**4**) cervix (**5**) ovary.

Table 3
Sonographic features of ectopic pregnancy

Sonographic Signs	Comments
Absence of an IUGS with a serum beta hCG above the discriminatory level (1,000 mIU/L)	Evaluation of adnexa for ectopic location of GS
Pseudogestational sac	Absence of a DDS sign
Extraovarian complex adnexal mass	Most common sign
Adnexal tubal ring sign	Mimics an exophytic corpus luteum cyst
Echogenic free fluid	Indicates hemorrhage and may or may not be associated with rupture of the ectopic gestation

Abbreviations: DDS, double decidual sac sign; IUGS, intrauterine gestational sac.

intravascular coagulation and infertility because of endometrial osseous metaplasia.[56] The appearance of retained products of conception is highly variable. A GS with a nonviable embryo or an irregular GS may be identified. Any endometrial mass or complex fluid collection irrespective of vascularity on Doppler evaluation should be considered as retained products of conception.[56,57] Color flow and pulsed Doppler is useful in identification of retained trophoblastic tissue, as it demonstrates low-resistance arterial flow (**Fig. 15**). A thick endometrial lining of more than 10 mm is a less sensitive sign of retained products and should be correlated with clinical presentation and serial quantitative beta hCG.[58,59] The retained products of conception are occasionally identified either in the endocervical canal or vagina, indicating an abortion in progress (**Fig. 16**).

UTERINE ARTERIOVENOUS MALFORMATIONS

Uterine AVMs were first described by Dubriel and Loubat in 1926.[60] They are either congenital or acquired in nature and are an uncommon but a potentially life threatening cause of vaginal bleeding. They are rarely associated with first trimester bleeding and spontaneous abortion. Congenital vascular malformations result from arrested vascular development and are composed of multiple vascular channels of variable caliber with fistulous communications within the myometrium. The acquired AVMs are the result of arteriovenous fistula between a single artery and single vein. The acquired arteriovenous fistulae result from previous trauma, infection, or malignancy. Previous trauma can be from abortion, dilation, and curettage, cesarian section, or IUCD. The malignant causes include cervical carcinoma, endometrial carcinoma, and gestational trophoblastic.[61,62]

Sonographic Features of Arteriovenous Malformations

The gray scale US features of AVM are variable. The most common finding is a spongy appearance of the myometrium because of multiple tubular and cystic anechoic spaces (**Fig. 17**A). They may

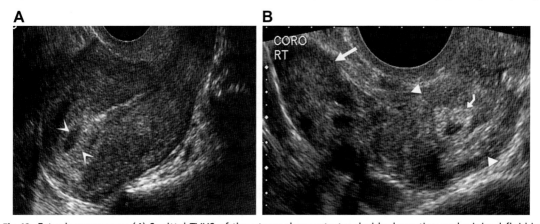

Fig. 19. Ectopic pregnancy. (*A*) Sagittal TVUS of the uterus demonstrates decidual reaction and minimal fluid in the endometrial cavity (*arrowheads*) and no intrauterine gestational sac. (*B*) Coronal TVUS of the right adnexa shows ovary (*arrow*) and an extra ovarian adnexal mass (*arrowheads*) with a gestational sac (*curved arrow*).

occasionally present as a focal myometrial mass resembling a fibroid. A polypoidal endometrial mass may be present.[62]

Color flow Doppler for AVM demonstrates a mosaic pattern color signal within the cystic spaces (**Fig. 17**B). Spectral analysis of these vascular spaces demonstrates high velocity and low resistance flow in the arteries, and pulsatile high velocity venous flow (**Fig. 17**C). Large AVMs are associated with prominent parametrial vessels.[60–62] There is considerable overlap of US features of AVM with those of retained products of conception following a spontaneous abortion and gestational trophoblastic disease (GTD).[10,63] Correlation with serum quantitative beta hCG is important to differentiate AVM from these two entities. This differentiation is crucial as management of an AVM by dilatation and curettage (see 17 D and C) can be catastrophic. MR imaging with intravenous gadolinium is useful in large congenital AVMs to assess the extent of myometrial and parametrial involvement.[62] Management of AVM is by selective arterial embolization and hysterectomy. An acquired AVM fistula is more amenable for arterial embolization because of a single or few feeding arteries.[60,61,64,65]

ECTOPIC PREGNANCY

Ectopic pregnancy remains an important cause of maternal mortality, accounting for 9% of all pregnancy-related deaths in 1992. The incidence of ectopic pregnancy has increased from 4.5 per 1,000 pregnancies in 1970 to 19.7 per 1,000 pregnancies in 1992.[66] This increased incidence is partly because of additional risk factors, but mostly the result of improvement in diagnostic methods. Ectopic pregnancy is defined as implantation of the fertilized ovum outside the uterine cavity. Approximately 97% of ectopic pregnancies occur in the fallopian tube and the remaining 3% occur in the cervix, ovary, or abdominal cavity. Ampulla is the most common site of tubal pregnancy, seen in 55% of all tubal pregnancies. The isthmus and fimbrial ends are less common sites of tubal pregnancy, accounting for 25% and 17%, respectively (**Fig. 18**).[67] The risk factors for ectopic pregnancy include pelvic inflammatory disease, previous ectopic pregnancy, endometriosis, previous tubal surgery, uterotubal anomalies, in utero exposure to diethylstilbestrol, and cigarette smoking.[68,69] Previous ectopic pregnancy is a significant risk factor, with a recurrence rate of 15% to 20% following

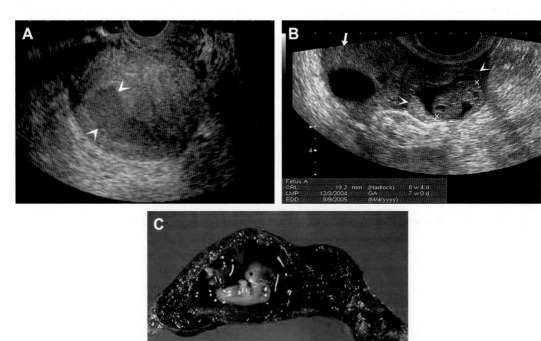

Fig. 20. Ectopic pregnancy. (A) TVUS of the uterus shows fluid in the endometrial cavity with thin decidual reaction representing pseudo gestational sac (*arrowheads*). (B) TVUS image of the right adnexa demonstrates right ovary (*arrow*) and ectopic tubal gestational sac (*arrowheads*) with an embryo (*cursors*). (C) Photograph of the salpingectomy specimen demonstrates a fallopian tube with ectopic gestational sac and an embryo (*arrow*).

treatment of an ectopic pregnancy.[70–72] Abdominal pain and vaginal bleeding or spotting with a history of amenorrhea is the most common presentation of ectopic pregnancy. This presentation is nonspecific and can be seen with threatened or spontaneous abortion. More specific signs are localized adnexal pain and tenderness, peritoneal signs with pain radiating to the shoulder, and hypovolemic shock are less commonly seen. Therefore, a high index of clinical suspicion and diagnostic work-up with serum beta hCG and US is the key to the early diagnosis of ectopic pregnancy.

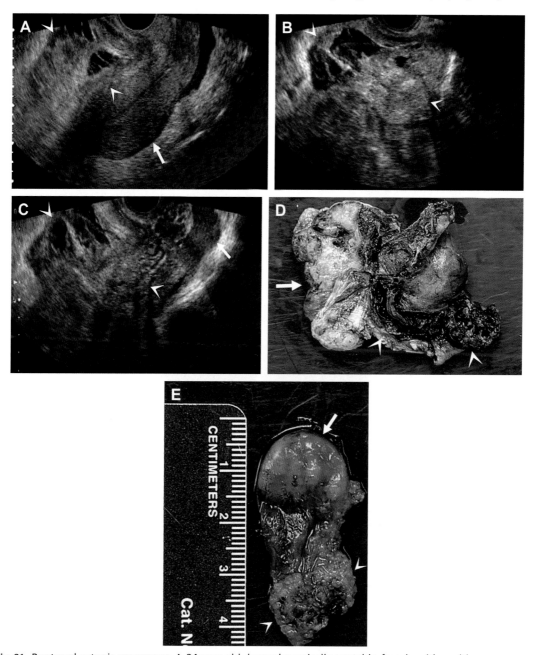

Fig. 21. Ruptured ectopic pregnancy. A 24-year-old, hemodynamically unstable female with positive pregnancy test and severe abdominal pain. (*A*) Sagittal TVUS image shows an empty uterus (*arrow*) and a large complex mass (*arrowheads*) adjacent to the uterus. (*B, C*) TVUS images show complex adnexal mass (*arrowheads*) with mixed anechoic and echogenic components and echogenic free fluid (*arrow*) in the cul-de-sac. No discrete ectopic gestational sac is identified. (*D*) Photograph of the gross specimen shows ruptured fallopian tube with hematosalpinx (*arrowheads*) and the adjacent ovary (*arrow*). (*E*) Gross specimen photograph of the extracted embryo (*arrow*) and the trophoblastic tissue (*arrowheads*).

Sonographic Features of Ectopic Pregnancy

A summary of sonographic findings of ectopic pregnancy is shown in **Table 3**. When the serum beta hCG is above the discriminatory level of 1,500 IU and no intrauterine GS is identified, a careful search of the adnexa with TVUS is mandatory for an extrauterine GS.[4,6] In the absence of an intrauterine GS associated with serum beta hCG below the discriminatory level, follow-up with serial quantitative beta hCG and US is necessary until a conclusive diagnosis is made.[25] A pseudogestational sac is seen in 10% to 20% of ectopic pregnancies because of decidual reaction of the endometrial lining and fluid in the endometrial cavity (**Fig. 19**A, **Fig. 20**A). Differentiation from a true GS is made by absence of "double decidual sac" sign and presence of a YS or embryo.[5,6,73] The most common sonographic finding is an extra ovarian complex adnexal mass with or without free fluid in the pelvis.[67,74] This adnexal mass is because of a combination of a dilated fallopian tube with a GS, with or without a hematosalpinx and surrounding hematoma (see **Fig. 19**). This extra ovarian adnexal mass has a sensitivity of 84.4%, specificity of 98.9%, and positive predictive value (PPV) of 96.3%.[73] The appearance of pelvic fluid in addition to the adnexal mass further increases the sensitivity and specificity. The presence of echogenic fluid in the pelvis because of hemoperitoneum has a much higher predictive value, and a moderate amount of echogenic fluid in the pelvis can be an isolated finding of an ectopic pregnancy.[75] The echogenic fluid in the pelvis represents either tubal abortion or rupture (**Fig. 21**).[76] The most definitive sign of ectopic pregnancy is the demonstration of an extrauterine GS with a YS or embryo (see **Fig. 20**). However, a YS and embryo are less commonly seen. The extrauterine GS is most often seen as an empty cystic structure, which has to be differentiated from the more common ovarian corpus luteum cyst. The ectopic GS has a 2-mm to 4-mm thick echogenic rim and represents the tubal ring sign of ectopic pregnancy (**Fig. 22**).[77] The tubal ring of an ectopic gestation is more echogenic than the ovarian parenchyma and the endometrial lining.[78,79] The corpus luteum cyst has a wide range of sonographic appearance and can have a thick echogenic rim similar to the ectopic GS. Color

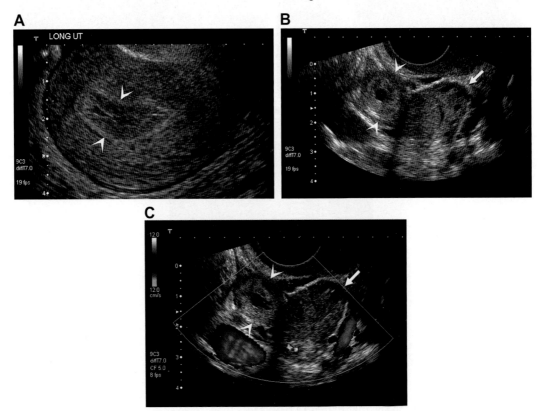

Fig. 22. Tubal ring sign of ectopic pregnancy. (*A*) Sagittal TVUS of the uterus demonstrates minimal fluid in the endometrial cavity with surrounding decidual reaction (*arrowheads*) representing a pseudogestational sac. (*B, C*) Gray scale and color flow Doppler TVUS images of the right adnexa show ovary (*arrow*) and an extra ovarian anechoic focus with surrounding thick echogenic rim (*arrowheads*) representing the "tubal ring sign" of an early ectopic tubal gestation.

flow Doppler is not useful in differentiating these two, as both can demonstrate increased vascularity, giving the "ring of fire" appearance.[79,80] Spectral Doppler and measurement of the resistive index (RI) may be useful in differentiating these two. The RI of the corpus luteum cysts is reported to vary from 0.39 to 0.7 and the RI of the ectopic GS is either less than 0.39 or greater than 0.7. This has a reported specificity and PPV of 100% in the diagnosis of ectopic pregnancy.[80] The above described sonographic signs are those seen in the more common tubal ectopic pregnancy. Interstitial, cervical, and ovarian ectopic pregnancies have more distinctive sonographic appearances.

Interstitial Pregnancy

The interstitial segment of the fallopian tube is the proximal portion of the tube that is within the myometrial wall of the uterus (see **Fig. 18**). It is about 1 cm to 2 cm in length and 0.7-mm wide. It is highly vascular because of the combined vascular supply from the uterine and ovarian vessels. Interstitial pregnancy is a rare type of ectopic pregnancy, accounting for 2% to 4% of all tubal pregnancies, but has high maternal mortality because of catastrophic hemorrhage. The high vascularity of this region and delayed rupture because of the surrounding protective myometrial wall are responsible for the high mortality of these patients. The ultrasound findings include an eccentric GS near the uterine cornual region with surrounding myometrial mantle. The surrounding myometrial mantle is thin, incomplete, and is generally 5-mm thick (**Fig. 23**).[81–83] The "interstitial line" sign, because of a linear echogenic endometrial lining extending to the edge of the eccentric GS, is reported to be highly sensitive and specific for the diagnosis of interstitial ectopic pregnancy (**Fig. 24**). The interstitial line sign has a sensitivity of 80% and specificity of 98% as compared with eccentric GS location (sensitivity, 40%; specificity, 88%) and thin myometrial mantle (sensitivity, 40%; specificity, 93%) for the diagnosis of interstitial pregnancy.[84] An eccentric location of intrauterine GS because of uterine contraction, uterine leiomyomas, or a GS within the horn of a bicornuate uterus can mimic an interstitial ectopic pregnancy. Angular pregnancy is an intrauterine pregnancy in the lateral angle of the uterine cavity medial to the uterotubal junction, and can be mistaken for an interstitial ectopic gestation because of eccentric position of the GS.[85,86] Three-dimensional US and MR imaging may be used when two-dimensional US findings of interstitial pregnancy are equivocal.[87–90]

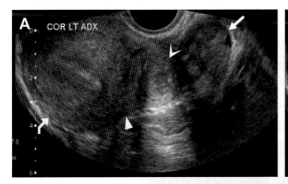
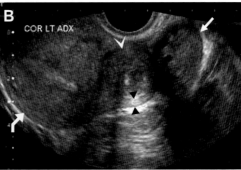
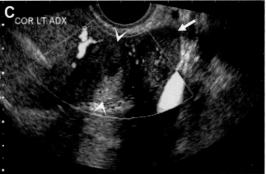

Fig. 23. Interstitial pregnancy. (*A, B*) Coronal TVUS images of the left adnexa show an ectopic gestational sac (*arrowhead*) between the left ovary (*arrow*) and uterus (*curved arrow*) with myometrial extension (*solid arrowhead*) and myometrial mantle (*black arrowheads*) surrounding the gestational sac. (*C*) Corresponding color flow Doppler image demonstrates combined ovarian and uterine vascular supply to the ectopic gestation.

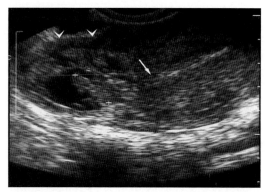

Fig. 24. Interstitial pregnancy. Coronal TVUS demonstrates an eccentric right interstitial gestational sac with embryo (*within calipers*). The endometrial lining extending to the edge of the gestational sac, "interstitial line" sign (*arrow*) and the surrounding myometrial mantle (*arrowheads*) are well demonstrated.

Ovarian Pregnancy

Ovarian pregnancy is an uncommon ectopic pregnancy with a reported incidence varying from 1 in 6,000 to 1 in 40,000 pregnancies.[91] The ratio of ovarian pregnancy to all other ectopic pregnancies is 1% to 6%.[92] There are few reports of multiple ovarian gestations.[92,93] The risk factors for ovarian pregnancy are similar to those of tubal pregnancy, which include pelvic inflammatory disease, IUCD usage, previous surgery, and endometriosis.[92–94] Spiegelberg in 1878 set four criteria for the diagnosis of ovarian pregnancy: normal tube on the affected side, GS located at the anatomic site of the ovary, GS connected to the uterus by the utero-ovarian ligament, and ovarian tissue demonstrated in the GS wall.[95] The GS may be within the substance of the ovary or on its surface and will appear as an echogenic ring with central sonolucent area (**Fig. 25**). In the absence of a YS and embryo, it may be mistaken for a hemorrhagic cyst on both TVUS and at surgery.[96–98] The diagnosis in such cases is usually made by the pathologist.[97] The risk of rupture and hemorrhage in ovarian pregnancy is similar to tubal pregnancy.

Cervical Pregnancy

Cervical pregnancy is an uncommon intrauterine ectopic pregnancy caused by implantation of the

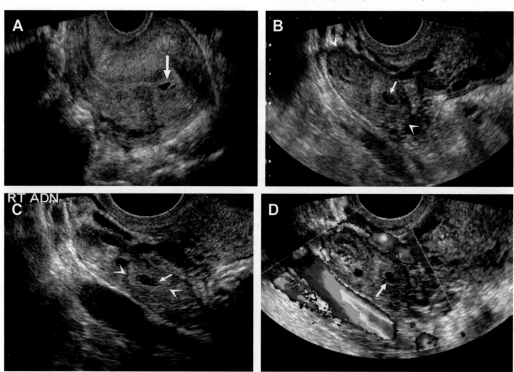

Fig. 25. Ovarian pregnancy. A patient with positive pregnancy test and a serum beta hCG of 1,200 IU presents with pelvic pain and vaginal spotting. (*A*) Sagittal TVUS of the uterus shows a pseudo gestational sac (*arrow*). (*B*) TVUS image of the right adnexa shows a small anechoic focus with thick echogenic wall (*arrow*) within the right ovary (*arrowheads*). No other adnexal mass was identified. Patient had curettage of the endometrial contents, which revealed decidual reaction and no chorionic tissue. (*C*) Follow-up TVUS because of persistent elevation of beta hCG revealed persistent suspicious gestational sac (*arrowheads*) within the right ovary with suggestion of a yolk sac (*arrow*). (*D*) Corresponding color flow Doppler TVUS image of the right ovary with suspicious gestational sac (*arrow*). Laparoscopic surgery and pathology confirmed ectopic right ovarian gestation.

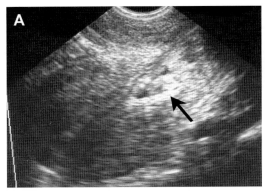 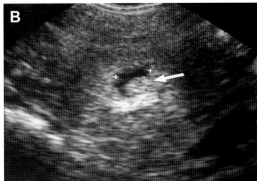

Fig. 26. Cervical pregnancy. Sagittal (*A*) and coronal (*B*) TVUS images of the uterus demonstrate a gestational sac with embryo (*arrow*) implanted within the cervix.

GS in the endocervical canal. It is potentially life threatening because of the increased risk of bleeding.[99] It has to be differentiated from the more common products of conception in the cervical canal during spontaneous abortion. The GS of a cervical pregnancy is round or oval and may demonstrate a YS or an embryo (**Fig. 26**). The GS in the products of conception during an abortion is collapsed and crenated.[100–102] Demonstration of trophoblastic flow in the cervix by color Doppler is more suggestive of a cervical pregnancy. There is always some evidence of decidual reaction or hemorrhagic products in the endometrial cavity with an open internal os of the cervix in patients with abortion in progress (see **Fig. 16**). A sliding motion of the GS against the cervical canal by gentle pressure with the endovaginal probe described as the "sliding sign" is seen in spontaneous abortion, where as the GS is fixed in cervical pregnancy.[103] There are reports of potential advantages of MR imaging in the diagnosis of cervical pregnancy, when US findings are inconclusive.[104,105]

Management of Ectopic Pregnancy

There are several treatment options for ectopic pregnancy, including expectant treatment, systemic methotrexate injection, US-guided local injection of methotrexate or potassium chloride, and surgery. Surgical management can be either a salpingectomy or a salpingostomy with preservation of the tube. The criteria for medical management include a hemodynamically stable patient who is compliant for posttreatment follow-up, pretreatment beta hCG of greater than 5,000 IU and the absence of embryonic cardiac activity.[106,107] After the first injection of methotrexate, weekly serum beta hCG follow-up is mandatory. A second dose of methotrexate is administered if there is less than a 15% decline in the serum beta hCG.[108–110] Cervical, interstitial, and cesarean

scar pregnancies may be treated by US-guided local injection of methotrexate or potassium chloride.[111]

GESTATIONAL TROPHOBLASTIC DISEASE

GTD encompasses a spectrum of conditions derived from the placental trophoblasts, including hydatidiform mole, invasive mole, choriocarcinoma, and placental site trophoblastic tumor. GTD is characterized by abnormal proliferation of the trophoblastic tissue with varying degree of malignant potential and increased beta hCG production.[112,113] Classification of GTD is displayed in **Box 2**.

Hydatidiform Mole

The incidence of molar pregnancy is higher in Asian countries than in the United States and Europe. The reported incidence of molar pregnancy in the United States is 1 in 1,000 deliveries. The incidence of molar pregnancy is also higher in teenage women and after age 35.[114–116] Maternal age and previous molar pregnancy are the two major risk factors. The hydatidiform mole is classified into complete molar pregnancy and partial molar pregnancy, based on the absence or presence of a fetus. The complete molar pregnancy has

Box 2
Classification of gestational trophoblastic disease

Hydatidiform mole
  Partial mole
  Complete mole

Gestational trophoblastic neoplasia
  Invasive mole
  Choriocarcinoma
  Placental site trophoblastic tumor

no fetus and partial molar pregnancy is associated with a fetus. Both types are characterized by abnormal proliferation of trophoblastic cells and hydropic villi. The karyotype in a complete mole is 46XX, with both chromosomes of paternal origin, and is referred to as "androgenesis." The karyotype of a partial mole is triploid (69, XXY) or even tetraploid (92, XXXY), with one paternal chromosome and the rest of maternal origin.[117,118] A complete mole is a result of fertilization of a defective ovum by a sperm and all chromosomes are derived from the sperm. The gross appearance of

a complete mole consists of a cluster of edematous vesicles 5 mm to 2 cm in size and in varying degrees of hemorrhage and necrosis.[119] The clinical presentation of molar pregnancy in the early first trimester is indistinguishable from a normal pregnancy or a threatened abortion. The classic presentation of vaginal bleeding, enlarged uterus, absent fetal tone, and hyperemesis are seen in the late first trimester and second trimester of pregnancy. Pregnancy-induced hypertension before 20 weeks and thyrotoxicosis are other clinical presentations. Serum beta hCG levels are elevated

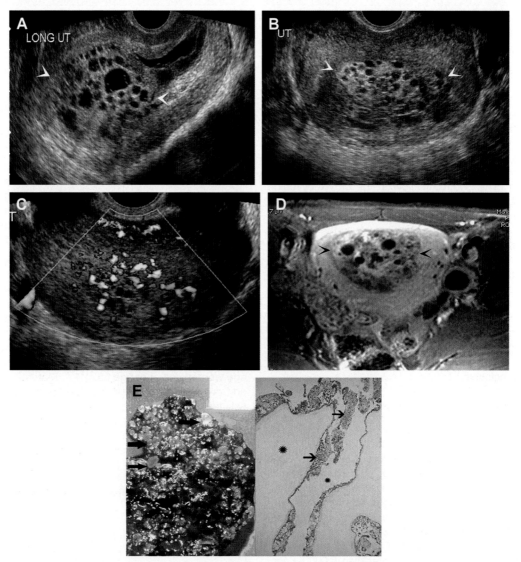

Fig. 27. Complete hydatidiform mole. A 40-year-old female with vaginal bleeding and a serum beta hCG of 200,000 mIU/mL. Sagittal (A) and coronal (B) TVUS images of the uterus show a complex mass (arrowheads) with multiple anechoic cystic foci corresponding to hydropic villi of molar pregnancy. There is no associated embryo. (C) Coronal TVUS with power Doppler demonstrates typical trophoblastic flow within the mass. (D) Corresponding T1-weighted postgadolinium axial image of the uterus demonstrates multiple well-defined hypointense lesions representing the hydropic villi of molar pregnancy. (E) Specimen photograph shows cystic villi (arrows) and photomicrograph shows hydropic villi (flowers) and trophoblastic hyperplasia (arrows).

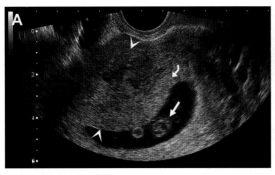 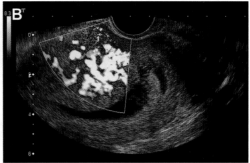

Fig. 28. Partial mole. A 35-year-old female with past history of molar pregnancy, presenting with hyperemesis and a serum beta hCG of 185,000 mIU/mL. (*A*) TVUS of the uterus shows an intrauterine gestational sac (*curved arrow*) with an embryo (*straight arrow*). A complex mass (*arrowheads*) with multiple anechoic foci in the myometrium corresponds to an associated hydatidiform mole. (*B*) TVUS with power Doppler demonstrates typical trophoblastic flow within the complex mass.

and are usually over 100,000 mIU/mL. Serum beta hCG levels are higher in complete mole than in partial mole. Because of the regular practice of first trimester US, molar pregnancy is diagnosed by US before the patient has typical clinical presentation.[120]

Sonographic Features of Molar Pregnancy

TVUS is the imaging modality for the diagnosis and follow up of molar pregnancy. The sonographic appearance is variable and depends upon the size of the vesicles, associated hemorrhage, and necrosis. The classic appearance is a mass in the endometrial cavity composed of multiple cystic anechoic spaces, which vary in size from 1 mm to 30 mm. The size of the cystic spaces is larger with advancing gestational age. The mass appears more echogenic and solid with small cystic spaces.[121,122] Color flow Doppler demonstrates some of the cystic spaces to be vascular with a high velocity and low resistance flow (**Fig. 27**). The degree of invasion of the myometrium by the molar tissue is variable. Doppler evaluation improves the accuracy of the depth of myometrial invasion by the molar tissue.[123,124] Comparing the sonographic features with serum beta hCG is useful to differentiate molar pregnancy from retained products of conception and blood clots in a patient with spontaneous abortion. Retained trophoblastic tissue with hydropic degeneration closely resembles molar pregnancy on US. Increased myometrial involvement is a feature of molar pregnancy and myometrial invasion of more than one-third of its depth is useful in differentiating molar pregnancy from retained products of conception.[125] In a partial molar pregnancy, a GS with an embryo is seen in addition to the molar tissue (**Fig. 28**). About 25% to 60% of cases with molar pregnancy have thecaleutin cysts because of hyperstimulation of the ovaries by the increased hCG. The ovaries are enlarged, with multiple cysts replacing the entire ovary, and have a "soap bubble" or "spoke-wheel" appearance (**Fig. 29**).[121,126]

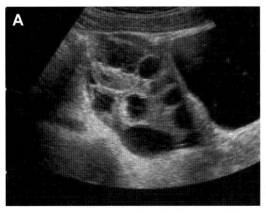 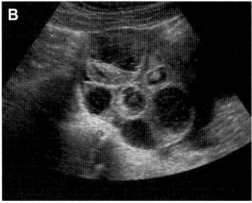

Fig. 29. Thecaleutin cysts. (*A*, *B*) Transabdominal US images of bilateral ovaries in a patient with molar pregnancy demonstrates enlarged ovaries with multiple cysts of varying sizes.

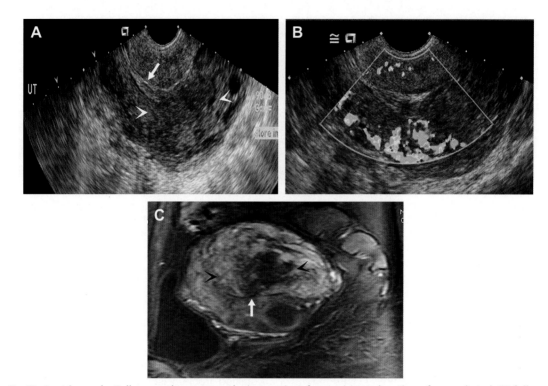

Fig. 30. Invasive mole. Follow-up ultrasonography in a patient for persistent elevation of serum beta hCG following evacuation of a complete hydatidiform mole. (*A*) Sagittal TVUS of the uterus demonstrates an illdefined mass (*arrowheads*) in the myometrium extending from the endometrial cavity (*arrow*). (*B*) Corresponding color Doppler image of the uterus shows vascularity of the infiltrating myometrial mass. (*C*) Axial postgadolinium T1-weighted image of the uterus demonstrates endometrial cavity (*arrow*) and the infiltrating mass in the myometrium (*black arrowheads*).

Gestational Trophoblastic Neoplasia

Gestational trophoblastic neoplasia (GTN) includes invasive molar pregnancy and choriocarcinoma. The invasive mole is characterized by local invasion of the myometrium without distant hematogenous metastases (**Fig. 30**). The choriocarcinoma is a malignant form of molar pregnancy, with distant hematogenous metastases to the lungs, liver, brain, and other organs. MR imaging is more accurate in demonstrating the depth of myometrial invasion by the molar tissue than US. The distant metastases in choriocarcinoma are better evaluated by CT scan. Choriocarcinoma is preceded by hydatidiform mole in 50% of cases, spontaneous abortion in 25%, normal pregnancy in 22.5%, and ectopic pregnancy in 2.5%. Choriocarcinoma is suspected in all patients with persistent elevation of serum beta hCG after evacuation of a molar pregnancy.[121,122,127]

SUMMARY

First trimester vaginal bleeding is a common clinical presentation to the emergency department. Clinical assessment of the viability of the pregnancy is unreliable at this early stage of pregnancy. TVUS is an essential imaging modality to confirm an intrauterine gestation and a living embryo. Knowledge of the normal sonographic milestones of early intrauterine gestation helps differentiate a normal from abnormal intrauterine gestation in the pre-embryonic stage and a pseudogestational sac of ectopic pregnancy from a true intrauterine GS. TVUS also plays a crucial role in the diagnosis of ectopic gestation and its suitability for conservative management. Follow-up of postabortion patients with persistent bleeding is performed with TVUS to identify retained products of conception. TVUS is also useful to identify rare causes of first trimester bleeding, such as GTD and AVM of the uterus.

ACKNOWLEDGMENTS

The authors thank Joseph Molter for his assistance in preparation of figures for this article.

REFERENCES

1. Nyberg DA, Laing FC, Filly RA. Threatened abortion: sonographic distinction of normal and abnormal gestation sacs. Radiology 1986;158:397–400.

2. Barnhart KT, Simhan H, Kamelle SA. Diagnostic accuracy of ultrasound above and below the beta-hCG discriminatory zone. Obstet Gynecol 1999;94:583–7.

3. Nyberg DA, Filly RA, Mahony BS, et al. Early gestation: correlation of HCG levels and sonographic identification. AJR Am J Roentgenol 1985;144: 951–4.

4. Banhart K, Mennuti MT, Benjamin I, et al. Prompt diagnosis of ectopic pregnancy in an emergency department setting. Obstet Gynecol 1994;84: 1010–5.

5. Bradley WG, Fiske CE, Filly RA. The double sac sign of early intrauterine pregnancy: use in exclusion of ectopic pregnancy. Radiology 1982;143: 223–6.

6. Mahony BS, Filly RA, Nyberg DA, et al. Sonographic evaluation of ectopic pregnancy. J Ultrasound Med 1985;4:221–8.

7. Levi CS, Lyons EA, Lindsay DJ. Early diagnosis of nonviable pregnancy with transvaginal US. Radiology 1988;167:383–5.

8. Nyberg DA, Mack LA, Harvey D, et al. Value of the yolk sac in evaluating early pregnancies. J Ultrasound Med 1988;7:129–35.

9. Wiebe ER, Switzer P. Arteriovenous malformations of the uterus associated with medical abortion. Int J Gynaecol Obstet 2000;71:155–8.

10. Kido A, Togashi K, Koyama T, et al. Retained products of conception masquerading as acquired arteriovenous malformation. J Comput Assist Tomogr 2003;27:88–92.

11. Implementation of the principle of as low as reasonably achievable (ALARA) for medical and dental personnel. NRCP report 107. Bethesda (MD): National Council on Radiation Protection and Measurements; 1990.

12. Emerson DS, Cartier MS, Altieri LA, et al. Diagnostic efficacy of endovaginal color flow imaging in an ectopic pregnancy screening program. Radiology 1992;183:413–20.

13. Yeh HC, Goodman JD, Carr L, et al. Intradecidual sign: a US criterion of early intrauterine pregnancy. Radiology 1986;161:463–7.

14. Rowling SE, Coleman BG, Langer JE, et al. First-trimester US parameters of failed pregnancy. Radiology 1997;203:211–7.

15. Coulam CB, Britten S, Soenksen DM. Early (34–56 days from last menstrual period) ultrasonographic measurements in normal pregnancies. Hum Reprod 1996;11:1771–4.

16. Goldstein SR, Wolfson R. Transvaginal ultrasonographic measurement of early embryonic size as a means of assessing gestational age. J Ultrasound Med 1994;13:27–31.

17. Wisser J, Dirschedl P, Krone S. Estimation of gestational age by transvaginal sonographic measurement of the greatest embryonic length in dated human embryos. Ultrasound Obstet Gynecol 1994;4:457–62.

18. Goldstein SR. Significance of cardiac activity on endovaginal ultrasound in very early embryos. Obstet Gynecol 1992;80:670–2.

19. Levi CS, Lyons EA, Zheng XH, et al. Endovaginal US: demonstration of cardiac activity in embryos of less than 5.0 mm in crown rump length. Radiology 1990;176:71–4.

20. Hertzberg BS, Mahony BS, Bowie JD. First trimester fetal cardiac activity. Sonographic documentation of a progressive early rise in heart rate. J Ultrasound Med 1988;7:573–5.

21. Yeh HC, Rabinowitz JG. Amniotic sac development: ultrasound features of early pregnancy—the double bleb sign. Radiology 1988;166(1 Pt 1):97–103.

22. Ulm B, Ulm MR, Bernaschek G. Unfused amnion and chorion after 14 weeks of gestation: associated fetal structural and chromosomal abnormalities. Ultrasound Obstet Gynecol 1999;13:392–5.

23. Bromley B, Shipp TD, Benacerraf BR. Amnion-chorion separation after 17 weeks' gestation. Obstet Gynecol 1999;94:1024–6.

24. Ljunger E, Cnattingius S, Lundin C, et al. Chromosomal anomalies in first-trimester miscarriages. Acta Obstet Gynecol Scand 2005;84:1103–7.

25. Condous G, Kirk E, Lu C, et al. Diagnostic accuracy of varying discriminatory zones for the prediction of ectopic pregnancy in women with a pregnancy of unknown location. Ultrasound Obstet Gynecol 2005;26:770–5.

26. Levi CS, Lyons EA, Lindsay DJ. Ultrasound in the first trimester of pregnancy. Radiol Clin North Am 1990;28:19–38.

27. Bernard KG, Cooperberg PL. Sonographic differentiation between blighted ovum and early viable pregnancy. AJR Am J Roentgenol 1985;144: 597–602.

28. McKenna KM, Feldstein VA, Goldstein RB, et al. The empty amnion: a sign of early pregnancy failure. J Ultrasound Med 1995;14:117–21.

29. Nyberg DA, Mack LA, Laing FC, et al. Distinguishing normal from abnormal gestational sac growth in early pregnancy. J Ultrasound Med 1987;6:23–7.

30. Levi CS. Prediction of early pregnancy failure on the basis of mean gestational sac size and absence of a sonographically demonstrable yolk sac. Radiology 1995;195:873.

31. Lindsay DJ, Lovett IS, Lyons EA, et al. Yolk sac diameter and shape at endovaginal US: predictors of pregnancy outcome in the first trimester. Radiology 1992;183:115–8.

32. Stampone C, Nicotra M, Muttinelli C, et al. Transvaginal sonography of the yolk sac in normal and abnormal pregnancy. J Clin Ultrasound 1996;24: 3–9.

33. Harris RD, Vincent LM, Askin FB. Yolk sac calcification: a sonographic finding associated with intrauterine embryonic demise in the first trimester. Radiology 1988;166:109–10.

34. Jauniaux E, Jurkovic D, Henriet Y, et al. Development of the secondary human yolk sac: correlation of sonographic and anatomical features. Hum Reprod 1991;6:1160–6.

35. Szabo J, Gellen J, Szemere G, et al. Significance of hyper-echogenic yolk sac in first-trimester screening for chromosome aneuploidy. Orv Hetil 1996;137:2313–5.

36. Reece EA, Scioscia AL, Pinter E, et al. Prognostic significance of the human yolk sac assessed by ultrasonography. Am J Obstet Gynecol 1988;159:1191–4.

37. Kurtz AB, Needleman L, Pennell RG, et al. Can detection of the yolk sac in the first trimester be used to predict the outcome of pregnancy? A prospective sonographic study. AJR Am J Roentgenol 1992;158:843–7.

38. Laboda LA, Estroff JA, Benacerraf BR. First trimester bradycardia. A sign of impending fetal loss. J Ultrasound Med 1989;8:561–3.

39. Doubilet PM, Benson CB. Outcome of first-trimester pregnancies with slow embryonic heart rate at 6–7 weeks gestation and normal heart rate by 8 weeks at US. Radiology 2005;236:643–6.

40. Bromley B, Harlow BL, Laboda LA, et al. Small sac size in the first trimester: a predictor of poor fetal outcome. Radiology 1991;178:375–7.

41. Devi Wold AS, Pham N, Arici A. Anatomic factors in recurrent pregnancy loss. Semin Reprod Med 2006;24:25–32.

42. Propst AM, Hill JA 3rd. Anatomic factors associated with recurrent pregnancy loss. Semin Reprod Med 2000;18:341–50.

43. Raga F, Bauset C, Remohi J, et al. Reproductive impact of congenital mullerian anomalies. Hum Reprod 1997;12:2277–81.

44. Benson CB, Chow JS, Chang-Lee W, et al. Outcome of pregnancies in women with uterine leiomyomas identified by sonography in the first trimester. J Clin Ultrasound 2001;29:261–4.

45. Ouyang DW, Economy KE, Norwitz ER. Obstetric complications of fibroids. Obstet Gynecol Clin North Am 2006;33:153–69.

46. Exacoustos C, Rosati P. Ultrasound diagnosis of uterine myomas and complications in pregnancy. Obstet Gynecol 1993;82:97–101.

47. Koetsawang S, Rachawat D, Piya-Anant M. Outcome of pregnancy in the presence of intrauterine device. Acta Obstet Gynecol Scand 1977;56:479–82.

48. Fallon JH. Pregnancy with IUD in situ. Kans Med 1985;86:322–4.

49. Mermet J, Bolcato C, Rudigoz RC, et al. Outcome of pregnancies with an intrauterine devices and their management. Rev Fr Gynecol Obstet 1986;81:233–5.

50. Abu-Yousef MM, Bleicher JJ, Williamson RA, et al. Subchorionic hemorrhage: sonographic diagnosis and clinical significance. AJR Am J Roentgenol 1987;149:737–40.

51. Bennette GL, Bromley B, Lieberman E, et al. Subchorionic hemorrhage in first-trimester pregnancies: prediction of pregnancy outcome with sonography. Radiology 1996;200:803–6.

52. Sauerbrei EE, Pham DH. Placental abruption and subchorionic hemorrhage in the first half of pregnancy: US appearance and clinical outcome. Radiology 1986;160:109–12.

53. Bloch C, Altchek A, Levy-Ravetch M. Sonography in early pregnancy: the significance of subchorionic hemorrhage. Mt Sinai J Med 1989;56:290–2.

54. Pedersen JF, Mantoni M. Prevalence and significance of subchorionic hemorrhage in threatened abortion: a sonographic study. AJR Am J Roentgenol 1990;154:535–7.

55. Maso G, D'Ottavio G, De Seta F, et al. First-trimester intrauterine hematoma and outcome of pregnancy. Obstet Gynecol 2005;105:339–44.

56. Kurtz AB, Shlansky-Goldberg RD, Choi HY, et al. Detection of retained products of conception following spontaneous abortion in the first trimester. J Ultrasound Med 1991;10:387–95.

57. Wong SF, Lam MH, Ho LC. Transvaginal sonography in the detection of retained products of conception after first-trimester spontaneous abortion. J Clin Ultrasound 2002;30:428–32.

58. Alcazar JL. Transvaginal ultrasonography combined with color velocity imaging and pulsed Doppler to detect residual trophoblastic tissue. Ultrasound Obstet Gynecol 1998;11:54–8.

59. Durfee SM, Frates MC, Luong A, et al. The sonographic and color Doppler features of retained products of conception. J Ultrasound Med 2005;24:1181–6.

60. Polat P, Suma S, Kantarcy M, et al. Color Doppler US in the evaluation of uterine vascular abnormalities. Radiographics 2002;22:47–53.

61. O'Brien P, Neyastani A, Buckley AR, et al. Uterine arteriovenous malformations: from diagnosis to treatment. J Ultrasound Med 2006;25:1387–92.

62. Huang MW, Muradali D, Thurston WA, et al. Uterine arteriovenous malformations: gray-scale and Doppler US features with MR imaging correlation. Radiology 1998;206:115–23.

63. Jain K, Fogata M. Retained products of conception mimicking a large endometrial AVM: complete resolution following spontaneous abortion. J Clin Ultrasound 2007;35:42–7.

64. Vedantham S, Goodwin SC, McLucas B, et al. Uterine artery embolization: an underused method of controlling pelvic hemorrhage. Am J Obstet Gynecol 1997;176:938–48.

65. Maleux G, Timmerman D, Heye S, et al. Acquired uterine vascular malformations: radiological and clinical outcome after transcatheter embolotherapy. Eur Radiol 2006;16:299–306.

66. Centers for Disease Control. Current trends ectopic pregnancy: United States, 1990–1992. MMWR Morb Mortal Wkly Rep 1995;44:46–8.

67. Atri M, Leduc C, Gillett P, et al. Role of endovaginal sonography in the diagnosis and management of ectopic pregnancy. Radiographics 1996;16:755–74.

68. Chavkin W. The rise in ectopic pregnancy-exploration of possible reasons. Int J Gynaecol Obstet 1982;20:341–50.

69. Bouyer J, Coste J, Shojaei T, et al. Risk factors for ectopic pregnancy: a comprehensive analysis based on a large case-control, population-based study in France. Am J Epidemiol 2003;157:185–94.

70. Urman B, Zouves C, Gomel V. Fertility outcome following tubal pregnancy. Acta Eur Fertil 1991;22:205–8.

71. Uotila J, Heinonen PK, Punnonen R. Reproductive outcome after multiple ectopic pregnancies. Int J Fertil 1989;34:102–5.

72. Gervaise A, Masson L, de Tayrac R, et al. Reproductive outcome after methotrexate treatment of tubal pregnancies. Fertil Steril 2004;82:304–8.

73. Brown DL, Doubilet PM. Transvaginal sonography for diagnosing ectopic pregnancy: positivity criteria and performance characteristics. J Ultrasound Med 1994;13:259–66.

74. Braffman BH, Coleman BG, Ramchandani P, et al. Emergency department screening for ectopic pregnancy: a prospective US study. Radiology 1994;190:797–802.

75. Nyberg DA, Hughes MP, Mack LA, et al. Extrauterine findings of ectopic pregnancy of transvaginal US: importance of echogenic fluid. Radiology 1991;178:823–6.

76. Frates MC, Brown DL, Doubilet PM, et al. Tubal rupture in patients with ectopic pregnancy: diagnosis with transvaginal US. Radiology 1994;191:769–72.

77. Fleischer AC, Pennell RG, McKee MS, et al. Ectopic pregnancy: features at transvaginal sonography. Radiology 1990;174:375–8.

78. Frates MC, Visweswaran A, Laing FC. Comparison of tubal ring and corpus luteum echogenicities: a useful differentiating characteristic. J Ultrasound Med 2001;20:27–31.

79. Stein MW, Ricci ZJ, Novak L, et al. Sonographic comparison of the tubal ring of ectopic pregnancy with the corpus luteum. J Ultrasound Med 2004;23:57–62.

80. Atri M. Ectopic pregnancy versus corpus luteum cyst revisited: best Doppler predictors. J Ultrasound Med 2003;2:1181–4.

81. Graham M, Cooperberg PL. Ultrasound diagnosis of interstitial pregnancy: findings and pitfalls. J Clin Ultrasound 1979;7:433–7.

82. Chen GD, Lin MT, Lee MS. Diagnosis of interstitial pregnancy with sonography. J Clin Ultrasound 1994;22:439–42.

83. Kaakaji Y, Nghiem HV, Nodell C, et al. Sonography of obstetric and gynecologic emergencies: part I, obstetric emergencies. AJR Am J Roentgenol 2000;174:641–9.

84. Ackerman TE, Levi CS, Dashefsky SM, et al. Interstitial line: sonographic finding in interstitial (cornual) ectopic pregnancy. Radiology 1993;189:83–7.

85. Jansen RP, Elliott PM. Angular intrauterine pregnancy. Obstet Gynecol 1981;58:167–75.

86. Tarim E, Ulusan S, Kilicdag E, et al. Angular pregnancy. J Obstet Gynaecol Res 2004;30:377–9.

87. Harika G, Gabriel R, Carre-Pigeon F, et al. Primary application of three-dimensional ultrasonography to early diagnosis of ectopic pregnancy. Eur J Obstet Gynecol Reprod Biol 1995;60:117–20.

88. Izquierdo LA, Nicholas MC. Three-dimensional transvaginal sonography of interstitial pregnancy. J Clin Ultrasound 2003;31:484–7.

89. Takeuchi K, Yamada T, Oomori S, et al. Comparison of magnetic resonance imaging and ultrasonography in the early diagnosis of interstitial pregnancy. J Reprod Med 1999;44:265–8.

90. Nishino M, Hayakawa K, Kawamata K, et al. MRI of early unruptured ectopic pregnancy: detection of gestational sac. J Comput Assist Tomogr 2002;26:134–7.

91. Marcus SF, Brinsden PR. Primary ovarian pregnancy after in vitro fertilization and embryo transfer: report of seven cases. Fertil Steril 1993;60:167–9.

92. Tuncer R, Sipahi T, Erkaya S, et al. Primary twin ovarian pregnancy. Int J Gynaecol Obstet 1994;46:57–9.

93. Marret H, Hamamah S, Alonso AM, et al. Case report and review of the literature: primary twin ovarian pregnancy. Hum Reprod 1997;12:1813–5.

94. de Vries K, Shapiro I, Degani S, et al. Ovarian pregnancy in association with an intrauterine device. Int J Gynaecol Obstet 1983;21:65–70.

95. Sergent F, Mauger-Tinlot F, Gravier A, et al. Ovarian pregnancies: reevaluation of diagnostic criteria. J Gynecol Obstet Biol Reprod (Paris) 2002;31:741–6.

96. Camstock C, Huston K, Lee W. The ultrasonographic appearance of ovarian ectopic pregnancies. Obstet Gynecol 2005;105:42–5.

97. Hallat JG. Primary ovarian pregnancy: a report of twenty-five cases. Am J Obstet Gynecol 1982; 143:55–60.

98. Han M, Kim J, Kim H, et al. Bilateral ovarian pregnancy after in vitro fertilization and embryo transfer in a patient with tubal factor infertility. Obstet Gynecol 2005;105:42–5.

99. Leeman LM, Wendland CL. Cervical ectopic pregnancy. Diagnosis with endovaginal ultrasound examination and successful treatment with methotrexate. Arch Fam Med 2000;9:72–7.

100. Werber J, Prasadarao PR, Harris VJ. Cervical pregnancy diagnosed by ultrasound. Radiology 1983; 149:279–80.

101. Vas W, Suresh PL, Tang-Barton P, et al. Ultrasonographic differentiation of cervical abortion from cervical pregnancy. J Clin Ultrasound 1984;12: 553–7.

102. Guerrier C, Wartanian R, Boblet V, et al. Cervical pregnancy. Contribution of ultrasonography to diagnosis and therapeutic management (in French). Rev Fr Gynecol Obstet 1995;90:355–9.

103. Jurkovic D, Hacket E, Campbell S. Diagnosis and treatment of early cervical pregnancy: a review and a report of two cases treated conservatively. Ultrasound Obstet Gynecol 1996;8:373–80.

104. Rafal RB, Kosovsky PA, Markisz JA. MR appearance of cervical pregnancy. J Comput Assist Tomogr 1990;14:482–4.

105. Jung SE, Byun JY, Lee JM, et al. Characteristic MR findings of cervical pregnancy. J Magn Reson Imaging 2001;13:918–22.

106. Kirk E, Bourne T. The nonsurgical management of ectopic pregnancy. Curr Opin Obstet Gynecol 2006;18:587–93.

107. Barnhart KT, Gosman G, Ashby R, et al. The medical management of ectopic pregnancy: a meta-analysis comparing "single dose" and "multidose" regimens. Obstet Gynecol 2003;101:778–84.

108. Gabbur N, Sherer DM, Hellmann M, et al. Do serum beta-human chorionic gonadotropin levels on day 4 following methotrexate treatment of patients with ectopic pregnancy predict successful single-dose therapy? Am J Perinatol 2006;23:193–6.

109. Tawfiq A, Agameya AF, Claman P. Predictors of treatment failure for ectopic pregnancy treated with single-dose methotrexate. Fertil Steril 2000; 74:877–80.

110. Menon S, Colins J, Barnhart KT. Establishing a human chorionic gonadotropin cutoff to guide methotrexate treatment of ectopic pregnancy: a systematic review. Fertil Steril 2007;87:481–4.

111. Kirk E, Condous G, Haider Z, et al. The conservative management of cervical ectopic pregnancies. Ultrasound Obstet Gynecol 2006;27:430–7.

112. Committee on Practice Bulletins-Gynecology. American College of Obstetricians and Gynaecologists. ACOG Practice Bulletin #53. Diagnosis and treatment of gestational trophoblastic disease. Obstet Gynecol 2004;103:1365–77.

113. Soper JT, Mutch DG, Schink JC. American College of Obstetricians and Gynecologists. Diagnosis and treatment of gestational trophoblastic disease: ACOG Practice Bulletin No. 53. Gynecol Oncol 2004;93:575–85.

114. Grimes DA. Epidemiology of gestational trophoblastic disease. Am J Obstet Gynecol 1984;150: 309–18.

115. Bracken MB. Incidence and aetiology of hydatidiform mole: an epidemiological review. Br J Obstet Gynaecol 1987;94:1123–35.

116. Buckley JD. The epidemiology of molar pregnancy and choriocarcinoma. Clin Obstet Gynecol 1984; 27:153–9.

117. Lawler SD, Fisher RA. Genetic studies in hydatidiform mole with clinical correlations. Placenta 1987;8:77–88.

118. Lawler SD, Fisher RA, Dent J. A prospective genetic study of complete and partial hydatidiform moles. Am J Obstet Gynecol 1991;164(5 Pt 1): 1270–7.

119. Wells M. The pathology of gestational trophoblastic disease: recent advances. Pathology 2007;39: 88–96.

120. Garner EI, Goldstein DP, Feltmate CM, et al. Gestational trophoblastic disease. Clin Obstet Gynecol 2007;50:112–22.

121. Wagner BJ, Woodward PJ, Dickey GE. From the archives of the AFIP. Gestational trophoblastic disease: radiologic-pathologic correlation. Radiographics 1996;16:131–48.

122. Allen SD, Lim AK, Seckl MJ, et al. Radiology of gestational trophoblastic neoplasia. Clin Radiol 2006;61:301–13.

123. Zhou Q, Lei XY, Xie Q, et al. Sonographic and Doppler imaging in the diagnosis and treatment of gestational trophoblastic disease: a 12-year experience. J Ultrasound Med 2005;24:15–24.

124. Jain KA. Gestational trophoblastic disease: pictorial review. Ultrasound Q 2005;21:245–53.

125. Betel C, Atri M, Arenson AM, et al. Sonographic diagnosis of gestational trophoblastic disease and comparison with retained products of conception. J Ultrasound Med 2006;25:985–93.

126. Montz FJ, Schlaerth JB, Morrow CP. The natural history of theca lutein cysts. Obstet Gynecol 1988;72:247–51.

127. Ha HK, Jung JK, Jee MK, et al. Gestational trophoblastic tumors of the uterus: MR imaging-pathologic correlation. Gynecol Oncol 1995;57:340–50.

Sonography of Adnexal Masses

Mukund Joshi, MD, FAMS*, Karthik Ganesan, DNB,
Harsha Navani Munshi, DNB, Subramania Ganesan, MD,
Ashwin Lawande, DNB

KEYWORDS

- Ultrasound • Ovarian neoplasm • Endometriosis
- Fibroma

Transabdominal and transvaginal sonography are the community standard for the performance of pelvic sonography. Since their introduction, transvaginal probes have become the principal tools for evaluating the female pelvis.[1] Transabdominal imaging provides a global anatomic survey, whereas transvaginal imaging provides improved texture determination and characterization of the internal architecture of the ovary, vascular anatomy, and adnexal area. The location, size, consistency, and origin of adnexal masses may be defined with a combination of transvaginal and transabdominal scanning.[2,3] Transrectal ultrasound is performed whenever there is a contraindication to transvaginal scan, such as in the evaluation of the pediatric pelvis or in women who have never been sexually active. Transperineal scans also have a role to play in determining the origin and extent of some tumors. This article presents grayscale, color, and power Doppler features of common and uncommon benign and malignant adnexal masses.

SONOGRAPHIC EVALUATION OF THE ADNEXAL MASS

The benefit of ultrasound lies in its ability to characterize the mass and give significant insight as to its probable nature. Correlation of sonographic images with pathologic findings has led to a substantial understanding of adnexal abnormalities. The development of scoring systems to characterize and define ovarian lesions, first based on morphologic characteristics and later including color Doppler flow data, brought us closer to a relatively reliable distinction between benign and malignant lesions, or at least to a negative predictive value in the range of 97% to 99%. The use of grayscale ultrasound morphology to characterize a pelvic mass is based on "pattern recognition." Subjective evaluation of ovarian masses based on pattern recognition can achieve sensitivity of 88% to 100% and specificity of 62% to 96%. Such subjective evaluation is found to be superior to scoring systems. Pattern recognition is superior to all other ultrasound methods (eg, simple classification systems, scoring systems, and mathematical models for calculating the risk of malignancy) for discrimination between benign and malignant extrauterine pelvic masses.[4,5]

Benign Adnexal Lesions

The majority of ovarian masses are simple cysts (**Fig. 1**), most of which are benign. In this context, it is important to remember that the diagnosis of a "simple cyst" is based purely on ultrasound findings.

Functional ovarian cysts

Functional ovarian cysts result when a mature follicle does not rupture and the follicle continues to grow. Functional cysts include follicular cysts, serous inclusion cysts, corpus luteum, corpus albicans cysts, hemorrhagic cysts, and theca lutein cysts.[2,3,6] Most of these are simple cysts. Sonographically they appear unilocular, round, and anechoic with an imperceptible wall and posterior

This article originally appeared in the Januray 2007 issue of Ultrasound Clinics.
Dr. Joshi's Imaging Clinic, 809 Harjivandas Estate, Dr. Ambedkar Road, Next to Babubhai Jagjivandas, Dadar T.T, Mumbai 400014, Maharashtra, India
* Corresponding author.
E-mail address: drmukundjoshi@gmail.com (M. Joshi).

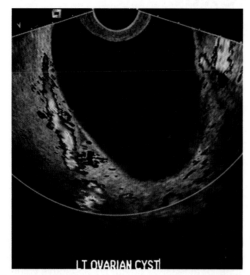

Fig. 1. Simple ovarian cyst. Transvaginal color flow Doppler image demonstrates a large simple ovarian cyst.

through transmission.[4] Functional cysts can become quite large but are usually less than 10 cm in size. These may produce discomfort or delayed menses but can be observed to regress within two menstrual cycles, although some persist for several months.

Corpus luteum cysts occur in the secretory phase of the menstrual cycle. Corpus luteal cyst in pregnancy reaches its maximum size by 7 weeks, and resolution occurs by 16 weeks. The corpus luteum can have a wide range of appearances on ultrasound (US) in the first trimester of

pregnancy. The most common appearance is that of a round, thin-walled hypoechoic structure that demonstrates diffuse, homogeneous, low-level echoes. Other reported grayscale appearances (in order of decreasing frequency) include a cyst with a thick wall and anechoic center, a cyst that contains scattered internal echoes (**Fig. 2**A), and a thin-walled simple cyst that is similar in appearance to a follicular cyst.[7] On color flow Doppler sonography, it shows a typical "ring of fire" (**Fig. 2**B), and spectral Doppler examination reveals prominent diastolic flow.[8] The "ring of fire" appearance is secondary to increased vascularity in the periphery and is a nonspecific sign, because this may be seen in a mature Graafian follicle as well. Corpus luteal cyst of pregnancy is very vascular because of its hormonal status and may present with hemorrhage (known as a hemorrhagic corpus luteum), but the physiologic features are the same regardless of size.[2,3,9]

Any functional cyst may hemorrhage within and present as a hemorrhagic cyst (HC). The internal echo pattern varies with the stage of hemorrhage and the amount of fluid within the cyst. Evidence of posterior through transmission is typically present because of the cystic composition.[10,11]

The average diameter of an HC is 3.0 to 3.5 cm (range: 2.5–8.5 cm). The cyst wall is thin (2–3 mm), well defined, and regular.[12] US appearance of HC may have diffuse echogenic material within, diffuse echoes with visible fibrin strands, retracting thrombus, or a fluid–fluid level. Jain[13] described the occurrence of fibrin strands within an HC as a "fishnet" appearance (**Fig. 3**A). The presence

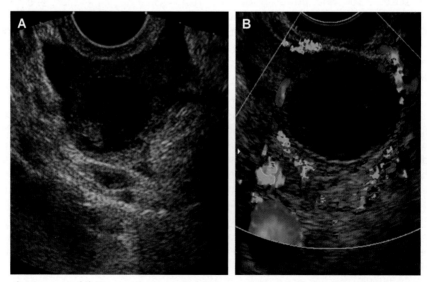

Fig. 2. Corpus luteum cyst. (*A*) Transvaginal grayscale image of the left ovary demonstrates a cyst with debris within, suggestive of hemorrhage in a corpus luteum cyst. (*Courtesy of* A. Khurana, MD, India). (*B*) Corresponding color flow Doppler image demonstrates peripheral vascularity—called the "ring of fire."

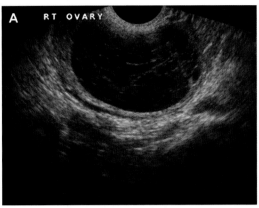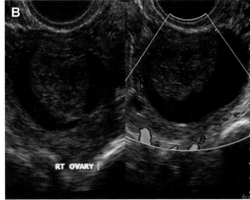

Fig. 3. Hemorrhagic ovarian cyst. (*A*) Transvaginal grayscale image of the right ovary demonstrates a typical "fishnet" appearance. (*B*) Grayscale and color flow Doppler image of the right ovarian cyst with a retracting blood clot adherent to the cyst wall and absent vascularity.

of a retracting thrombus adhering to the wall of a cyst is an additional sonographic feature. This finding may be occasionally confused with a focal mural nodule. A retracting clot typically has a concave margin, whereas mural nodules have convex margins. Retracting clots also appear to have a variable central echogenic pattern, whereas most mural nodules appear isoechoic in relation to the wall of the cyst. Okai and colleagues[14] serially followed 28 cases of hemorrhagic ovarian cysts that regressed spontaneously within 8 weeks. Color Doppler flow studies do not reveal any blood flow within a retracting clot or the fibrin strands (**Fig. 3**B).[2,3,9]

Theca lutein cysts (also called lutein cysts, *hyperreactio luteinalis*) are luteinized follicle cysts that form as a result of overstimulation from high hCG levels or hypersensitivity to human chorionic gonadotrophin (hCG) in normal pregnancy. Bilateral multiseptated cystic adnexal masses in a woman who has gestational trophoblastic disease (**Fig. 4**), multiple gestation, ovarian hyperstimulation, or a pregnancy complicated by fetal hydrops are likely to represent theca lutein cysts, rather than malignancy. Theca lutein cysts are reported with complete hydatidiform moles 14% to 30% of the time.[15] In normal pregnancy, the cysts gradually resolve weeks to months after the source of hCG is eliminated. Complications include torsion, infarction, and hemorrhage.

Endometriosis

Endometriosis is defined as the presence of functional endometrial tissue outside the uterine cavity and the myometrium. The most common site of involvement in endometriosis is the ovary, followed by the uterine ligaments (posterior broad ligament, uterosacral ligament), pelvic cul-de-sac,

pelvic peritoneum, fallopian tubes, rectosigmoid, and bladder. Endometriotic cysts (endometriomas) usually occur within the ovaries and result from repeated cyclic hemorrhage. More than 90% of endometriomas are pseudocysts formed by invagination of the ovarian cortex, which is sealed off by adhesions. Endometriomas may completely replace normal ovarian tissue. Cyst walls are usually thick and fibrotic, frequently with dense fibrous adhesions and areas of discoloration. Cyst content generally is composed of thick, dark, degenerate blood products, and this appearance has been called "chocolate cyst".[12]

The sonographic features of endometriomas are varied, ranging from anechoic cysts to cysts with diffuse low-level echoes to solid-appearing

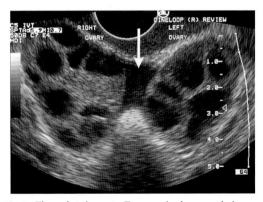

Fig. 4. Theca lutein cysts. Transvaginal grayscale image of the pelvis demonstrates multiple simple bilateral ovarian cysts in this patient with a hydatidiform mole. A pocket of free fluid is present between the two ovaries (*arrow*). (*From* Webb EM, Green GE, Scoutt LM. Adnexal mass with pelvic pain. Radiol Clin North Am 2004;42:335; with permission.)

masses. Fluid–fluid or debris–fluid levels may also be seen. They may be unilocular or multilocular with thin or thick septations.[7]

One of the more common appearances of endometrioma is that of an adnexal mass with diffuse low-level echoes (**Fig. 5**A). This appearance is seen in 95% of endometriomas.[16] Typical endometriomas do not show any vascularity.[17] The presence of hyperechoic wall foci (punctate peripheral echogenic foci) on sonographic examination is very specific for endometriomas. Echogenic wall foci differ from wall nodularity and are an important discriminating feature. A mass with low-level internal echoes, hyperechoic wall foci, and no neoplastic features is 32 times more likely to be an endometrioma than another adnexal mass. This echogenic wall focus was found to be the highest single predictor of endometrioma and is believed to represent cholesterol deposits.[12,16]

In a recent study, the appearance of "kissing ovaries" is suggested as an indirect sign of endometriosis, especially in diagnosing adhesions and the most severe form of the disease, which is significant pelvic extension of the endometriosis with dense adhesions. The diagnosis of kissing ovaries is made when both ovaries are joined behind the uterus in the cul-de-sac and cannot be separated by pushing the transvaginal probe or by manipulating the uterus transabdominally (**Fig. 5**B). The detection of kissing ovaries by US is strongly associated with the presence of endometriosis and is a marker of the most severe form of this disease.[18]

Certain reports have suggested that solid areas or polypoid projections are suggestive of malignancy in an endometrioma. Malignant transformation has been documented in 0.3% to 0.8% of patients who have ovarian endometriosis. For a high level of sonographic confidence in detection of endometriomas, attention must be focused on assessment of wall nodularity to exclude a malignancy.[2,3,9,19]

Hydrosalpinx

Hydrosalpinx is characterized by obliteration of the fimbriated end and dilatation of the fallopian tube, usually the ampullary and infundibular portions. If the ovary is first involved by tubo-ovarian adhesions, the dilated tube may compress the ovary. The tube usually contains clear, serous fluid. Most cases of hydrosalpinx have a typical appearance and may be easily distinguished from ovarian abnormalities. Hydrosalpinges are tubular, elongated, extraovarian structures, and some show longitudinal folds (**Fig. 6**).

Tessler and colleagues[20] described a tubular structure with folded configuration and incomplete septations as the most consistent sonographic feature in 12 cases of hydrosalpinx. Timor-Tritsch and colleagues[21] also analyzed the shape of the mass, wall structure, wall thickness, and ovarian involvement. They suggested that many hydrosalpinges appear as ovoid or pear-shaped fluid collections with incomplete septae, multiple hyperechoic mural nodules (beads-on-a-string sign), and short linear projections (cogwheel sign). A waist sign has been described in cases of hydrosalpinges, representing the diametrically opposed indentations along the wall of the mass lesion.

Patel[22] reported that the combination of the waist sign and tubular shape of the mass had no false positives for diagnosis of hydrosalpinx, leading to a calculated likelihood ratio exceeding 18:9. In their study, incomplete septations and short linear projections were findings predictive of hydrosalpinx; however, independently each sign was less predictive than the tubular shape of the mass or the waist sign. They suggested that incomplete septations were less useful as

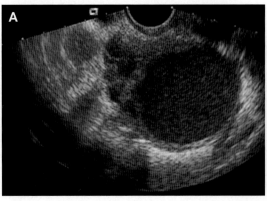
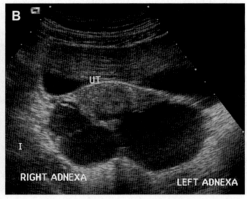

Fig. 5. Endometrioma. (*A*) Transvaginal grayscale image demonstrates a left ovarian cyst with low-level echoes. (*B*) Transabdominal grayscale image of the pelvis with bilateral endometriomas demonstrates the "kissing ovaries" sign. (UT, uterus.)

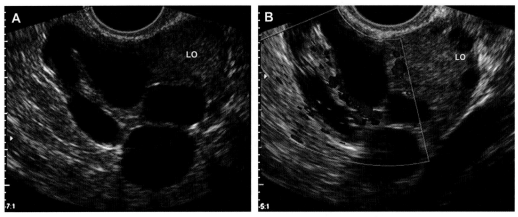

Fig. 6. Hydrosalpinx. Transvaginal grayscale (*A*) and color flow Doppler (*B*) images of the left adnexa demonstrate serpiginous, tubular, anechoic, and avascular structures in the left adnexa. (LO, left ovary.)

a diagnostic sign, because these can also be detected in some cystic tumors. The sonographic detection of a normal-appearing ovary ipsilateral to a cystic adnexal mass aids in accurate diagnosis of the mass as representing a hydrosalpinx rather than an ovarian mass. However, in some cases the ovary may also be involved in the disease process, extending to form a chronic tubo-ovarian mass.

Pelvic inflammatory disease

Pelvic inflammatory disease (PID) is one of the most common causes of acute pelvic pain in women, and imaging findings vary with the stage of disease. The sonographic findings may be normal early in the course of the disease. Sonographic markers for tubal inflammatory disease have been described as 1) thickening of the tube wall of 5 mm or more; 2) the cogwheel sign, defined as a sonolucent, cogwheel-shaped

structure visible in a cross-section of a tube with thick walls, correlating with inflammatory changes in acute salpingitis; 3) incomplete septa, correlating with folds or kinks in the dilated tube, which may be sonolucent or contain low-level echoes (**Fig. 7**A); 4) the beads-on-a-string sign, defined as hyperechoic mural nodules (about 2–3 mm) seen on the cross-section of a fluid-filled, distended structure; 5) Tubo-ovarian complex, in which the ovaries and tubes are recognized, but the ovary cannot be separated from the tube; 6) tubo-ovarian abscess with marked probe tenderness, formation of a conglomerate mass, or fluid collection; and 7) cul-de-sac fluid.

A tubo-ovarian abscess may present as an asymptomatic probable adnexal mass that did not completely resolve previously. The US appearance varies according to its appearance at the time of stabilization of the inflammatory process. The mass may be purely cystic, have multiple

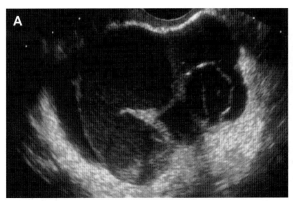 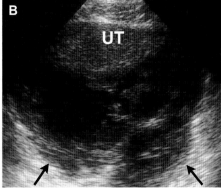

Fig. 7. Pelvic inflammatory disease. (*A*) Transvaginal grayscale image demonstrates debris within the dilated fallopian tube. (*B*) Transabdominal grayscale image in patient with fever and confirmed PID reveals pelvic abscess (*arrows*). (UT, uterus.)

loculations, have thick septations, and contain complex debris (**Fig. 7B**). Much less common than a tubo-ovarian abscess is an abscess confined to the ovary. An ovarian abscess is typically a result of direct or lymphatic spread of organisms from a nongynecologic pelvic inflammatory process (eg, diverticulitis, appendicitis, infection following pelvic surgery).[2,4,9] Presence of any free fluid is worrisome, and the possibility of pus must be considered. Although the combination of sonographic and clinical findings is often quite specific for PID, there are several other common diagnoses in the differential diagnosis. The most common alternative diagnoses, with findings that simulate PID by the presence of an indistinct uterus and complex pelvic fluid, are ruptured endometrioma or HC and perforated appendicitis.[23] Perihepatitis associated with PID is known as Fitz-Hugh-Curtis Syndrome.[23]

Mature cystic teratoma

Mature cystic teratoma constitutes 20% to 25% of pelvic masses. Mean age of presentation is 30 years, and 12% are bilateral. Mature cystic teratomas grow slowly at an average rate of 1.8 mm each year, prompting some investigators to advocate nonsurgical management of smaller (<6 cm) tumors. The presence of fat opacity or fat signal intensity in an ovarian lesion is highly specific for a teratoma. Mature cystic teratomas are predominantly cystic with dense calcifications, whereas immature teratomas are predominantly solid with small foci of lipid material and scattered calcifications. Although dermoids have a wide spectrum of sonographic appearances, depending on the elements present (ectoderm, mesoderm, or endoderm), certain distinct features occur with a degree of consistency. Among these are dermoid mesh with hyperechoic calcifications, indicating the presence of bone, teeth, or other ectodermal derivatives in a predominantly cystic medium, hyperechoic solid mural components, and hair–fluid levels.[2–4,24]

Sonographic appearance, in order of decreasing frequency, is cystic lesion with a densely echogenic tubercle (Rokitansky nodule); diffusely or partially echogenic mass, with the echogenic area usually demonstrating sound attenuation; and multiple thin echogenic bands caused by hair in the cyst. These sonographic criteria have 58% sensitivity and 99% specificity.[25] Sometimes the presence of echogenic focus (secondary to calcification) results in a curvilinear interface with acoustic shadowing and may obscure the visualization of mature cystic teratoma; hence this is called the "tip of the iceberg" sign (**Fig. 8**).

Unusual findings in mature cystic teratoma may result in occasional diagnostic difficulties. Multiple spherical structures (fat balls) floating free in a large cystic mass is one of the rarer patterns that can be mistaken for malignancy. The sonographic feature of intracystic floating echogenic balls is probably pathognomonic for mature teratoma and is easily detected in most cases.[26] In cases with sonographic features simulating malignancy, color Doppler mapping may be helpful. Color Doppler sonography is helpful in differentiating these benign nodules (small balls) from malignant tumor.[26] The most common tumor associated with ovarian torsion is mature cystic teratoma.[27]

Parovarian/paratubal cysts

Parovarian/paratubal cysts may arise from mesonephric (Wolffian) structures, paramesonephric (Mullerian) structures, or mesothelial inclusions. The hydatid of Morgagni is by far the most common paramesonephric cyst and is found arising from the fimbrial end of the fallopian tube. Sonographically, these have thin, deformable walls that are not surrounded by ovarian stroma and appear as simple cysts adjacent to the ovary (**Fig. 9**). They may be easily missed or mistaken for ovarian cysts but are confirmed by separating the cyst from the ovary on transvaginal examination. These cysts can arise anywhere in the adnexal structures; if they are large, their point of origin may not be clear. Their size does not change with the hormone cycle.[2,3]

Peritoneal inclusion cysts

Although fairly common, peritoneal inclusion cysts are less well-recognized entities on imaging of the female pelvis. Peritoneal inclusion cysts, also known as peritoneal pseudocysts and inflammatory cysts of the pelvic peritoneum, present with a variety of imaging appearances, which can be

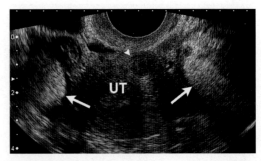

Fig. 8. Bilateral mature cystic teratoma. Transverse grayscale image demonstrates bilateral mature cystic teratomas (*arrows*). This image also shows the "tip of the iceberg" sign. Incidentally seen is a fibroid (*arrowhead*) in the anterior wall of the uterus (UT). (*Courtesy of* V. Dogra, MD, Rochester, NY.)

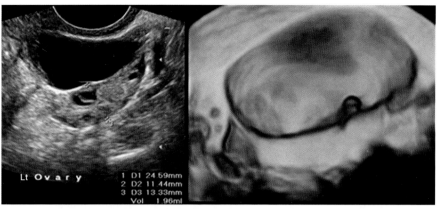

Fig. 9. Parovarian cyst. Transvaginal grayscale image demonstrates a left parovarian cyst with a corresponding four-dimensional US reformatted image that demonstrates better delineation and extent of the cyst. (*Courtesy of* A. Khurana, MD, India.)

confused with various adnexal masses of the female pelvis.

Peritoneal inclusion cysts occur predominantly in premenopausal women who have a history of previous abdominal surgery, trauma, PID, or endometriosis.[28] Peritoneal adhesions extend to the surface of the ovary and may distort the ovarian contour but not penetrate the ovarian parenchyma. When the adhesions surround the ovary, and fluid accumulates, complex cystic masses form. The entrapped ovary appears like a spider in a web and may be mistaken for a solid nodular portion of the tumor with surrounding septations. Sometimes the ovary is eccentrically located to the adhesions. This is called spider-web pattern (entrapped ovary) (**Fig. 10**).[29] These cysts may simulate hydrosalpinx, pyosalpinx, or even an

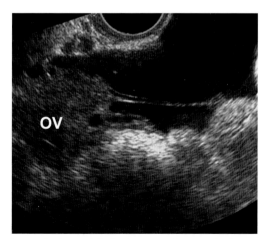

Fig. 10. Peritoneal inclusion cyst. Transvaginal grayscale image of the right adnexa demonstrates a spider-web pattern with presence of loculated fluid and an eccentric right ovary (OV).

ovarian mass. Sonographic diagnosis depends on the presence of normal ipsilateral ovary with surrounding loculated fluid conforming to the peritoneal space.[29] The fluid is usually anechoic but may contain echoes in some compartments, owing to hemorrhage or proteinaceous fluid. Peritoneal inclusion cyst must be differentiated from parovarian cysts and hydrosalpinx.[2,3]

Polycystic ovaries
Polycystic ovaries occur in approximately 17% of women of reproductive age. The classic signs and symptoms result from excessive androgen production, inappropriate gonadotropin secretion, and chronic anovulation and are manifested by acne, hirsutism, and menstrual irregularity.[30] Polycystic ovarian disease (PCOD), or Stein-Leventhal syndrome, is a common cause of infertility that is accompanied by secondary amenorrhea, hirsutism, and/or obesity.[31] The morphologic hallmark of the disease is mild enlargement of both ovaries, which contain multiple small cysts. Discrete cysts, however, are not sonographically visible in the majority of patients[32], and as many as 30% of patients who have PCOD have ovaries that are within normal size limits.[33] The number of follicles necessary to establish the diagnosis of polycystic ovaries has been reported to vary from more than five to 10 or at least 15.[34–36] In a study by Pache and colleagues[37], a maximum of 11 follicles could be detected in normal ovaries, and a considerable number of ovaries in patients who had PCOD contained fewer than 11 follicles. Increased ovarian echogenicity is an additional criterion for diagnosing PCOD but is very subjective. A combination of follicular size and ovarian volume is the most sensitive objective parameter. It has a sensitivity of 92% and a specificity of 97% (**Fig. 11**).

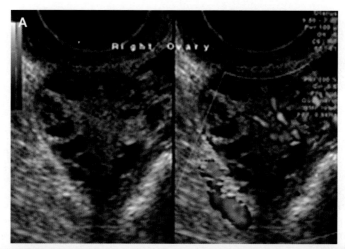

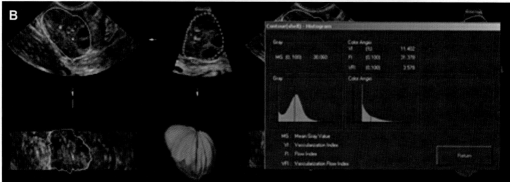

Fig. 11. Polycystic ovarian disease. (A) Power Doppler image of bilateral ovaries demonstrates multiple follicles. (B) Corresponding four-dimensional images demonstrate ovarian volume calculation in polycystic ovaries. (*Courtesy of* A. Khurana, MD, India.)

Postmenopausal cysts

Small simple cysts are common in postmenopausal patients.[38] Fifteen percent of postmenopausal women may show simple cystic adnexal structures as large as 5 cm (**Fig. 12**). A cystic structure that is less than 30 mm in size, unilateral, and unilocular, has no internal echoes, solid areas, or nodules, and is avascular on color flow mapping may be re-evaluated 6 and 12 weeks later and then annually if it does not increase in size or change in morphology. A simple unilocular cyst without solid components is highly unlikely to be malignant. Any mass with abnormal vascularity and all masses greater than 50 mm in size warrant surgical evaluation. All masses associated with a rising CA-125 level warrant surgical exploration.[39]

Ectopic pregnancy

Ectopic pregnancy is one of the most common gynecologic emergencies that presents as vaginal bleeding or abdominal pain. Ectopic pregnancy most commonly (95%) occurs in the ampullary or isthmic portions of the fallopian tube. An ectopic pregnancy can be diagnosed with confidence when an adnexal mass that contains a yolk sac or viable embryo is identified (**Fig. 13**A). In the absence of a visualized yolk sac or fetal pole, the so-called "echogenic adnexal" (or tubal) ring sign is the second most specific US finding for ectopic pregnancy.[40] It may be difficult to differentiate the tubal ring of an ectopic pregnancy from an exophytic corpus luteal cyst. An anechoic structure with an echogenic, vascular rim truly located within the ovary is statistically much more likely to be a corpus luteal cyst, because true intraovarian ectopic pregnancies are rare.[7]

Differentiation between an ectopic pregnancy and an exophytic corpus luteal cyst can be aided by gently tapping on the ovary with the transducer. Independent movement of the ovary indicates an extraovarian location of the adnexal ring, which confirms ectopic pregnancy.[7] The demonstration of the embryonic cardiac activity confirms intrauterine pregnancy. (However, gestations earlier

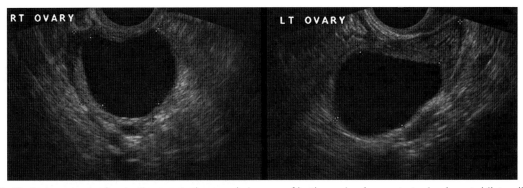

Fig. 12. Postmenopausal cysts. Transvaginal grayscale images of both ovaries demonstrate simple cysts bilaterally in a postmenopausal woman.

than 5 to 6 weeks may not show evidence of cardiac activity.)

As many as 20% of patients who have ectopic pregnancy demonstrate an intrauterine pseudo-gestational sac, which should be differentiated from the double decidual sac of an intrauterine pregnancy. The pseudogestational sac does not contain a living embryo or yolk sac and is located in the center of the endometrial cavity (unlike the burrowed gestational sac, which is placed eccentrically). Color Doppler imaging plays an important role in differentiating an ectopic pregnancy from a corpus luteum (CL). Both demonstrate abundant vascularity at the periphery—"ring of fire" on color flow imaging (**Fig. 13**B)—which is by itself a nonspecific sign and may also be seen around a mature ovarian follicle or HC.

It has been found that low (<0.39) and high (>0.7) resistive indices (RIs) are specific for ectopic pregnancy (100% specificity and positive predictive

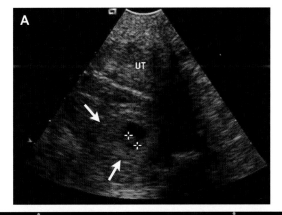

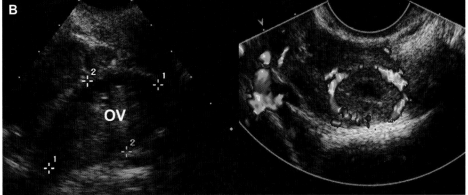

Fig. 13. Ectopic pregnancy. (A) Transvaginal grayscale image demonstrates an extraovarian mass with an embryonic pole (*within calipers*) and a tubal ring sign (*arrows*). (B) Grayscale and color flow Doppler image demonstrates a nonovarian adnexal mass with tubal ring sign and peripheral vascularity (ring of fire). (OV, ovary.)

value). A higher RI suggests the presence of less active trophoblasts and therefore a spontaneous resolution of the ectopic pregnancy. Color Doppler evaluation of the endometrium may help discriminate between ectopic pregnancy and CL. Ectopic pregnancies may show endometrial blood flow, but the RI is usually greater than 0.55, and peak systolic velocity (PSV) is less than 15 cm/s. Demonstration of the presence of trophoblastic tissue in the endometrium, even in the absence of a visible double decidual sac, is suggestive of an intrauterine pregnancy and excludes ectopic pregnancy. Trophoblastic tissue is identified by the detection of low resistance flow in the endometrium with RI less than 0.55 and PSV greater than or equal to 15 cm/s. Screening of the upper abdomen as a routine part of the pelvic examination is mandatory to search for free fluid in Morison's pouch or along the flanks. Echogenic free fluid does not always mean a ruptured ectopic pregnancy, although the greater the quantity of fluid, the greater the chance of finding a ruptured ectopic pregnancy.[3,9,41,42]

The sonographer should remember that in as many as 26% of ectopic pregnancies, no intrauterine pregnancy or adnexal abnormality may be detectable by endovaginal sonography. Clinical correlation and close follow-up are of paramount importance.[43]

Ovarian remnant syndrome

Ovarian remnant syndrome, a complication of oophorectomy, usually occurs in patients who have distorted anatomy resulting from adhesions and endometriosis, making surgical dissection difficult. Residual ovarian tissue under hormone stimulation can become functional and produce pelvic pain, extrinsic compression of the distal ureter, or both. These cysts can be significantly symptomatic despite their small size because of the surrounding adhesions. Seen as complex cystic masses on ultrasonography, the cysts vary from small to relatively large completely cystic or complex masses. A thin rim of ovarian tissue is usually present in the wall of the cyst (**Fig. 14**).[2,3] Laparoscopic ultrasonography has been reported to be a useful tool adjunct in laparoscopic surgery for ovarian remnant syndrome.

Serous cystadenoma

Serous cystadenoma is a very common tumor and may mimic a physiologic cyst or, occasionally, an atypical mature cystic teratoma that lacks the characteristic eccentric mural nodule. Serous cystadenomas arise from the surface epithelium of the ovary and are lined by cuboidal epithelium. They constitute 20% of all benign ovarian neoplasms

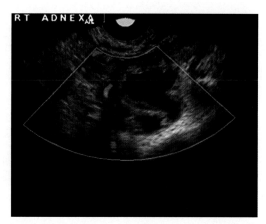

Fig. 14. Ovarian remnant syndrome. Transvaginal color flow Doppler image of right adnexa in a patient with history of oophorectomy demonstrates an ovarian cystic structure with surrounding ovarian tissue secondary to hormone stimulation.

and are usually encountered during the reproductive years. In 7% to 12% of patients, these tumors are bilateral. They are thin walled and uni- or multilocular and range in size from 5 cm to more than 20 cm (**Fig. 15**). They may have fine septa. The inner lining may be smooth or have areas with grossly visible papillary projections. Color Doppler flow studies obtained from the mural nodule may detect low resistance flow pattern.[2–4,44]

Mucinous cystadenoma

Mucinous cystadenoma is a less common, almost always simple or septate, thin-walled multilocular cyst; it may be large (**Fig. 16**). In many of these tumors, the imaging appearance of the individual locules may vary as a result of differences in degree of hemorrhage or protein content, often with internal echoes, with compartments differing in echogenicity. Apart from the septa that divide the cavities of the masses into smaller independent compartments, no solid areas are seen.[2–4] The sonographic detection of variable echogenicity in the contents of an adnexal multilocular cyst strongly suggests a mucinous tumor.[45] The difference in the chemical composition of fluids, rather than the difference in viscosity, is responsible for the different sonographic echogenicities. This sign may not appear in all mucinous tumors, because some may have small differences in the chemical composition of the contents of the different cavities that are undetectable on sonography.[45]

Furthermore, some of the tumors are unilocular and have one type of mucin. Preoperative knowledge of the mucinous nature of the tumor is of crucial importance, because many of these tumors are resected laparoscopically, and spillage may

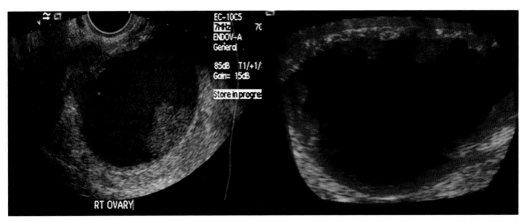

Fig. 15. Surgically confirmed serous cystadenoma. Transvaginal grayscale and corresponding three-dimensional US image of the right ovary demonstrate a complex cystic mass with a mural nodule that shows vascularity on the three-dimensional image.

occur. Spillage should be prevented, to avert both the potential spread of cells (in the event tumor turns out to be malignant) and pseudomyxoma peritoneii.[4]

Fibromas

Fibromas are the most common benign, solid neoplasms of the ovary. Their malignant potential is low, less than 1%. These tumors compose approximately 5% of benign ovarian neoplasms and approximately 20% of all solid tumors of the ovary. Fibromas occur at all ages but are most frequently seen in middle-aged women.

These tumors are commonly misdiagnosed as exophytic fibroids or primary ovarian malignancy. Meigs' syndrome is the association of an ovarian fibroma, ascites, and hydrothorax. Both the ascites and the hydrothorax resolve after removal of the ovarian tumor.[2] The diameter of a fibroma is important clinically, because the incidence of

associated ascites is directly proportional to the size of the tumor. Ascites is present in 10% to 15% of cases of ovarian fibromas greater than 10 cm in diameter. On sonography, fibromas appear as solid, typically hypoechoic masses, but hyperechoic appearance has been reported with attenuation of the acoustic beam. Dense calcifications are known to occur in fibromas, which produce extensive posterior acoustic shadowing. Less than 10% of fibromas have calcifications or small areas of hyaline or cystic degeneration. Bilateral ovarian fibromas are commonly found in women who have rare, genetically transmitted basal cell nevus syndrome.

Malignant Adnexal Masses

Considerable overlap in morphologic characteristics and corresponding imaging features may prevent definitive preoperative characterization of

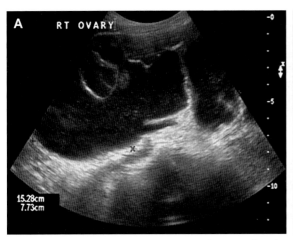
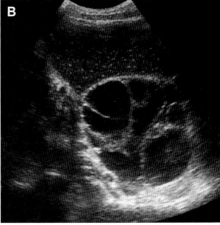

Fig. 16. Surgically confirmed mucinous cystadenoma. (A, B) Grayscale images in two different patients demonstrate multiloculated cystic lesion with septations.

ovarian masses as benign or malignant. Nonetheless, features suggestive of malignant epithelial tumors include a thick, irregular wall; thick septa; papillary projections; and a large soft tissue component with necrosis (**Fig. 17**A, B).[4,44] Calcifications may be present. Solid elements or bilateral tumors[46] suggest malignancy. Ascites form secondary to peritoneal surface implantation (**Fig. 17**C). The tumor may spread to the lymph nodes (ie, the periaortic, mediastinal, supraclavicular, or peritoneum) (**Fig. 17**D).[4,47,48]

Other features supporting malignancy include papillary protrusions greater than 2 to 3 mm in thickness. The mass may show solid cystic components with bizarre, irregular vessels, with changing calibers and occasional vascular "lakes".[49] The presence of a mural nodule is an additional feature supporting the diagnosis of malignancy and may demonstrate internal blood flow on color flow Doppler.

Descriptive morphologic scoring may overcome the subjectivity of interpretation of morphologic characteristics in small masses and, at the same time, may incorporate criteria that prevent simplistic description of a complex mass (**Table 1**).

With a score of 8 or higher, the likely ratio of malignancy was 3.61, sensitivity was 92%, specificity was 76.9%, and positive predictive value was 25.6%. Thus, sonographic morphologic characteristics could represent a cornerstone of the differential diagnosis of small adnexal masses from their first observation.[50] Approximately 90% of primary ovarian cancers are epithelial tumors, arising from the surface epithelium, and the rest arise from stromal and germ cells.[51]

Rulin and Preston[52] analyzed 150 adnexal tumors in women older than 50 and noted 103 benign and 47 malignant tumors. Only one tumor of 32 that was smaller than 5 cm proved to be malignant, whereas 6 of 55 tumors 5 to 10 cm in size and 40 of 63 tumors larger than 10 cm were malignant. The majority of the malignant tumors in this age group were epithelial, and most were greater than 10 cm. The size criteria for malignancy and benignity are based on this study; in a reproductive age group, a tumor smaller than 5 cm is usually benign, and a tumor larger than 5 cm needs further investigation, irrespective of age.

Cystadenocarcinomas

Serous cystadenocarcinoma is the most common malignant tumor seen in all age groups but is rare before age 40. Serous cystadenocarcinomas are bilateral in more than 50% of cases, with peak age of presentation being 70 to 75 years. The typical imaging finding is a large-volume ascites out of proportion to the size of bilateral complex adnexal masses, of irregular shape with polypoid excrescences on the surface. Widespread peritoneal carcinomatosis with omental infiltration by the tumor (so-called "omental caking") is invariably present in cases of serous papillary carcinoma.[51]

Mucinous cystadenocarcinoma neoplasms are seen in older patients with a peak age of 75 to 80 years. These tumors manifest as large, unilateral, multiseptated masses with a variable ratio of solid to cystic components. The presence of an enhancing solid component within a multicystic mass is a strong indicator of malignant cause. These tumors may be associated with pseudomyxoma peritonei (**Fig. 18**). Pseudomyxoma peritonei appear as loculated ascites with mass effect; on sonography they appear as hypoechoic fluid with bright punctate echoes.[4]

Less common varieties of epithelial tumors are endometrioid, clear cell, Brenner, and undifferentiated carcinoma. These cannot be distinguished sonographically. Endometrioid cancers are usually bilateral mixed solid and cystic masses, which may be associated with endometrial hyperplasia and even concomitant endometrial carcinoma. Clear cell tumor manifests at the younger age of 55 to 59 years and has the typical appearance of a solitary complex cystic mass with a vascular solid mural nodule. It is associated with endometriosis and occasionally may arise within endometriomas.[53,54]

Malignant germ cell tumors include dysgerminoma and endodermal sinus tumors. Dysgerminomas are the most common malignant ovarian germ cell tumor, and they are the female equivalent of testicular seminomas.[55] If diagnosed when less than 10 cm in size, they have a good prognosis for a cure with surgical resection. Dysgerminomas are bilateral in 10% to 20% of cases.[56] These are large, predominantly solid masses that are more common in younger women (second and third decades of life) (**Fig. 19**). These tumors manifest as a large, solid, round, oval or lobulated, slightly glistening fibrous capsule and can be as large as 50 cm. Calcification may be present in a speckled pattern. Characteristic imaging findings include multilobulated solid masses with prominent fibrovascular septa.[2,3] Patients treated conservatively should be closely followed with periodic pelvic US or CT imaging evaluations, or both. Occasionally the serum lactic dehydrogenase is elevated as a nonspecific tumor marker.[57]

Ovarian metastasis

Approximately 5% to 30% of malignant ovarian tumors are metastatic in origin. The ovary is a common site of tumor metastasis from the bowel (Krukenberg tumor) (**Fig. 20**), breast, and

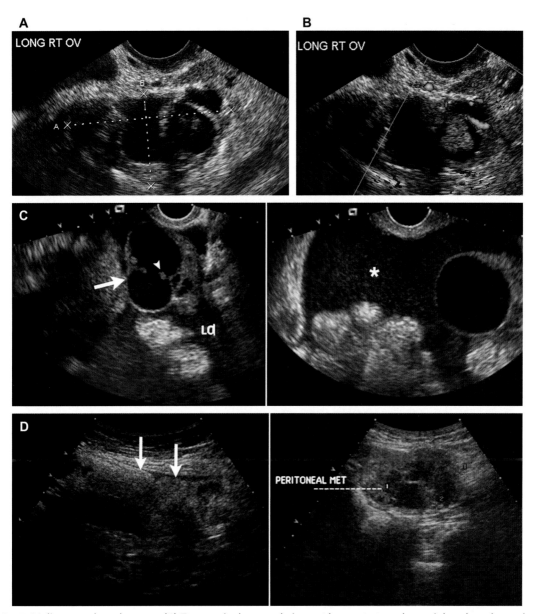

Fig. 17. Malignant adnexal masses. (*A*) Transvaginal grayscale image demonstrates a large right adnexal complex mass with solid and cystic components. (*B*) Corresponding power Doppler image shows increased vascularity within the septae. Spectral Doppler (not shown) confirmed resistive index of less than 0.4, suggesting an ovarian carcinoma. (*C*) Mucinous cystadenocarcinoma. Transvaginal grayscale images of left adnexa demonstrate a cystic left ovarian mass (*arrow*) with mural nodulations (*arrowhead*) and low-level echoes with complex free fluid (*asterisk*), consistent with malignant ascites. (*D*) Omental and peritoneal metastases. Grayscale US of the abdomen demonstrates omental caking (*arrows*) and peritoneal metastasis in a known case of ovarian carcinoma.

endometrium, as well as from melanoma and lymphoma. The most common gastrointestinal tract origin for these tumors is the stomach, and the next most frequent is the large intestine. At least 80% of Krukenberg tumors are bilateral.

Metastatic disease to the ovaries is often associated with ascites. Metastatic lesions are usually solid or have a "moth-eaten" cystic pattern. The

presence of a purely solid tumor indicates a higher probability of metastatic carcinoma than of primary ovarian cancer. However, with the use of grayscale and color Doppler sonography, it is difficult to differentiate primary ovarian carcinomas from metastatic tumors to the ovary.[58] Metastases are frequently bilateral and, at imaging, they range from solid enhancing lesions with different

Table 1
Sonographic morphologic score for adnexal masses

Score	Capsule	Septa	Papillary Excrescences	Echogenicity
1	<3 mm	Absent	Absent	Anechoic
2	>3 mm	Thin (≤3 mm)	...	Low echogenicity/ ground glass
3	...	Thick (>3 mm)	...	...
4	Irregular, solid	...	<3 mm	With solid areas
5	Irregular, not applicable	...	<3 mm	Inhomogeneous, solid

Data from Ferrazzi E, Lissoni AA, Dordoni D, et al. Differentiation of small adnexal masses based on morphologic characteristics of transvaginal sonographic imaging: a multicenter study. J Ultrasound Med 2005;24:1469.

degrees of necrosis to complex cystic masses of various sizes. Although multilocularity at US or MR imaging favors the diagnosis of primary rather than secondary neoplasm, accurate distinction between primary and secondary ovarian tumor is difficult.[59]

Other (Nongynecologic) Pelvic Masses

Not all pelvic masses are gynecologic in origin: others include postoperative masses such as abscesses, hematomas, lymphoceles, urinomas, seromas, and postpartum complications (**Fig. 21**). Bladder flap hematoma is a common complication following cesarean section. It may be diagnosed sonographically as a complex or anechoic mass located adjacent to the scar and between the lower uterine segment and posterior bladder wall; echogenicity varies depending on the degree of organization within the hematoma. Presence of air inside is highly suggestive of an

infected hematoma. Subfascial hematomas are extraperitoneal in location, contained within the prevesical space and caused by disruption of the inferior epigastric vessels or their branches during cesarean section or traumatic vaginal delivery. Sonographically, a complex or cystic mass is seen anterior to the bladder, although CT is the initial imaging modality of choice for postoperative complications such as pelvic abscess and hematoma. Uterine perforation may result from dilatation and curettage or occur after delivery and may appear as an enhancing parametrial fluid collection and discontinuity of the uterus.[3]

Adnexal Masses in Pregnancy

Occasionally an adnexal mass, such as an ovarian or parovarian cyst or a dermoid, may be coexistent in a gravid woman. US features of an ovarian cyst or a dermoid may occasionally be seen with the pregnancy.

Mimics of an Adnexal Mass

Subserosal leiomyomas are the exophytic fibroids that protrude from the outer surface of the uterus. Leiomyomas create a uterine contour abnormality and may mimic an adnexal mass (**Fig. 22**).[41] Leiomyomas usually demonstrate a peripheral rim of vascularity in the pseudocapsule (covering almost three fourths of the circumference); this feature aids in the identification of isoechoic intramural myomas and the diagnosis of subserosal myomas.

The presence of multiple vessels between the uterus and the presumed adnexal mass is called the vascular bridging sign (VBS). Demonstration of a VBS or a vascular pedicle between the uterus and the periuterine mass helps one to differentiate a subserosal leiomyoma from a true adnexal mass.[41] The VBS is secondary to recruitment of multiple vessels feeding the exophytic uterine

Fig. 18. Pseudomyxoma peritoneii. Transabdominal grayscale image of the pelvis in a known case of mucinous cystadenocarcinoma demonstrates presence of loculated ascites. (UB, urinary bladder.)

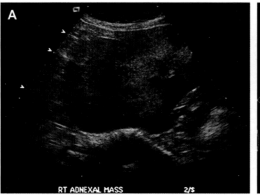 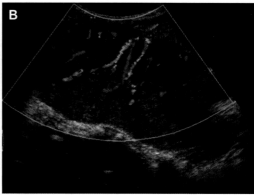

Fig. 19. Dysgerminoma. Grayscale (A) and color flow Doppler (B) images of the right ovary demonstrate a solid mass with increased vascularity.

fibroid and confirms the origin of the vascular blood supply in uterine fibroids from the uterine arteries, implying that the tissue is uterine, not ovarian. Color flow Doppler may also demonstrate a solitary vessel originating from the uterine artery that supplies the subserosal leiomyoma, called the vascular pedicle sign. Demonstration of a common source of blood for the mass and the uterus implies the mass originates in the uterus.[41]

ROLE OF THREE-DIMENSIONAL ULTRASOUND

Three-dimensional ultrasound (3D US) and real-time 3D US are increasingly used to understand spatial relations and vascular morphology. The qualitative and quantitative assessment of sonographic volume data is now possible with the use of several analysis tools, such as multiplanar imaging, surface and volume rendering, and

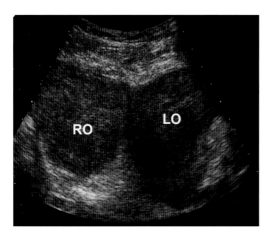

Fig. 20. Krukenberg tumors. Grayscale US image of the pelvis demonstrates bilateral solid ovarian tumors in a known case of stomach cancer. (LO, left ovary; RO, right ovary.)

semiautomated volume calculation using a technique known as virtual organ computer-aided analysis.[60] Virtual organ aided analysis overcomes some limitations of conventional two-dimensional sonography, allowing a more detailed assessment of morphologic features of the object studied, with no restriction on the number and orientation of the scanning planes.[61]

3D US is particularly superior for (1) evaluating for papillary projections, (2) showing characteristics of cystic walls, (3) identifying the extent of capsular infiltration of tumors, and (4) calculating ovarian volume (**Fig. 23A**). 3D US may also be used to assess the location of masses in relation to normal ovarian tissue.[62] It assists in identification of tumor vascularity and tumor angiogenesis, thereby distinguishing between normal and tumor vessels in benign and malignant tumors. Precise evaluation of tumor morphology and vascular patterns is obtained without a significant increase in scan times. The 3D approach allows visualization of multiple overlapping tumor vessels, the vascular network, and the relationship of the mass to the vessels (**Fig. 23B**).[63,64]

ROLE OF COLOR FLOW DOPPLER

Doppler examination should be performed when any abnormality of the ovary is detected. In cysts, color Doppler is helpful in differentiating an echo-free potential cyst from adjacent vascular structures. Using "color as morphology" and understanding its meaning can support a diagnosis or rule out the structure as benign (eg, the lack of color signals in benign cystic teratomas, simple cysts, or endometriomas) or as physiologic (eg, the characteristic "ring of fire" of a CL) (see **Fig. 2B**).

Color may also be used to localize flow for pulsed Doppler, which should be obtained on all

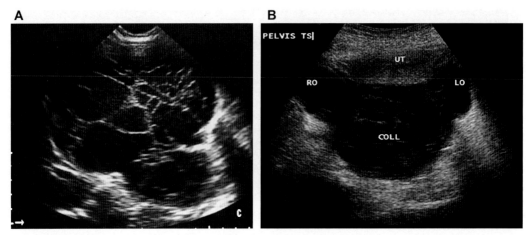

Fig. 21. Nongynecologic pelvic masses. (*A*) Lymphocele. Grayscale image of the pelvis demonstrates a complex septated fluid collection. (*B*) Postpartum collection. Grayscale image of the pelvis demonstrates a complex collection (coll) in the cul-de-sac, consistent with hemorrhage. (LO, left ovary; RO, right ovary; UT, uterus.)

ovarian masses. Pulsed Doppler of the adnexal branch of the uterine artery, the ovarian artery, or intratumoral flow is performed to determine the RI or pulsatility index (PI). Patients who have normal menstrual cycles are best scanned in the first 10 days of the cycle to avoid confusion with normal changes in intraovarian blood flow, because high diastolic flow occurs in luteal phase around the CL.

A debate exists in the literature regarding the value of the RI in distinguishing between benign and malignant adnexal masses. The largest study in the literature uses a cut-off point of greater than 0.4 as a normal RI in a nonfunctioning ovary; others describe a PI of greater than 1 as normal. Intratumoral vessels, low-resistance flow, and absence of a normal diastolic notch in the Doppler waveform are all worrisome signs for malignancy;

however, abnormal waveforms can be seen in inflammatory masses, in metabolically active masses (including ectopic pregnancy), and in corpus luteum. The most significant problem with the use of RI is that it is not a sensitive indicator of malignancy: a low RI is seen in only 25% of malignant lesions.

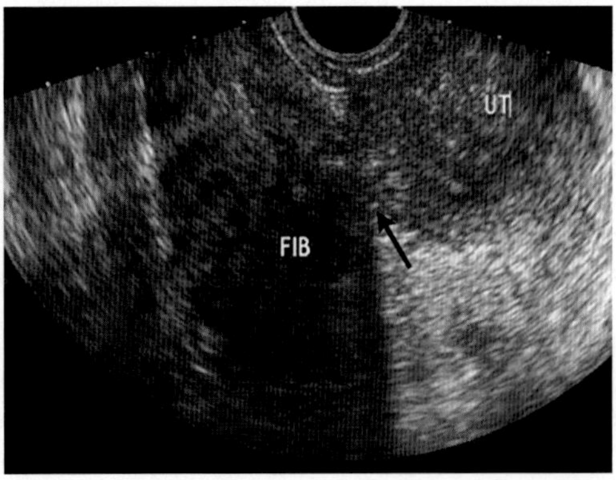

When a large number of erratic vessels with changing calibers, unusual anastomoses, and vascular lakes are seen entering an adnexal structure with centrally located flow within the mass, regardless of the RI, these findings may be considered highly suggestive of malignancy. The same may be said of the detection of blood vessels in papillae. If the papillary protrusions show blood flow, are 3 mm or larger, and are observed to be numerous, these findings should also raise the possibility of malignancy. On color Doppler, tumors tend to have vessels with low impedance, because of the lack of muscular media in the vessel wall and arteriovenous shunts, and the vessels tend to be clustered.[41,65–68]

Power Doppler Imaging

Though spectral Doppler sonography and color Doppler US have been used successfully in the evaluation of adnexal tumor vascularity, they have inherent limitations, such as lack of sensitivity to slow flow, angle dependency, and aliasing. Further contributors to the confusion are a nonuniversal selection of Doppler parameters (RI or PI), the choice of highest, lowest, or mean impedance values, and the selection of vessels for investigations, together with operator variance and system sensitivity.

Fig. 22. Subserosal fibroid. Transvaginal grayscale US image of the pelvis demonstrates a large solid adnexal lesion (Fib) arising from the uterus (*arrow*). (UT, uterus.)

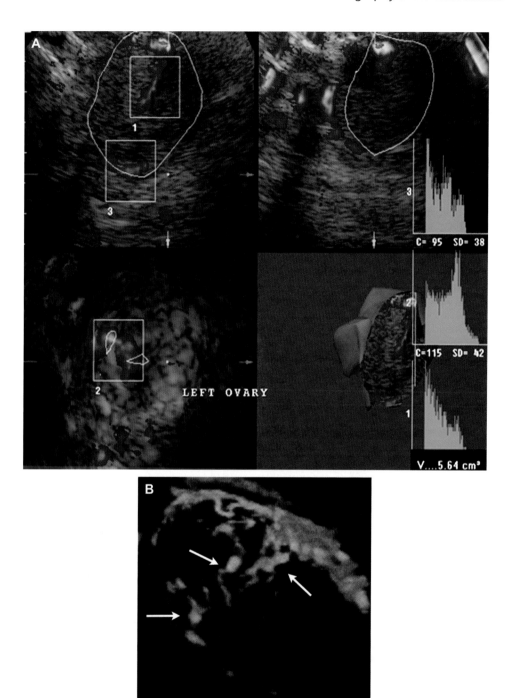

Fig. 23. 3D US. (*A*) Multiple 3D US images of the left ovary being used to calculate the ovarian volume. (*B*) 3D US also helps better to demonstrate the tumor vascularity (*arrows*).

Power Doppler improves visualization of intra-tumoral vascularity, which may aid in detection of malignant adnexal tumors. Tumor vasculature consists of vessels recruited from the pre-existing network of host vasculature and vessels grown from the host vessels under the influence of the angiogenic factors. The organization of this tumor vasculature is completely different from that of the host vasculature, depending on the tumor's type, growth rate, and location. The architecture differs among various tumor types and also between the primary tumor and its transplants. It is possible with three-dimensional power Doppler to visualize vessel continuity more completely (in three orthogonal projections) and to demonstrate vessel branching more clearly (three-dimensional vascular reconstruction) (**Fig. 24**).

Physiologic angiogenesis is seen in folliculogenesis, embryogenesis, and implantation and in some benign neoplasms. The mesovarium vessels entering the hilum can be depicted as extending gradually to the stroma with increasing numbers and branches of fine vessels during the preovulatory phase. After ovulation, luteal cyst formation may be seen. The luteal vessels are usually fewer and seldom have complicated branching patterns or encircle the cyst, in contrast to the findings in malignant neoplasms. In endometriotic cysts, the vessels are usually straight and regularly branching; they generally emerge from a hilar vessel and run along the surface of a tumor.

Tumor vasculature consists of vessels recruited from a pre-existing network of vasculature and vessels produced by neoangiogenesis under the influence of angiogenic factors produced by tumor cells. Within a tumor, variable territories exhibiting one or the other type of vascular pattern may be visualized on color Doppler studies. Tumor vascularity can be differentiated from a normal vascular network by certain characteristics. These include a single elongated and coiled branch, variable incaliber, a nonhierarchical vascular network, absence of normal precapillary architecture with dichotomous branching, absence of decrease in diameter of the higher-order branches, and an incomplete vascular wall with multiple breaks in the endothelial lining and basement membrane. Tumor vessels may also appear tortuous or saccular and may contain tumor cells within these walls. Tumor blood flow is commonly associated with anomalous veno–veno communications and arteriovenous shunts.[49,69]

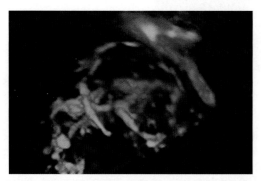

Fig. 24. Three-dimensional power Doppler. Three-dimensional reconstruction of power Doppler image of the ovarian mass demonstrates better vascular continuity and branching.

Quantitated color Doppler sonography

Progressive improvement and development of the technology has led to three-dimensional quantification of blood flow using three-dimensional color histograms that measure the color percentage and flow amplitudes in the region of interest.[70] Quantitative sonographic criteria for tumor vascularity analyzed include the vascularity index (VI) (which quantifies the difference between the total number of pixels and the number of pixels containing no color divided by the total $\times$ 100) and the power-weighted pixel density (PWPD), which weights the strength of the signal divided by the total. With a VI of greater than 2.3, a sensitivity of 75% and specificity of 90% were obtained for malignancies. When this was combined with a PWPD of greater than 4555, sensitivity improved to 88% and specificity improved to 93%—as compared with morphologic analysis, which had a sensitivity of 72% and specificity of 76% for malignancies.[71] Additional indices such as flow index (FI) and vascularization flow index are being studied to provide the insight needed to differentiate benign from malignant adnexal masses. VI and FI are suspected to be reliable predictors for tumoral neoangiogenesis. This method has been found helpful in distinguishing benign from malignant ovarian masses.[70]

Contrast-enhanced, three-dimensional power Doppler

Use of US contrast agents may aid in distinguishing benign from malignant ovarian masses. Intravascular sonographic contrast agents enhance depiction of tumor vessels by providing a stronger Doppler signal.[72] Contrast agents may improve the diagnostic ability of sonography to identify early microvascular changes that are known to be associated with early-stage ovarian cancer, but only a few small published studies have used contrast agents for gynecologic purposes. Use of a contrast agent makes it possible to gain a more accurate map of the vascular anatomy by enhancing the signal strength from power Doppler sonography, increasing the number of large vessels and allowing recruitment of small vessels.[73–75] Tumors have a longer wash-out time, perhaps a reflection of the presence of tumor angiogenesis.

The vascular distribution in adnexal masses may be classified into three patterns using three-dimensional power Doppler US: pattern 0, no signal pattern (no detectable vessels); pattern 1, peripheral pattern (blood vessels are peripheral and surround the lesion); pattern 2, penetrating pattern (blood vessels arise outside the lesion and course toward its center); and pattern 3, mixed penetrating and peripheral pattern. The pattern of irregularly branching penetrating vessels in an adnexal mass, with or without contrast enhancement, is an important factor in predicting the likelihood of malignancy. The use of a US contrast agent with three-dimensional power Doppler sonography increases the diagnostic efficiency of nonenhanced three-dimensional power Doppler sonography from 86.7% to 95.6%.[69]

SUMMARY

Transabdominal sonography combined with high-frequency endovaginal US is considered the community standard for the performance of pelvic US for evaluation of an adnexal mass.[36,46,76] Subjective evaluation of ovarian masses based on pattern recognition can achieve a sensitivity of 88% to 100% and specificity of 62% to 96%. Addition of color and power Doppler to grayscale imaging for pelvic mass evaluation increases the specificity

in the range of 82% to 97% and increases the positive predictive value to 63% to 91%[4], aiding in subsequent evaluation and management.[5] Pelvic sonography can confidently diagnose most of the benign adnexal masses and helps with triage of patients for surgical management in collaboration with tumor markers. The key points of adnexal masses are presented in **Box 1**.[77]

ACKNOWLEDGMENTS

The authors are extremely thankful to Vikram Dogra, MD, and Shweta Bhatt, MD, for their editorial advice and assistance in preparation of this manuscript. They would also like to express their sincere thanks to Dr. Ashok Khurana, MD, for his contribution.

REFERENCES

1. Timor-Tritsch IE, Goldstein SR. The complexity of a "complex mass" and the simplicity of a "simple cyst." J Ultrasound Med 2005;24:255–8.
2. Dill-Macky MJ, Atri M. Ovarian sonography. 4th edition. Philadelphia: W.B.Saunders; 2000.
3. Salem S, Wilson SR. Gynecologic ultrasound. 3rd edition. St. Louis (MO): Mosby; 2005.
4. Arger PH. Asymptomatic palpable adnexal masses. New York: Thieme; 2000.
5. Valentin L. Use of morphology to characterize and manage common adnexal masses. Best Pract Res Clin Obstet Gynaecol 2004;18:71–89.
6. de Kroon CD, van der Sandt HA, van Houwelingen JC, et al. Sonographic assessment of non-malignant ovarian cysts: does sonohistology exist? Hum Reprod 2004;19:2138–43.
7. Webb EM, Green GE, Scoutt LM. Adnexal mass with pelvic pain. Radiol Clin North Am 2004;42:329–48.
8. Durfee SM, Frates MC. Sonographic spectrum of the corpus luteum in early pregnancy: gray-scale, color, and pulsed Doppler appearance. J Clin Ultrasound 1999;27:55–9.
9. Pellerito JS. Acute pelvic pain. New York: Thieme; 2000.
10. Nemoto Y, Ishihara K, Sekiya T, et al. Ultrasonographic and clinical appearance of hemorrhagic ovarian cyst diagnosed by transvaginal scan. J Nippon Med Sch 2003;70:243–9.
11. Swire MN, Castro-Aragon I, Levine D. Various sonographic appearances of the hemorrhagic corpus luteum cyst. Ultrasound Q 2004;20:45–58.
12. Bhatt S, Kocakoc E, Dogra VS. Endometriosis: sonographic spectrum. Ultrasound Q 2006;22:273–80.
13. Jain KA. Sonographic spectrum of hemorrhagic ovarian cysts. J Ultrasound Med 2002;21:879–86.
14. Okai T, Kobayashi K, Ryo E, et al. Transvaginal sonographic appearance of hemorrhagic functional

ovarian cysts and their spontaneous regression. Int J Gynaecol Obstet 1994;44:47–52.

15. Montz FJ, Schlaerth JB, Morrow CP. The natural history of theca lutein cysts. Obstet Gynecol 1988;72: 247–51.

16. Patel MD, Feldstein VA, Chen DC, et al. Endometriomas: diagnostic performance of US. Radiology 1999;210:739–45.

17. Alcazar JL, Laparte C, Jurado M, et al. The role of transvaginal ultrasonography combined with color velocity imaging and pulsed Doppler in the diagnosis of endometrioma. Fertil Steril 1997;67:487–91.

18. Ghezzi F, Raio L, Cromi A, et al. "Kissing ovaries": a sonographic sign of moderate to severe endometriosis. Fertil Steril 2005;83:143–7.

19. Woodward PJ, Sohaey R, Mezzetti TP Jr. Endometriosis: radiologic–pathologic correlation. Radiographics 2001;21:193–216 [questionnaire: 288–94].

20. Tessler FN, Perrella RR, Fleischer AC, et al. Endovaginal sonographic diagnosis of dilated fallopian tubes. AJR Am J Roentgenol 1989;153:523–5.

21. Timor-Tritsch IE, Lerner JP, Monteagudo A, et al. Transvaginal sonographic markers of tubal inflammatory disease. Ultrasound Obstet Gynecol 1998;12:56–66.

22. Patel MD. Practical approach to the adnexal mass. Ultrasound Clinics 2006;1:335–56.

23. Horrow MM. Ultrasound of pelvic inflammatory disease. Ultrasound Q 2004;20:171–9.

24. Outwater EK, Siegelman ES, Hunt JL. Ovarian teratomas: tumor types and imaging characteristics. Radiographics 2001;21:475–90.

25. Mais V, Guerriero S, Ajossa S, et al. Transvaginal ultrasonography in the diagnosis of cystic teratoma. Obstet Gynecol 1995;85:48–52.

26. Tongsong T, Wanapirak C, Khunamornpong S, et al. Numerous intracystic floating balls as a sonographic feature of benign cystic teratoma: report of 5 cases. J Ultrasound Med 2006;25:1587–91.

27. Rha SE, Byun JY, Jung SE, et al. CT and MR imaging features of adnexal torsion. Radiographics 2002;22: 283–94.

28. Sohaey R, Gardner TL, Woodward PJ, et al. Sonographic diagnosis of peritoneal inclusion cysts. J Ultrasound Med 1995;14:913–7.

29. Jain KA. Imaging of peritoneal inclusion cysts. AJR Am J Roentgenol 2000;174:1559–63.

30. Dolz M, Osborne NG, Blanes J, et al. Polycystic ovarian syndrome: assessment with color Doppler angiography and three-dimensional ultrasonography. J Ultrasound Med 1999;18:303–13.

31. Ginsburg J, Havard CW. Polycystic ovary syndrome. Br Med J 1976;2:737–40.

32. Hann LE, Hall DA, McArdle CR, et al. Polycystic ovarian disease: sonographic spectrum. Radiology 1984;150:531–4.

33. Parisi L, Tramonti M, Derchi LE, et al. Polycystic ovarian disease: ultrasonic evaluation and correlations with clinical and hormonal data. J Clin Ultrasound 1984;12:21–6.

34. Yeh HC, Futterweit W, Thornton JC. Polycystic ovarian disease: US features in 104 patients. Radiology 1987;163:111–6.

35. Adams J, Franks S, Polson DW, et al. Multifollicular ovaries: clinical and endocrine features and response to pulsatile gonadotropin releasing hormone. Lancet 1985;2:1375–9.

36. Fox R, Corrigan E, Thomas PA, et al. The diagnosis of polycystic ovaries in women with oligo-amenorrhoea: predictive power of endocrine tests. Clin Endocrinol (Oxf) 1991;34:127–31.

37. Pache TD, Wladimiroff JW, Hop WC, et al. How to discriminate between normal and polycystic ovaries: transvaginal US study. Radiology 1992;183:421–3.

38. Wolf SI, Gosink BB, Feldesman MR, et al. Prevalence of simple adnexal cysts in postmenopausal women. Radiology 1991;180:65–71.

39. Khurana A, Jha U. Ultrasound for pelvic assessment in menopausal women. New Delhi (India): Jaypee brothers; 2004.

40. Brown DL, Doubilet PM. Transvaginal sonography for diagnosing ectopic pregnancy: positivity criteria and performance characteristics. J Ultrasound Med 1994;13:259–66.

41. Bhatt S, Dogra V. Doppler imaging of the uterus and adnexae. Ultrasound Clinics 2006;1:201–21.

42. Levine D. Ectopic pregnancy. 4th edition. Philadelpia: W.B.Saunders; 2000.

43. Russell SA, Filly RA, Damato N. Sonographic diagnosis of ectopic pregnancy with endovaginal probes: what really has changed? J Ultrasound Med 1993;12:145–51.

44. Fried AM. Family history of ovarian carcinoma. New York: Thieme; 2000.

45. Caspi B, Hagay Z, Appelman Z. Variable echogenicity as a sonographic sign in the preoperative diagnosis of ovarian mucinous tumors. J Ultrasound Med 2006;25:1583–5.

46. Lee SI. Radiological reasoning: imaging characterization of bilateral adnexal masses. AJR Am J Roentgenol 2006;187:S460–6.

47. Jeong YY, Outwater EK, Kang HK. Imaging evaluation of ovarian masses. Radiographics 2000;20:1445–70.

48. Woodward PJ, Hosseinzadeh K, Saenger JS. From the archives of the AFIP: radiologic staging of ovarian carcinoma with pathologic correlation. Radiographics 2004;24:225–46.

49. Kurjak A, Kupesic S, Breyer B. The assessment of ovarian tumor angiogenesis by three dimensional power Doppler. New York: Parthenon publishing; 2000.

50. Ferrazzi E, Lissoni AA, Dordoni D, et al. Differentiation of small adnexal masses based on morphologic characteristics of transvaginal sonographic imaging: a multicenter study. J Ultrasound Med 2005; 24:1467–73 [quiz: 1475–6].

51. Mironov S, Akin O, Pandit-Taskar N, et al. Ovarian cancer. Radiol Clin North Am 2007;45:149–66.

52. Rulin MC, Preston AL. Adnexal masses in postmenopausal women. Obstet Gynecol 1987;70:578–81.

53. Green GE, Mortele KJ, Glickman JN, et al. Brenner tumors of the ovary: sonographic and computed tomographic imaging features. J Ultrasound Med 2006;25:1245–51 [quiz: 1252–4].

54. Wu TT, Coakley FV, Qayyum A, et al. Magnetic resonance imaging of ovarian cancer arising in endometriomas. J Comput Assist Tomogr 2004;28:836–8.

55. Stepanian M, Cohn DE. Gynecologic malignancies in adolescents. Adolesc Med Clin 2004;15:549–68.

56. Chen VW, Ruiz B, Killeen JL, et al. Pathology and classification of ovarian tumors. Cancer 2003;97:2631–42.

57. Schwartz PE, Morris JM. Serum lactic dehydrogenase: a tumor marker for dysgerminoma. Obstet Gynecol 1988;72:511–5.

58. Alcazar JL, Galan MJ, Ceamanos C, et al. Transvaginal gray scale and color Doppler sonography in primary ovarian cancer and metastatic tumors to the ovary. J Ultrasound Med 2003;22:243–7.

59. Brown DL, Zou KH, Tempany CM, et al. Primary versus secondary ovarian malignancy: imaging findings of adnexal masses in the Radiology Diagnostic Oncology Group Study. Radiology 2001;219:213–8.

60. Benacerraf BR, Benson CB, Abuhamad AZ, et al. Three- and 4-dimensional ultrasound in obstetrics and gynecology: Proceedings of the American Institute of Ultrasound in Medicine Consensus Conference. J Ultrasound Med 2005;24:1587–97.

61. Alcazar JL, Galan MJ, Garcia-Manero M, et al. Three-dimensional sonographic morphologic assessment in complex adnexal masses: preliminary experience. J Ultrasound Med 2003;22:249–54.

62. Pretorius DH, Nelson TR, Lev-Toaff AS. Three dimensional ultrasound in obstetrics and gynecology. 4th edition. Philadelphia: W.B.Saunders; 2000.

63. Downey DB, Fenster A. Vascular imaging with a three-dimensional power Doppler system. AJR Am J Roentgenol 1995;165:665–8.

64. Kurjak A, Kupesic S, Sparac V, et al. Three-dimensional ultrasonographic and power Doppler characterization of ovarian lesions. Ultrasound Obstet Gynecol 2000;16:365–71.

65. Alcazar JL, Ruiz-Perez ML, Errasti T. Transvaginal color Doppler sonography in adnexal masses: which parameter performs best? Ultrasound Obstet Gynecol 1996;8:114–9.

66. Timor-Tritsch LE, Lerner JP, Monteagudo A, et al. Transvaginal ultrasonographic characterization of ovarian masses by means of color flow–directed Doppler measurements and a morphologic scoring system. Am J Obstet Gynecol 1993;168:909–13.

67. Valentin L, Sladkevicius P, Marsal K. Limited contribution of Doppler velocimetry to the differential diagnosis of extrauterine pelvic tumors. Obstet Gynecol 1994;83:425–33.

68. Zanetta G, Vergani P, Lissoni A. Color Doppler ultrasound in the preoperative assessment of adnexal masses. Acta Obstet Gynecol Scand 1994;73: 637–41.

69. Kupesic S, Kurjak A. Contrast-enhanced, three-dimensional power Doppler sonography for differentiation of adnexal masses. Obstet Gynecol 2000;96: 452–8.

70. Pairleitner H. Three dimensional color histogram using three dimensional power Doppler. New York: Parthenon publishing; 2000.

71. Wilson WD, Valet AS, Andreotti RF, et al. Sonographic quantification of ovarian tumor vascularity. J Ultrasound Med 2006;25:1577–81.

72. Deng CX. Contrast agents for ultrasound imaging. In: Dogra V, Rubens DJ, editors. Ultrasound secrets. Philadelphia: Hanley & Belfus; 2004. p. 23–9.

73. Abramowicz JS. Ultrasonographic contrast media: has the time come in obstetrics and gynecology? J Ultrasound Med 2005;24:517–31.

74. Orden MR, Jurvelin JS, Kirkinen PP. Kinetics of a US contrast agent in benign and malignant adnexal tumors. Radiology 2003;226:405–10.

75. Marret H, Tranquart F, Sauget S, et al. Sonographic diagnosis of ovarian tumors: pre-operative Doppler evaluation. J Radiol 2003;84:1725–31.

76. Fogata ML, Jain KA. Degenerating cystic uterine fibroid mimics an ovarian cyst in a pregnant patient. J Ultrasound Med 2006;25:671–4.

77. Pelvic and lower abdominal masses. In: Stenchever MS, Droegemueller W, Herbst A, et al, editors. Comprehensive gynecology. 4th edition. Saint Loius: Mosby, Inc.; 2001. p. 70–2.

Postmenopausal Bleeding

Ismail Mihmanli, MD*, Fatih Kantarci, MD

KEYWORDS

- Ultrasonography • Postmenopausal bleeding
- Endometiral cancer • Polyps • Tamoxifen

Postmenopausal bleeding (PMB) may be defined as recurrent vaginal bleeding in a menopausal woman at least 1 year after cessation of cycles. It may also occur as unscheduled bleeding in women on hormone replacement therapy. There is a broad spectrum of diseases that may cause PMB (**Box 1**). Of them probably the most important differential diagnosis includes the malignancies of the female genital tract, which may present with irregular or excessive vaginal bleeding. Endometrial cancer may be found in 10% of women with unexpected PMB, depending on age and risk factors.[1,2] Bleeding occurs in 80% to 90% of women with endometrial cancer, and the prevalence of endometrial cancer among women who present with PMB has been reported to range from 1% to 60%.[3] All women who present with postmenopausal bleeding should be evaluated for potential malignancy such as endometrial cancer, premalignant atypical endometrial hyperplasia, or cervical cancer. Vaginal bleeding, however, may be attributable to many causes other than cancer and is a common problem in postmenopausal women, occurring in as many as 1 per 10 women older than 55 years.[4,5]

Evaluation of vaginal bleeding in a postmenopausal woman may be accomplished by dilatation of the cervix and curettage of the endometrium (D&C), outpatient endometrial biopsy, ultrasonography (**Table 1**), and outpatient hysteroscopy. Despite the accepted advantages of outpatient investigation, there remains uncertainty regarding the best sequence or combination of these tests in PMB. A cost-effectiveness study showed that women presenting for the first time with PMB should undergo initial evaluation with transvaginal ultrasonography (TVUS) or endometrial biopsy (EMB).[6] The choice between initial testing with EMB or TVUS will depend on the patient's age and preference, disease prevalence, and the availability of high-quality US scanner, which may use a threshold of 4 or 5 mm to define abnormal results. However, the actual sensitivity rate for endometrial biopsy remains unknown. Studies have shown that TVUS has similar (or slightly lower) false-negative rates for cancer detection when compared with endometrial tissue sampling.[5] Because up to 90% of PMB has a benign cause, questions have arisen regarding the appropriateness of performing biopsies on all patients with bleeding. Subsequently, imaging techniques, mainly TVUS, have been explored to help determine which patients are at higher risk of malignancy and would benefit from tissue sampling and which are more likely to have a benign cause for the bleeding.

TECHNIQUE

Ultrasonography must be performed according to the following standards to exclude malignancy. It should be performed preferentially by transvaginal route with a 5- to 10-MHz transducer and an empty bladder. Transverse/coronal (short-axis) and longitudinal/sagittal (long-axis) images of the uterus should be obtained in each examination and should also include images of the cervix and fundal and cornual portions of the endometrium. The uterus and adnexa should be imaged in each examination, although it is understood that the ovaries may not be visible in all postmenopausal women. Endometrial thickness should

Department of Radiology, Istanbul University, Cerrahpasa Medical Faculty, 34098-Istanbul, Turkey
* Corresponding author.
E-mail address: mihmanli@yahoo.com (I. Mihmanli).

Ultrasound Clin 3 (2008) 391–397
doi:10.1016/j.cult.2008.08.001

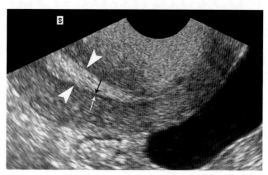

Fig. 1. Longitudinal ultrasound image. The endometrial thickness measurement should include the thickest portion (*between white arrowheads*) of the endometrium. The inner myometrium (*between arrows*) should not be included in the measurement.

be measured on a sagittal (long-axis) image of the uterus, and the measurement should be performed on the thickest portion of the endometrium (**Fig. 1**). The endometrial thickness should be reported as the "double-thickness" measurement. A small amount of fluid will be found in the endometrial canal of some postmenopausal women without abnormalities. This fluid should not be included in the endometrial measurement (**Fig. 2**). In these cases, the reported endometrial thickness should be the sum of the thickness of the two endometrial layers, excluding the fluid.

Saline infusion sonohysterography (SHG) can be performed in selected patients. Although a detailed description of the technique is mentioned in another article in this issue, it is worth briefly mentioning the technique of SHG here. It should be performed after routine TVUS examination with

a vaginal speculum positioned in the vagina while the woman is in the dorsal lithotomy position. A plastic pediatric feeding catheter is adjusted to the size of the uterus and filled with sterile saline solution. The catheter is then inserted into the cavity up to the fundus with the help of sterile forceps. The speculum is carefully removed, and the vaginal probe is then inserted in the fornix of the vagina from behind the catheter. After that, 5 to 40 mL of sterile saline is injected to expand the uterine cavity, and transverse and longitudinal images of the distended cavity are obtained by TVUS. Five to 10 mL of saline solution usually proved to be sufficient to distend the cavity. In the SHG procedure,

Table 1
Sonographic features of common conditions that cause postmenopausal bleeding

Causes of Bleeding	Sonographic Feature
Atrophic endometrium	• Endometrial thickness <4 mm on transvaginal examination
Tamoxifen therapy	• Hyperechoic or heterogeneous solid tissue with multiple cystic spaces
Endometrial carcinoma	• Distended or fluid-filled uterine cavity, enlarged or lobular uterus, prominent echogenicity of the endometrium (nonspecific signs) • Homogeneously thickened endometrium (>5 mm) without a focal abnormality • Focal endometrial abnormality • Indistinct endometrial margins
Uterine leiomyoma	• Area of increased echogenicity bulging into the endometrial cavity with echogenicity similar to that of the myometrium • Broad-based, hypoechoic, well-defined, solid masses with shadowing
Endometrial hyperplasia	• Endometrial thickness >10 mm on transvaginal examination • Asymmetric thickening with surface irregularity
Endometrial polyps	• Focal mass within the endometrial canal or nonspecific endometrial thickening • Sonohysterography: well-defined, homogeneous, polypoid lesion that is isoechoic to the endometrium

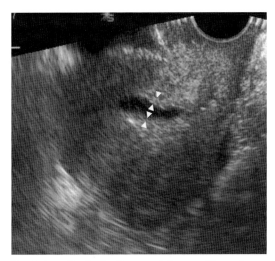

Fig. 2. Longitudinal ultrasound image. There is an-echoic fluid within the endometrial cavity. The thickness measurement should be reported as the sum of the two layers of the endometrium (*between white arrowheads*).

the endometrial cavity is observed as anechogenic because it is full of saline; a symmetric and flat endometrial shape is considered to be normal (**Fig. 3**).

NORMAL APPEARANCE OF ENDOMETRIUM IN POSTMENOPAUSAL WOMEN

The peri- and postmenopausal endometrial thickness is normally less than that in the pre-menopausal patient. During menopause, the endometrium primarily consists of a thin basalis

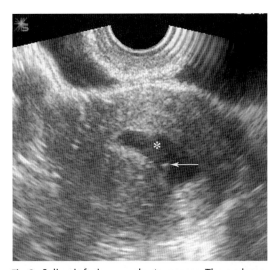

Fig. 3. Saline infusion sonohysterogram. The endometrial cavity is filled with sterile saline (*asterisk*) and appears anechoic. Note the catheter (*white arrow*) within the endometrial cavity.

layer, and the measurement of the endometrial echo complex represents the apposition of the two basal layers. Atrophic changes occurring in menopause demonstrate an endometrial echo complex less than 5-mm thick composed of sclerotic blood vessels and glands.[7] Normally 5- to 7-mm thick, the postmenopausal endometrial stripe may be nonpathologically increased to 8- to 10-mm thick if the patient is using hormone replacement therapy.[4,8–10] Although rare, small echogenic foci may be seen within the endometrium. Endometrial microcalcifications are the most common cause of the echogenic foci seen on US examinations. They appear to be stable or to regress with time and are associated mostly with benign endometrial conditions. Hormone use, intrauterine device use, interventions such as D&Cs, cesarean deliveries, therapeutic or spontaneous abortions, and infections are the most common conditions associated with endometrial microcalcifications.[11]

ATROPHIC ENDOMETRIUM

In patients with postmenopausal bleeding, if the endometrium measures less than 4 mm on transvaginal US scans (**Fig. 4**), endometrial atrophy is assumed to be the cause of the postmenopausal bleeding. In the absence of estrogen after menopause, the functional layer is inactive and atrophies, which leaves only the shallow basalis layer. However, if the patient continues to have abnormal bleeding, continued follow-up with transvaginal US or routine endometrial biopsy should be performed. The overall risk of carcinoma or atypical hyperplasia in this population is low. In women with postmenopausal bleeding, endometrial thickness 4 mm or less decreases the odds of malignancy 10-fold.[5]

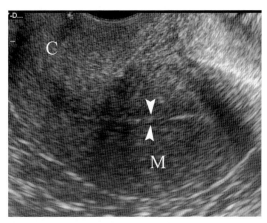

Fig. 4. Longitudinal ultrasound image. The endometrial echo complex is seen as thin echogenic line (*between white arrowheads*). C, cervix; M, myometrium.

ENDOMETRIAL HYPERPLASIA

Endometrial hyperplasia is a histologic diagnosis characterized by overgrowth of glands with or without stromal proliferation and is believed to result from prolonged estrogen stimulation of the endometrium. Up to one third of endometrial carcinoma is believed to be preceded by hyperplasia.[12] A definitive diagnosis can be made only with biopsy, and imaging cannot reliably allow differentiation between hyperplasia and carcinoma. The US appearance can simulate that of normal thickening during the secretory phase, sessile polyps, submucosal fibroids, cancer, and adherent blood clots, yielding potentially false-positive results.[13] Endometrial hyperplasia is considered whenever the endometrium appears to exceed 10 mm in thickness in postmenopausal patients,[14] although it can be reliably excluded in these patients only when the endometrium measures less than 6 mm. Endometrial hyperplasia may also cause asymmetric thickening with surface irregularity, an appearance that is suspicious for carcinoma. Because endometrial hyperplasia has a nonspecific appearance, any focal abnormality should lead to biopsy if there is a clinical suspicion for malignancy. At sonohysterography, endometrial hyperplasia typically appears as a diffuse thickening of the echogenic endometrial stripe without focal abnormality; however, focal endometrial hyperplasia can occasionally be seen. The latter form of hyperplasia is more difficult to differentiate from endometrial polyps at SHG because the characteristics of the focal endometrial thickening occurring in both conditions overlap.

ENDOMETRIAL POLYPS

An endometrial polyp is a circumscribed overgrowth of the endometrial mucosa and occasional stromal tissue that protrudes into the uterine cavity on a fibrovascular stalk. The polyps can be singular or multifocal. They are most often benign and, in postmenopausal women, can show the typical atrophic and cystic change of the rest of the endometrium on pathologic evaluation. Adenocarcinomas may grow in a polypoid fashion, however, or can arise within a polyp. A polyp that appears in a symptomatic postmenopausal woman warrants biopsy. Although endometrial polyps may be visualized on TVUS as nonspecific endometrial thickening, they are frequently identified as focal masses within the endometrial canal (**Fig. 5**). Polyps are best seen on SHG and the typical appearance of an endometrial polyp is a well-defined, homogeneous, polypoid lesion that is isoechoic to the endometrium (**Fig. 6**) with

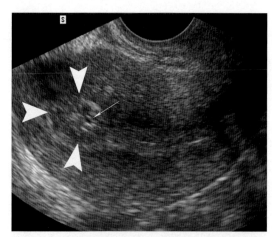

Fig. 5. Longitudinal ultrasound image. The endometrium is thickened at the fundal region with a heterogeneous hypoechoic lesion (*white arrowheads*) within the cavity. Note also small cystic degenerations (*thin white arrow*) inside of the polyp.

preservation of the endometrial-myometrial interface.[15] Color Doppler US may be used to image vessels within the stalk. On Doppler US, a single-vessel pattern, representing the vascularized polyp's pedicle, was described for the diagnosis of endometrial polyps.[16] Fibroids or foci of endometrial hyperplasia or carcinoma can mimic a sessile polyp, and foci of atypical hyperplasia are sometimes found within polyps.[17]

UTERINE LEIOMYOMAS

Uterine leiomyomas, frequently referred to as fibroids, are common benign neoplastic growths

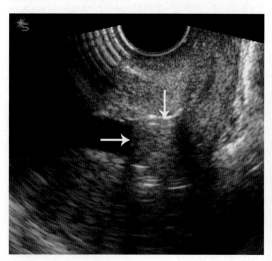

Fig. 6. Sonohysterogram shows a well-marginated polypoid mass (*white arrows*) projecting into the endometrial cavity.

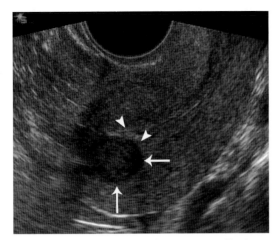

Fig. 7. Longitudinal ultrasound image. A small submucous well-defined fibroid (*white arrows*) is seen displacing the endometrium (*white arrow heads*).

of smooth muscle cells within the myometrium. Although their size and frequency increases with age, they may grow until menopause and then involute and are a cause of premenopausal uterine bleeding. In postmenopausal women, these benign tumors usually regress, and malignant degeneration is rare. In the presence of continued hormonal stimulation, however, they may continue to be symptomatic. Submucosal leiomyomas are the most likely to cause vaginal bleeding and may appear as an area of increased echogenicity bulging into the endometrial cavity with echogenicity similar to that of the myometrium (**Fig. 7**). At SHG, submucosal fibroids are typically broad-based, hypoechoic, well-defined, solid masses with shadowing.

ENDOMETRIAL CANCER

Endometrial cancer is the most common of the gynecologic malignancies. It also has the best prognosis. Presentation is usually painless vaginal bleeding in a postmenopausal woman and detection is usually done by a combination of US and pipette biopsy. Endometrial atrophy is the commonest cause of postmenopausal bleeding. Risk factors include increased age and prolonged exposure to unopposed estrogens. The endometrial thickness of postmenopausal women should not exceed 5 mm. A 4-mm threshold negligibly alters the sensitivity for cancer detection but substantially decreases the specificity (more false-positive results).[5] This threshold does not apply to an asymptomatic woman with an incidentally observed endometrium of greater than 5 mm. Among these postmenopausal women, a normal maximal endometrial thickness measurement has not yet been established. Women with thickened endometrial linings on US examination merit biopsy. Even in the presence of vaginal bleeding, however, endometrial thickness of less than 5 mm on US excludes endometrial cancer. Women taking hormone replacement therapy or tamoxifen may have slightly thicker endometrial linings (8 mm); however, 5 mm should still be taken as the upper limit of normal because these women are at a higher risk for endometrial carcinoma.[8,18,19] US signs of endometrial carcinoma include a distended or fluid-filled uterine cavity, an enlarged or lobular uterus, and prominent echogenicity of the endometrium. These signs are nonspecific and can be seen in endometrial hyperplasia as well as polyps, leading to biopsy of almost any irregularity in the setting of

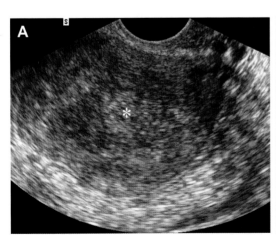
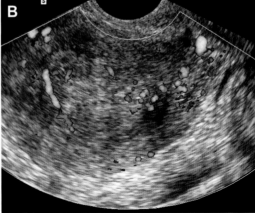

Fig. 8. Transverse ultrasound images. (*A*) Gray-scale US demonstrate diffuse endometrial thickening (*asterisk*) with indistinct margins. (*B*) Power Doppler US shows multiple vessels within the myometrium and endometrial mass lesion.

postmenopausal bleeding. However, polypoid tumors tend to cause more diffuse and irregular thickening than a polyp and more heterogeneity than endometrial hyperplasia.[20] The Society of Radiologists in Ultrasound Consensus Conference stated that there can be four different sonographic patterns in the diagnosis of endometrial cancer.[21] One pattern is a homogeneously thickened endometrium more than 5 mm without a focal abnormality. The endometrium should be visualized in its entirety. In the second pattern, the endometrium is not visualized in its entirety. This observation, found in approximately 5% to 10% of patients,[22–24] is not specific for disease, but an incompletely visualized endometrium cannot be interpreted as benign or reassuring. Because this appearance can occur with endometrial cancer, a nondiagnostic sonogram should lead to the further evaluation, similar to positive sonographic findings. A third pattern is focal endometrial abnormality, and the final pattern is indistinct endometrial margins (**Fig. 8**).

Transvaginal color and power Doppler sonography was introduced in an attempt to refine the diagnosis of endometrial disease when ultrasound is used. Many articles analyzing the role of pulsed and color Doppler sonography have reported conflicting results.[25–27] It has been suggested that low-impedance blood flow at Doppler US can be associated with malignancy.[28] Increased focal vascularity may be seen at color Doppler US in both benign and malignant diseases of the endometrium. Significant overlap in Doppler indices (ie, peak systolic velocity, resistive index, pulsatility index) in benign and malignant endometrial processes reduces the value of Doppler US in characterizing endometrial masses. Color and power Doppler US may occasionally aid in determining the presence and extent of tumor invasion and ensuring that biopsies are directed toward regions with increased blood flow.

TAMOXIFEN THERAPY

Women who are on tamoxifen therapy for breast cancer present with added difficulties in the assessment of PMB. Tamoxifen is a competitive inhibitor of the estrogen receptor and is well documented to increase the risk of endometrial hyperplasia and carcinoma.[29] The detection of endometrial abnormalities in the earliest stage in this population is essential. Any patient who develops bleeding while taking tamoxifen requires evaluation. Tamoxifen therapy may alter the sonographic appearance of the endometrium. Tamoxifen-induced changes include endometrial hyperplasia and endometrial polyps, which appear

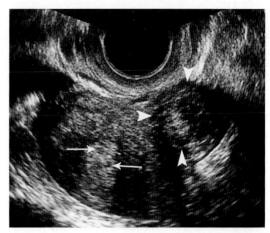

Fig. 9. Transverse ultrasound image. Postmenopausal woman with breast carcinoma on tamoxifen therapy. The endometrium appears echogenic with cystic structures (*white arrows*) inside. There is also subserous myoma (*white arrowheads*).

as hyperechoic or heterogeneous solid tissue with multiple cystic spaces (**Fig. 9**). An endometrial thickness of 6 mm in a postmenopausal woman on tamoxifen is considered normal. A high false-positive rate from screening of asymptomatic women on tamoxifen was observed because a physiologic thickened myometrium might be mistaken for endometrial hypertrophy by transvaginal sonography.[30]

SUMMARY

Transvaginal sonography can be used safely as the initial diagnostic test to evaluate the endometrial lining in a woman with PMB. If the sonogram shows a normal-appearing endometrium with a double-thickness measurement of less than 5 mm, the test can be considered negative for endometrial cancer. In women in whom office EMB is nondiagnostic, a thin endometrium can be used safely to obviate additional attempts at tissue sampling. SHG has a high diagnostic effectiveness and is a useful tool especially in anatomic lesions such as polyps and fibroids in the cavity.

REFERENCES

1. Lidor A, Ismajovich B, Confino E, et al. Histopathological findings in 226 women with post-menopausal uterine bleeding. Acta Obstet Gynecol Scand 1986; 65:41–3.
2. Reid PC, Brown VA, Fothergill DJ. Outpatient investigation of postmenopausal bleeding. Br J Obstet Gynaecol 1993;100:498.

3. Hawwa ZM, Nahhas WA, Copenhaver EH. Postmenopausal bleeding. Lahey Clin Found Bull 1970;19:61–70.

4. Karlsson B, Granberg S, Wikland M, et al. Transvaginal ultrasonography of the endometrium in women with postmenopausal bleeding—a Nordic multicenter study. Am J Obstet Gynecol 1995;172:1488–94.

5. Smith-Bindman R, Kerlikowske K, Feldstein VA, et al. Endovaginal ultrasound to exclude endometrial cancer and other endometrial abnormalities. JAMA 1998;280:1510–7.

6. Clark TJ, Barton PM, Coomarasamy A, et al. Investigating postmenopausal bleeding for endometrial cancer: cost-effectiveness of initial diagnostic strategies. BJOG 2006;113:502–10.

7. Bradley LD, Falcone T, Magen AB. Radiographic imaging techniques for the diagnosis of abnormal uterine bleeding. Obstet Gynecol Clin North Am 2000;27:245–76.

8. Levine D, Gosink BB, Johnson LA. Change in endometrial thickness in postmenopausal women undergoing hormone replacement therapy. Radiology 1995;197:603–8.

9. Lin MC, Gosink BB, Wolf SI, et al. Endometrial thickness after menopause: effect of hormone replacement. Radiology 1991;180:427–32.

10. Nasri MN, Shepherd JH, Setchell ME, et al. The role of vaginal scan in measurement of endometrial thickness in postmenopausal women. Br J Obstet Gynaecol 1991;98:470–5.

11. Duffield C, Gerscovich EO, Gillen MA, et al. Endometrial and endocervical micro echogenic foci: sonographic appearance with clinical and histologic correlation. J Ultrasound Med 2005;24:583–90.

12. Kurman RJ, Kaminski P, Norris HJ. The behavior of endometrial hyperplasia: a long-term study of "untreated" hyperplasia in 170 patients. Cancer 1985;56:403–12.

13. Sohaey R, Woodward P. Sonohysterography: technique, endometrial findings, and clinical applications. Semin Ultrasound CT MR 1999;20:250–8.

14. Malpani A, Singer J, Wolverson MK, et al. Endometrial hyperplasia: value of endometrial thickness in ultrasonographic diagnosis and clinical significance. J Clin Ultrasound 1990;18:173–7.

15. Davis PC, O'Neill MJ, Yoder IC, et al. Sonohysterographic findings of endometrial and subendometrial conditions. Radiographics 2002;22:803–16.

16. Alcázar JL, Ajossa S, Floris S, et al. Reproducibility of endometrial vascular patterns in endometrial disease as assessed by transvaginal power Doppler sonography in women with postmenopausal bleeding. J Ultrasound Med 2006;25:159–63.

17. Dubinsky TJ, Parvey HR, Gormaz G, et al. Transvaginal hysterosonography in the evaluation of small endoluminal masses. J Ultrasound Med 1995;14:1–6.

18. Hann LE, Giess CS, Bach AM, et al. Endometrial thickness in tamoxifen-treated patients: correlation with clinical and pathologic findings. AJR Am J Roentgenol 1997;168:657–61.

19. Ascher SM, Johnson JC, Barnes WA, et al. MR imaging appearance of the uterus in postmenopausal women receiving tamoxifen therapy for breast cancer: histopathologic correlation. Radiology 1996;200:105–10.

20. Fleischer AC. Transvaginal sonography of endometrial disorders: an overview. Radiographics 1998;18:923–30.

21. Goldstein RB, Bree RL, Benson CB, et al. Evaluation of the woman with postmenopausal bleeding: Society of Radiologists in Ultrasound-sponsored Consensus Conference Statement. J Ultrasound Med 2001;20:1025–36.

22. Karlsson B, Granberg S, Wikland M, et al. Endovaginal scanning of the endometrium compared to cytology and histology in women with postmenopausal bleeding. Gynecol Oncol 1993;50:173–8.

23. Garuti G, Sambruni I, Cellani F, et al. Hysteroscopy and transvaginal ultrasonography in postmenopausal women with uterine bleeding. Int J Gynaecol Obstet 1999;65:25–33.

24. Neele SJ, Marchien Van Baal W, Van Der Mooren MJ, et al. Ultrasound assessment of the endometrium in healthy, asymptomatic early postmenopausal women: saline infusion sonohysterography versus transvaginal ultrasound. Ultrasound Obstet Gynecol 2000;16:254–9.

25. Sladkevicius P, Valentin L, Marsal K. Endometrial thickness and Doppler velocimetry of the uterine arteries as discriminators of endometrial status in women with postmenopausal bleeding: a comparative study. Am J Obstet Gynecol 1994;171:722–8.

26. Aleem F, Predanic M, Calame R, et al. Transvaginal color and pulsed Doppler sonography of the endometrium: a possible role in reducing the number of dilatation and curettage procedures. J Ultrasound Med 1995;14:139–45.

27. Sheth S, Hamper UM, McCollum ME, et al. Endometrial blood flow analysis in postmenopausal women: can it help differentiate benign from malignant causes of endometrial thickening? Radiology 1995;195:661–5.

28. Bourne TH, Campbell S, Steer CV, et al. Detection of endometrial cancer by transvaginal ultrasonography with color flow imaging and blood flow analysis: a preliminary report. Gynecol Oncol 1991;40:253–9.

29. Fornander T, Cedarmark B, Mattson A, et al. Adjuvant tamoxifen in early breast cancer: occurrence of new primary cancers. Lancet 1989;1:117–20.

30. Liedman R, Lindahl B, Andolf E, et al. Disaccordance between estimation of endometrial thickness as measured by transvaginal ultrasound compared with hysteroscopy and directed biopsy in breast cancer patients treated with tamoxifen. Anticancer Res 2000;20:4889–91.

Endometriosis

Ercan Kocakoc, MD[a], Shweta Bhatt, MD[b], Vikram S. Dogra, MD[b],*

KEYWORDS

- Endometriosis • Ultrasound • Ovary

Ultrasound often is used as primary imaging technique in the evaluation of female pelvic pathologies. Pelvic pain and infertility are the most common problems affecting women of reproductive age. Endometriosis is a common gynecologic disorder affecting about 10% of women of reproductive age, and it is an important cause of infertility and pelvic pain. A recent study showed that 20% of women undergoing laparoscopic evaluation for infertility and 24% of women who had pelvic pain had endometriosis.[1] It is estimated that 30% to 50% of women who have endometriosis are infertile.[1,2] Fifty percent to 80% of patients who have endometriosis are symptomatic; symptoms can include the triad of dysmenorrhea, dyspareunia, and infertility.[3] Because endometriosis is a relatively common condition that may mimic other, more serious adnexal masses, it is important to recognize its diverse sonographic findings and to be able to recommend appropriate follow-up when necessary. The aim of this article is to familiarize the reader with the sonographic appearances of endometriosis. The pathophysiology, clinical presentations, and treatment of endometriosis are briefly reviewed also.

DEFINITION AND EPIDEMIOLOGY

Endometriosis is defined as the presence of functional endometrial glands and stroma outside the uterine cavity and the myometrium.[2,4,5] It may occur as endometrial implants along various peritoneal surfaces, or it may occur as a focal cystic collection, referred to as an "endometrioma." The terms "endometriosis" and "endometrioma" frequently are used interchangeably, but endometriomas are only a part of the disease process, which also may include endometriotic implants and adhesions.[2] Endometriosis is a common disease affecting millions of women worldwide.[6] The mean age at diagnosis is 25 to 29 years, but it is often greater in women who present with infertility rather than pelvic pain.[7] Adolescent endometriosis also occurs; the average age at presentation is about 16 years.[8] About 50% of women under 20 years of age who have chronic pelvic pain or dyspareunia have the disease.[2,8] Obstructive Müllerian duct anomalies of the cervix or vagina account for most cases of endometriosis in girls under the age of 17 years.[2,9] Approximately 5% of cases of endometriosis are seen in postmenopausal women; it has been suggested that exogenous estrogen replacement therapy plays a role in these cases.[2,10]

The prevalence varies according to geography and race; it is highest in Japanese women.[11] Endometriosis has been reported in 4.1% of asymptomatic women undergoing laparoscopy for tubal ligation,[1] but a high prevalence also has been reported in women being evaluated for infertility (20%–80%) and in women who have pelvic pain (15%–70%).[11] Estimates of prevalence vary widely (depending on the study population), but up to 15% of women may be affected.[6] There is a 10-fold increase in prevalence in women who have an affected first-degree relative.[12] A menstrual characteristic associated with endometriosis is a menstrual cycle length of less than 28 days.[13]

PATHOPHYSIOLOGY

The pathophysiology and causes of endometriosis are complex, and its origin remains controversial. Several theories to explain the evolution of endometriosis have been suggested, but no single theory explains all types and sites of endometriosis.[11]

a Department of Radiology, Faculty of Medicine, Firat University, 23119, Elazig, Turkey
b Department of Radiology, University of Rochester School of Medicine and Dentistry, Rochester, NY 14642, USA
* Corresponding author.
E-mail address: vikram_dogra@urmc.rochester.edu (V.S. Dogra).

Ultrasound Clin 3 (2008) 399–414
doi:10.1016/j.cult.2008.07.001
1556-858X/08/$ – see front matter © 2008 Published by Elsevier Inc.

Retrograde Menstruation and Implantation Theory (Sampson's Theory)

Since the 1920s, Sampson's theory has been the most widely accepted theory of development of endometriosis[11,14] This theory proposes the shedding of the endometrial glands during retrograde menstruation through the fallopian tubes to the peritoneum.[12] Sampson observed menstrual blood exiting tubal ostea in menstruating women during surgery. Reflux menstruation occurs in about 80% of women, but most of these women do not have endometriosis.[11] Impairment of the immune response to remove peritoneal menstrual debris has been suggested as an additional factor.[2] Women who have endometriosis have been found to have abnormalities of T-cell–mediated cytotoxicity, natural killer–cell activity, B-cell function, and complement deposition.[2,15]

Coelomic Metaplasia (Meyer's Theory) and the Induction Theory

The coelomic metaplasia theory postulates a conversion of peritoneal epithelium into endometrial epithelium by unknown mechanism.[12] Rising estrogen production induces these mature peritoneal or ovarian surface cells to undergo metaplasia into endometrial cells at puberty.[11] This theory has not been supported by scientific evidence. Metaplasia is an age-related process, which occurs with increasing frequency with advancing age; endometriosis occurs mostly during the reproductive years.[11]

Vascular and Lymphatic Metastasis (Halban's Theory)

Halban's theory suggests that distant endometriosis occurs via vascular or lymphatic spread of viable endometrial cells. This theory explains the rare endometriotic lesions occurring in extrapelvic sites (eg, brain, lung) but does not explain the more common pelvic lesions.[11]

Recent awareness of the increasing incidence of endometriosis in asymptomatic women has led to the hypothesis that endometrial implants are in fact physiologic and do not in themselves indicate a disease process until recurrent bleeding occurs in these implants, causing symptoms and progressive disease.[16]

Although the origin of endometriosis remains an enigma, most investigators agree that the persistence and progression of ectopic endometrial tissue is intimately connected with a local pelvic inflammatory process.[17,18] Thus, it has been demonstrated that women who have endometriosis have higher concentrations of proinflammatory cytokines in their peritoneal fluid than women who do not have endometriosis.[17,19]

PATHOLOGIC FEATURES AND PRESENTATIONS OF ENDOMETRIOSIS

Pathologic diagnosis requires microscopic demonstration of endometrial tissue, preferably both glands and stroma.[20] The most common site of involvement in endometriosis is the ovary, followed by the uterine ligaments (posterior broad ligament, uterosacral ligament), pelvic cul-de-sac, pelvic peritoneum, fallopian tubes, rectosigmoid, and bladder.[21,22]

The typical findings of endometriosis are endometriotic implants, endometriomas, and adhesions. Implants may measure a few millimeters to a few centimeters and may be superficial or deep. Endometriotic implants may change in appearance during the menstrual cycle, becoming more swollen and congested during menses and developing internal hemorrhage. Endometriotic implants are more noticeable during the late secretory phase of the menstrual cycle. Mature endometriotic foci initiate an inflammatory response, with areas of hemorrhage, fibrosis, and adhesion formation.[4,23]

Superficial Endometriosis

The term "superficial endometriosis" usually is used synonymously with "peritoneal endometriosis," although one of the most common superficial locations is the ovarian surface.[24]

Endometriotic Cysts (Endometriomas)

Endometriomas usually occur within the ovaries and result from repeated cyclic hemorrhage. More than 90% of endometriomas are pseudocysts formed by invagination of the ovarian cortex, which is sealed off by adhesions. Endometriomas may replace normal ovarian tissue completely. Cyst walls usually are thick and fibrotic and frequently have dense fibrous adhesions and areas of discoloration. Cyst content generally is composed of thick, dark, degenerate blood products, an appearance that has been called "chocolate cyst" (**Fig. 1**).[2] The preferential site for endometriomas is the left ovary.[25] Endometriomas are bilateral in approximately 50% of the cases and may be large, although they rarely exceed 15 cm in diameter.[23] Large lesions and lesions with wall nodularity should be considered suspicious and sampled to rule out malignancy. Endometriosis usually regresses substantially after menopause.[21]

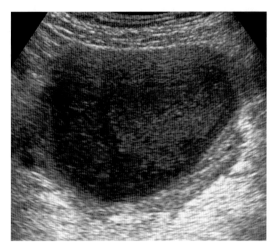

Fig. 1. Recurrent endometrioma ("chocolate cyst"). The patient had history of surgery for endometrioma 10 years ago. Transverse sonography of the pelvis shows an inhomogeneous, isoechoic-to-hypoechoic, large mass with a thick wall consistent with different-stage blood products.

Deep Pelvic Endometriosis

Deep pelvic or infiltrating endometriosis is defined by endometriotic lesions involving smooth muscle of uterosacral ligaments or the walls of hollow viscera typically associated with marked proliferation of smooth muscle cells and fibrosis.[25] Deep endometriotic lesions are located most often in the pouch of Douglas, the rectovaginal septum, and the uterosacral ligaments and more rarely in the vesico-uterine space and are responsible for pelvic pain. The intensity of pelvic pain is proportional to the depth of the lesions.[26] The bowel is a frequent location for deep retroperitoneal endometriosis.[26,27] Intestinal involvement occurs in 3% to 37% of the estimated 15% of menstruating women in whom endometriosis develops.[26,27] Intestinal lesions predominantly affect serosa, muscularis propria, and submucosa; the mucosa is rarely involved.[26,27]

Adhesions

Extensive adhesions can distort the normal pelvic anatomy and obliterate the pouch of Douglas.[23] Adhesions cannot be diagnosed easily by ultrasound. A recent study, however, suggested that the appearance described as "kissing ovaries" on ultrasound is associated with endometriosis, especially in patients who have adhesions and extensive pelvic extension of the endometriosis with dense adhesions, and is a marker for the most severe form of the disease (**Fig. 2**).[17] The diagnosis of kissing ovaries is made when the ovaries

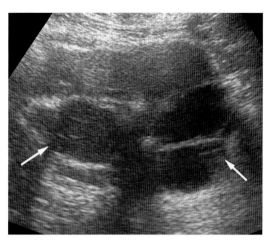

Fig. 2. Transverse sonogram reveals "kissing ovaries" (*arrow*) behind the uterus. Low-level echoes are seen in the right ovary, and the left ovary has a thick, multiseptated appearance. These lesions were confirmed surgically as different presentations of endometriomas.

are joined behind the uterus in the cul-de-sac and are not separable by pushing the transvaginal probe or by manipulating the uterus transabdominally.[17]

Extraperitoneal Endometriosis

Extraperitoneal sites include the lungs, pleura, skin, skeletal muscle, and central nervous system.[16,28] The extrapelvic implantation of endometrial tissue has been described in virtually every organ.[22,28]

CLINICAL PRESENTATION

Endometriosis usually presents with painful symptoms, such as menstrual period pain (dysmenorrhea), pain on intercourse (dyspareunia), or nonmenstrual pelvic pain.[6] It also may be found incidentally at surgery (eg, for sterilization) or during investigation for infertility.[6]

Endometriosis is classified according to the revised American Fertility Society classification (rAFS)[29] as minimal, mild, moderate, or severe endometriosis based on laparoscopic appearance. The severity of patients' symptoms do no correlate with rAFS stage.[30] All classification systems for endometriosis are subjective and correlate poorly with pain symptoms but may be of value in infertility prognosis and management.[26,27,31]

DIAGNOSIS
Endometrial and Serum Markers

Detection of aromatase P-450 protein in endometrial biopsy samples strongly correlates with the presence of endometriosis or adenomyosis, with a sensitivity of 91% and specificity of 100%.[32] Elevated levels of carcinoembryonic antigen 125 (CA125) in the peripheral blood have been detected in women with endometriosis,[20] but the CA125 level has low sensitivity and specificity as a screening test, and its usefulness for therapeutic monitoring is uncertain.[20] Harada and colleagues[33] suggested that CA19-9 is a useful marker for the severity of the disease. A recent study suggested that serum levels of interleukin-6, with a cut-off value of 2 pg/mL, could discriminate between patients with and without endometriosis.[34]

Physical Examination

Pelvic tenderness, a fixed retroverted uterus, tender uterosacral ligaments or enlarged ovaries on physical examination are suggestive of endometriosis.[31] If deeply infiltrating nodules are found on the uterosacral ligaments or in the pouch of the Douglas, and/or visible lesions are seen in the vagina or on the cervix, the diagnosis is more certain.[31]

Laparoscopy

Laparoscopy is the reference standard for the diagnosis of endometriosis.[5] It is the most sensitive examination, because only laparoscopy can identify superficial peritoneal implants.[21] Laparoscopy, however, is an invasive technique and should be performed only after imaging techniques prove insufficient for confident diagnosis.

The diagnosis is made by noting the presence of typical lesions consisting of blue-brown or black nodules or the presence of stains on peritoneal surfaces of the ovaries, fallopian tubes, uterus, uterosacral ligaments, and bowel. These lesions are the result of tissue bleeding and retention of blood pigments.[20] There are atypical lesions that lack the typical brown or black appearance but show histologic evidence of endometrial glands and stroma; these lesions require biopsy for confirmation of diagnosis.[20] Scarring of the peritoneum around endometrial implants is a typical finding. In addition to encapsulating an isolated implant, the scar may deform the surrounding peritoneum or result in development of adhesions.[35] Clinicians use the term "frozen pelvis" to indicate masking of the retro-uterine excavation by a block of tissue with lesions of the posterior pelvis, such as torus uteri, uterosacral ligaments, and vaginal and rectal wall invasion associated with extensive adnexal adhesions.[30] Severe dysmenorrhea and noncyclic chronic pelvic pain are suggestive of a frozen pelvis.[30]

Histology and Nonvisible Lesions

Positive histology confirms the diagnosis of endometriosis; negative histology does not exclude it. Visual inspection generally is adequate, but histologic confirmation of at least one lesion is ideal; histology is obtained to demonstrate endometriosis and to exclude rare instances of malignancy.[31]

Investigators have performed histologic studies to demonstrate nonvisible lesions.[36] Biopsies were taken from visually normal peritoneum from two groups of women without and with endometriosis who underwent laparoscopy for infertility.[36] In this study endometriotic tissue was present in 6% of infertile women who did not have endometriosis and in 13% of infertile women who had endometriosis.[36]

Ultrasonography (Gray-Scale and Doppler Ultrasound)

Ultrasound often is the initial screening test for endometrioma and for follow-up of known endometrioma. A transabdominal and endocavitary sonographic approach is required for the assessment of endometriosis.[4] Endorectal ultrasound can demonstrate the uterus and ovaries; in addition, it is useful for the evaluation of the rectal wall, the parametrium, and cul-de-sac. Guerriero and colleagues[37] reported the sensitivity and specificity of endovaginal ultrasound to be 83% and 89%, respectively, in differentiating endometriomas from other ovarian cysts.

Transvaginal ultrasound is more sensitive than transabdominal ultrasound for detecting endometriomas; however, small implants and adhesions usually are not detectable with transvaginal ultrasound.[4]

Endometrioma is the only form of endometriosis readily diagnosed with transvaginal ultrasound. Both transabdominal and transvaginal ultrasound should be performed to evaluate patients suspected of having endometriosis. Ovarian cystic lesions should be evaluated for internal echogenicity, wall morphology, and effects on surrounding organs. Transvaginal ultrasound is a useful tool for detecting and monitoring ovarian endometriomas that are larger than 10 mm in diameter.[38] Rectal ultrasound may offer a promising technique for assessing difficult forms (rectovaginal space and uterosacral ligament) of endometriosis.[6] In cases of severe endometriosis, 82% agreement has been reported between ultrasound and intraoperative evaluation.[39]

The sonographic features of endometriomas are varied and range from anechoic cysts to cysts with diffuse low-level echoes to solid-appearing masses. Fluid–fluid or debris–fluid levels can be seen also. They may be unilocular or multilocular with thin or thick septations (**Figs. 3** and **4**).[40]

The morphology of the endometriotic implant is heterogeneous. Nodular and/or cystic lesions differing in number and size or with a plaquelike appearance can be found. Endometriotic foci usually are nodular (secondary to reactive fibrosis) and hypoechoic in appearance or cystic (secondary to hemorrhage) (**Fig. 5**). Recently, Clarke and colleagues[41] proposed that acoustic streaming is useful for differentiating endometriomas from other benign cystic lesions. Acoustic streaming is defined as the bulk movement of fluid as the result of a sound field caused by energy transfer from a ultrasound wave to a fluid.[41] In essence, the energy of the ultrasound beam pushes the fluid in the direction of insonation (away from the transducer). Movements of fluid particles away from the transducer and in the direction of the beam result in acoustic streaming. This study demonstrates that, whereas 63% of cysts show acoustic streaming, endometriomas do not. Therefore, acoustic streaming seems to be a promising differentiating criterion for adnexal cystic lesions.

Adhesions usually are not visualized by any imaging modality unless fluid is present at both sides. In this circumstance, adhesions appear as an abnormal line or sheet within the pelvis.[30] Organ mobility may be checked using transvaginal probe during transvaginal ultrasound examination.[2] Pelvic adhesions are demonstrated in 81% of women who have surgically confirmed adhesions at three-dimensional ultrasound.[42] Angulation of bowel

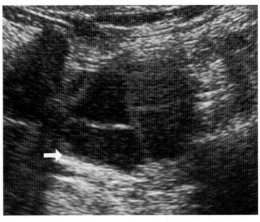

Fig. 4. Thick, multiseptated appearance of endometrioma. Transverse sonogram reveals multiseptated left ovarian endometrioma with low-level echoes (*arrow*) on some part of lesion.

loops, loculated fluid collections, and a hydrosalpinx are additional findings of adhesions.[43]

Doppler waveform analysis is not helpful in differentiating endometriomas from other masses: low-resistance waveforms resembling malignancy can be encountered in endometriomas.[25] Typical endometriomas do not show internal vascularity but may have perilesional flow (**Fig. 6**).[44] Alcazar and colleagues[44] found that the performance of ultrasound in the diagnosis of endometriomas was not improved by adding color flow Doppler. Similarly, Guerriero and colleagues[45] reported that endometriomas are associated with "poor" blood supply, whereas approximately 20% of non-endometriotic cysts are characterized by "rich"

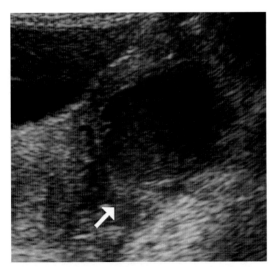

Fig. 3. Transverse sonogram shows a cystic left adnexal mass (*arrow*) with diffuse low-level echoes consistent with classic endometrioma.

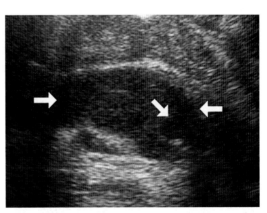

Fig. 5. Transverse gray-scale sonogram of the right ovary shows an enlarged cystic mass with diffuse low-level echoes (*horizontal arrows*) containing hypoechoic nodular area (*oblique arrow*) representing endometriotic foci.

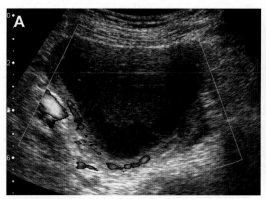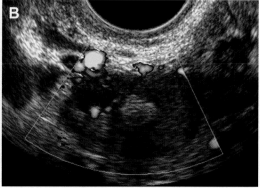

Fig. 6. (*A*) Transverse color Doppler sonogram shows peripheral vascularity of large endometrioma (same case as in **Fig.1**). (*B*) Transverse power Doppler sonogram shows moderate level peripheral and some internal vascularity of right ovarian endometrioma.

vascularization or the presence of arterial flow in the papillary structures or echogenic areas of the cyst.

Endometrioma with low-level echoes
Ninety-five percent of endometriomas have the appearance of an adnexal mass with diffuse low-level echoes (**Fig. 7**).[46] An adnexal mass with low-level internal echoes and absence of neoplastic features is 64 times more likely to be an endometrioma if multilocularity is present than if it is not and is 32 times more likely to be an endometrioma if hyperechoic wall foci are present (**Fig. 8**). The classic endometrioma has been described as a homogeneous hypoechoic focal lesion within the ovary with diffuse low-level internal echoes.[46] Absence of acoustic streaming also may support the diagnosis of endometriomas.[41]

Endometrioma as a simple cyst
Rarely, endometriomas may be anechoic, mimicking a functional ovarian cyst. At times, endometriosis may appear as a simple cyst with a thin wall and an anechoic center and exhibit enhanced through-transmission. The anechoic pattern has been found in 5.5% of the patients who have endometriomas.[47]

Endometrioma as a solid mass
Endometrioma also can appear as a complex solid adnexal mass, thereby raising the concern for malignancy (**Fig. 9**). Five percent to 10% of American women suspected of having an adnexal mass undergo surgery; only 13% to 21% of these masses prove to be malignant.[48] Unlike malignant lesions, endometriomas do not have internal vascularity. A typical vascular pattern for the endometrioma is described as a "pericystic flow" at the level of

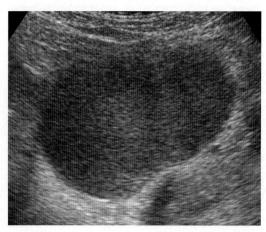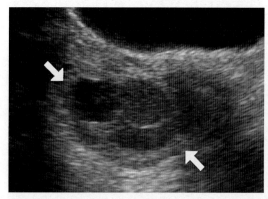

Fig. 7. Transverse gray-scale sonogram reveals a large cystic right adnexal mass with diffuse low-level echoes consistent with classic endometrioma.

Fig. 8. A slightly oblique transverse sonogram shows a right adnexal multiseptated cystic mass (*arrows*) containing low-level echoes confirmed surgically as endometrioma.

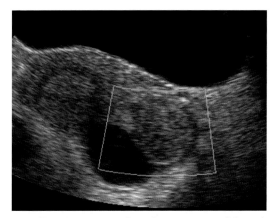

Fig. 9. Transverse power Doppler sonogram of the pelvic region shows a well-defined complex cystic mass containing a hyperechoic avascular solid component. The patient underwent MR examination that confirmed this mass as a typical left ovarian endometrioma.

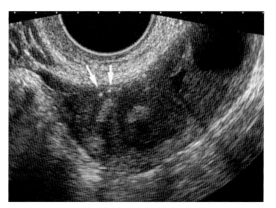

Fig. 10. Longitudinal transvaginal sonogram shows a large heterogeneous lesion with peripheral hyperechoic foci (*arrows*) confirmed as right ovarian endometrioma. Two other echogenic foci inside the lesion are consistent with old blood products.

the ovarian hilus.[44] The solid pattern has been found in 4.9% of endometriomas.[47]

Endometrioma with hyperechoic wall foci

The presence of hyperechoic wall foci (punctate peripheral echogenic foci) on sonographic examination is very specific for endometriomas. Echogenic wall foci differ from wall nodularity and are an important discriminating feature. In a study conducted by Patel and colleagues,[46] hyperechoic wall foci were found in 35% of the endometriomas studied but in only 6% of the masses that were not endometriomas. This echogenic wall focus was found to be the highest single predictor of endometrioma and is thought to represent cholesterol deposits (**Fig. 10**).[4,46] Brown and colleagues,[49] however, suggested that small echogenic foci in the ovaries are caused most commonly by hemosiderin or calcification and are not a reliable indicator of endometriosis. The authors' have not seen solid echogenic foci lining the endometrial wall but have observed cystic structures with hyperechoic margins lining the wall of the endometrioma.

Endometrioma with calcium deposits

As many as 10% of endometriomas may contain focal calcium deposits, a finding typically associated with mature cystic teratoma (**Fig. 11**).[50] The absence of other typical ultrasound features of teratoma is useful for the diagnosis of endometriosis.

CT

CT has been considered to lack specificity in the diagnosis of endometriosis,[51] but a CT study has shown that 15% of endometrial cysts (9 of 62

lesions) had a hyperdense round or crescent-shaped focus measuring 2 to 15 mm. This focus was located close to inner border of the cyst in eight cases and in the central part of the cyst in one case.[51] This hyperdense area, which seems to represent a blood clot on CT scans, was shown as a nonspecific hyperechogenic focus on sonograms in four or five cases and as a hypointense signal on T1 and/or T2-weighted MR images in four of five cases.[51]

MR Imaging

In the detection of ovarian endometrial cysts, MR imaging has demonstrated sensitivity of 90% and specificity of 98%.[52] A large endometrioma (> 1 cm in diameter) appears as a homogenously hyperintense mass on T1-weighted MR images and

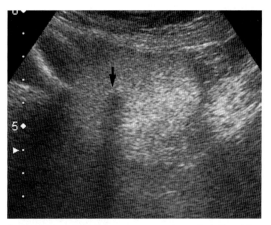

Fig. 11. Transverse sonogram reveals well-defined hyperechoic lesion containing central calcification with acoustic shadowing (*arrow*). This lesion considered an endometrioma and was confirmed on surgery.

as a mass with low signal intensity with areas of high signal intensity on T2-weighted images (**Fig. 12**).[20] The shading sign is a distinguishing feature of endometriotic cysts (endometriomas) in MR images and has been described as T2 shortening in an adnexal cyst that is hyperintense on T1-weighed images.[53] The hypointensity initially was described as either focal or diffuse; however, the most common manifestation is complete loss of signal intensity or dependent layering with a hypointense fluid level.[2,52,53] Endometriotic cysts are highly viscous and have a high concentration of protein and iron from recurrent hemorrhage. All these components can shorten T2 imaging and may contribute to the loss of signal intensity, which is described as "shading."[2,53] Marked loss of signal intensity on T2-weighted images usually is not seen with hemorrhagic cysts, because they do not bleed repeatedly.[53] Sometimes endometriosis may appear as multiple, homogeneously hyperintense cysts on T1-weighted MR images regardless of the signal intensity on T2-weighted images.[20]

After contrast administration, most endometriosis remain bright, and contrast enhancement of peritoneal surfaces subjacent to endometrial implants is seen frequently.[2,20]

Differential Diagnosis of Endometriosis

Teratomas usually present as echogenic masses with acoustic shadowing caused by hairballs or calcifications such as teeth or bone in the Rokitanski protuberance.[54] Layered lines and dots, fat–fluid level, and isolated bright echogenic foci with acoustic shadowing are characteristic sonographic findings of dermoid cysts (**Fig. 13**).[30,50,54]

Corpus luteum and hemorrhagic follicular cysts disappear or decrease in size at short-term follow-up.[4,30] Classically, fresh blood is anechoic. In subacute stages, when the clot forms, it becomes echogenic.[4] Hemorrhagic cyst wall is thin (2–3 mm), well defined, and regular. A fine reticular pattern or fishnet weave, which actually is caused by the retracting blood clot, is the most common

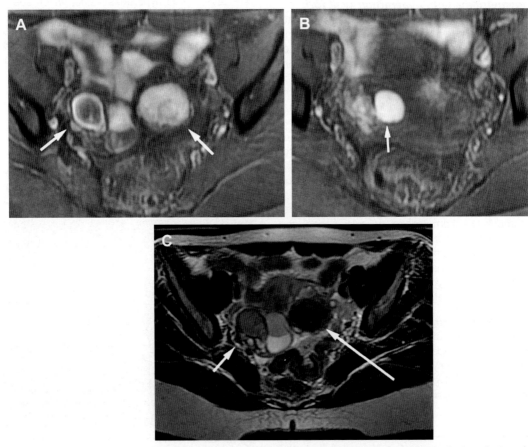

Fig. 12. (*A, B*) Transverse fat-saturated T1-weighted MR images reveal bilateral adnexal hyperintense lesions (*arrows*). (*C*) Transverse T2-weighted MR image shows complete loss of signal intensity in the left ovary (*long arrow*) and decreased signal intensity ("shading") in the right ovary (*short arrow*).

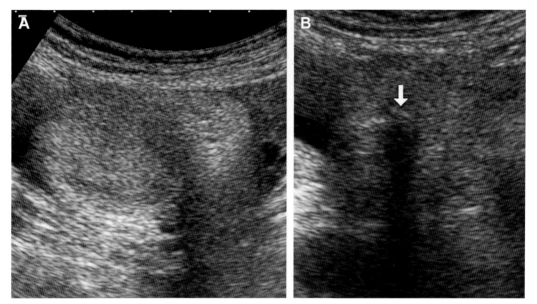

Fig. 13. (A) Longitudinal and (B) transverse sonograms show a homogenous hyperechoic mass lesion containing hyperechoic calcification (arrow). The patient underwent surgery, and pathology confirmed the mass to be a left ovarian mature cystic teratoma.

sonographic appearance of hemorrhagic ovarian cyst (Fig. 14).[55] Fibrin strands of hemorrhagic ovarian cysts can mimic the septation seen in endometrioma, but they usually are thinner and weaker reflectors than are true septations.[2] Color Doppler sonography shows no flow in these fine septations.[4] Ovarian fibromas show small vessels within a hypoechoic mass at color Doppler examination.[4,30] Tubo-ovarian abscesses present with fever and leucorrhea.[30] Ovarian cancer can be difficult to exclude if wall irregularities are present; absence of color Doppler flow within the cyst helps confirm the benign nature of the lesion.[30,56] If papillary structures protruding from the internal cyst wall are visualized, ovarian malignancy, such as endometrioid carcinoma, needs to be excluded (Fig. 15).[56] If a large number of irregular vessels with changing calibers, unusual anastomoses, and vascular lakes are seen entering an adnexal structure with centrally located flow within the mass, regardless of the resistive indices, the finding can be considered highly suggestive of malignancy.[57] Subserosal leiomyoma also may present as a solid-appearing mass in the adnexa; usually,

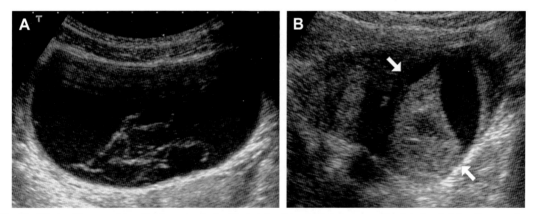

Fig. 14. (A) An 18-year-old patient presented with intolerable right lower quadrant pain. Pelvic ultrasound revealed a cystic adnexal mass with few septae. Laparoscopic surgery confirmed the lesion as a hemorrhagic ovarian cyst. (B) A 16-year-old patient had left lower quadrant pain. The pelvic sonogram showed a complex cystic mass containing triangular hyperechoic component consistent with clot retraction (arrows). This lesion had resolved completely on follow-up examination at 6 weeks.

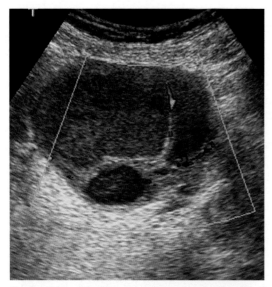

Fig. 15. A 39-year-old patient presented with vaginal bleeding. Transverse color Doppler examination shows multiseptated complex cystic mass with septal vascularization. This lesion was removed surgically and was confirmed to be a mucinous cystic ovarian tumor.

however, it is possible to demonstrate vascular connectivity with the uterine myometrium.[4] The presence of multiple vessels along the interface between the uterus and exophytic myomas on color and power Doppler ultrasound is known as the "bridging vascular sign" (**Fig. 16**).[58] Ovarian torsion also may mimic the appearance of endometrioma, but clinical presentation of torsion is acute and more painful than endometrioma (**Fig. 17**).

POSTMENOPAUSAL ENDOMETRIOSIS AND MALIGNANT TRANSFORMATION

Postmenopausal endometriosis is rare, with an incidence of about 2%.[59] Malignant change in endometriotic deposits, first described by Sampson in 1925, is very rare.[17] The rate of malign transformation is about 0.7% to 1%. Cancer can arise at any site of endometriosis but occurs most commonly in the ovary (in 79% of cases).[59] Clear-cell and endometrioid carcinoma are the most common types of tumor in the ovary; clear-cell adenocarcinoma and adenosarcoma seem to be the most common types of tumor in extraovarian endometriosis.[59] Patients who have endometriosis-associated ovarian cancers have a better overall survival than those who have ovarian cancer without endometriosis because of less advanced stage at diagnosis and lower-grade disease presentation.[59]

In pregnant women, ovarian endometrioma may mimic malignant ovarian tumor.[60] During pregnancy, decidualization involves hypertrophy of the stromal cells leading to thickening of the normal and ectopic endometrium and giving rise to the deciduas.[60] Decidualized tissue can grow during pregnancy to acquire a gross appearance that macroscopically mimics a malignant tumor.[60]

SCAR ENDOMETRIOSIS

Scar endometriosis is uncommon complication following cesarean sections, but it also can occur after episiotomy, laparotomy, and laparoscopy.[61] Scar endometriosis is very rare. A recent study found its incidence after cesarean section to be 0.8%, but the true incidence is likely to be higher, because cases may go undetected.[62] Scar endometriosis occurs via the iatrogenic transfer of endometrial cells into the

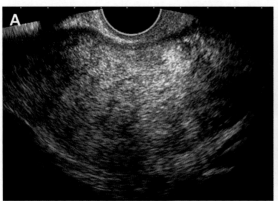
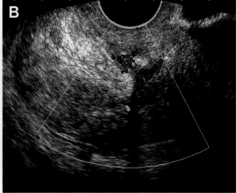

Fig. 16. (*A*) Longitudinal transvaginal sonogram reveals a large slightly heterogeneous hyperechoic mass located in the right adnexa. (*B*) Color Doppler sonogram shows multiple vascular channels bridging the space between the cervix and the exophytic mass (bridging vascular sign) suggestive of its origin from the cervix. This mass was removed surgically and was confirmed pathologically to be exophytic leiomyoma.

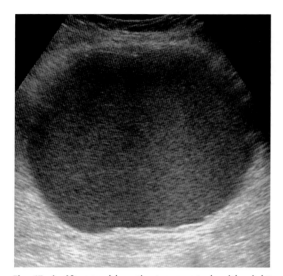

Fig. 17. A 40-year-old patient presented with right lower quadrant pain. The transverse pelvic sonogram demonstrates a large hypoechoic mass with low-level echoes. The patient underwent surgery, and this mass was confirmed to be right ovarian torsion without a distinctive cause.

surgical wound. The differential diagnosis includes scar hernia, endometrioma, primary cancer, metastasis, and desmoid tumor.[61] The mean period between the procedure and manifestation of symptoms is about 5 years.[61] The most frequent clinical presentation is a palpable subcutaneous mass near surgical scars associated with cyclic pain and swelling during menses.[63] The typical sonographic pattern has been reported to be a subcutaneous discrete nodule that is hypoechoic with scattered hyperechoic strands and irregular, often speculated, margins infiltrating the muscularis fascia, circumscribed by a complete or incomplete hyperechoic ring caused by a perilesional inflammatory reaction.[63] Small cystic areas may be detected in lesions larger than 3 cm, possibly caused by small blood lacunae of recent hemorrhage.[63] A single peripheral vascular pedicle with arterial flow entering the nodule can be shown by color Doppler, and with increasing size the intralesional vascularization is more readily visible (Fig. 18).[63] Fine-needle aspiration biopsy (for rapid diagnosis and to exclude malignancy) or excision biopsy can be performed for definitive diagnosis.[61] Wide excision of the scar endometrioma is a useful option that is both diagnostic and therapeutic. The success of medical therapy often is limited. Recurrence after excision is very rare, usually resulting from incomplete excision.[61]

URINARY TRACT AND BLADDER ENDOMETRIOSIS

Urinary tract involvement occurs in 16% to 24% of women who have endometriosis, but it is estimated that only 1% to 2% manifest urologic symptoms.[64] Ureteral obstruction is a rare but serious complication of deep pelvic endometriosis.[64] The most commonly affected organ of the urinary tract is the urinary bladder (84%), followed the ureter (7%–15%), kidneys (4%), and urethra (2%).[64,65] Clinical manifestations of bladder endometriosis are menouria and urethral and pelvic pain syndrome occurring cyclically.[64] Bladder implants typically develop at the vesicouterine pouch.[28] They can grow through the muscle into the submucosa, producing an obtuse bulge into the bladder lumen; rarely, endometriosis can grow through the mucosa and produce a polypoid mass that mimics bladder cancer (Fig. 19).[28] The bladder trigone and dome are the most commonly affected sites.[64] Small lesions may exhibit no symptoms and are diagnosed incidentally during a gynecologic examination for other conditions. Lesions affecting detrusor manifest symptoms in 75% of cases, almost always in cyclical manner, being more intense during the premenstrual period.[64] Despite the evidence of cyclical symptoms in most cases, the mean delay for correct diagnosis is about 4 to 5 years.[28,64,65] Nearly half of patients have a history of pelvic surgery, particularly cesarean section, because disruption of the uterus produces endometrial seeding and subsequent infiltration of tissue surrounding the bladder, detrusor, and mucosa, respectively.[28,64] Transabdominal and transvaginal sonography, CT, or MR imaging may show endometriotic bladder masses but are not specific.[64] CT and especially MR imaging define and more precisely delineate the area affected and the depth of the bladder wall lesion and serve as an extended study, identifying additional foci, particularly in the pelvic region.[64] The most cost-effective examination is cystoscopy. The cystoscopic image of endometriosis varies over the menstrual cycle, being clearer and more characteristic during menstruation when the lesions are larger and more congestive. If only the bladder adventitia is affected, cystoscopy will not provide a diagnosis. Diagnosis is confirmed histologically after cold biopsy or transurethral resection of the mass.[64] When the bladder mass or lesion has been documented by imaging techniques and/or cystoscopy, bladder carcinoma, angiomas, leiomyoma, cystopathies (amyloidosis, malakoplakia, glandular cystitis, and nephrogenic adenoma), and extravesical processes such as diverticulitis should be considered in the differential diagnosis, and histologic study is needed in almost all cases.[64,65]

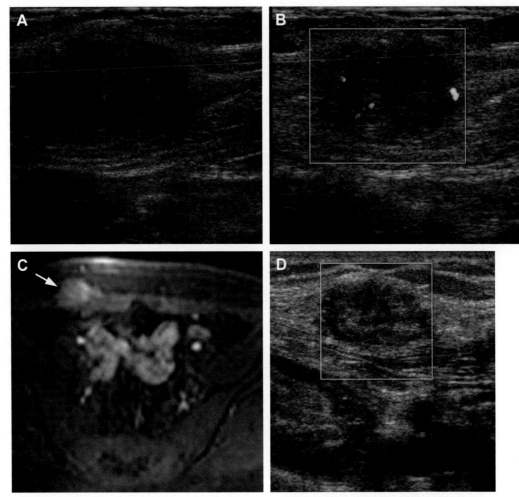

Fig. 18. Cesarean scar endometriomas in two different patients. Both patients had previous history of cesarean section (3.5 years ago and 8 years ago, respectively) and cyclic pain and swelling during menses. (*A*) Abdominal sonogram reveals a hypoechoic mass in the anterior abdominal wall. (*B*) Power Doppler sonogram shows intra-lesional vascularization. (*C*) Dynamic contrast-enhanced fat-saturated T1-weighted image shows marked contrast enhancement of the lesion (*arrow*). (*D*) Power Doppler sonogram of the second patient demonstrates hypoechoic mass without prominent vascularization.

MANAGEMENT AND THERAPY

Treatment should be individualized according to the patient's age, her desire for future pregnancies, the severity of the clinical symptoms, the location of the lesion, and the involvement of other organs.[64] Management can be medical (hormonal), surgical, or expectant.[2] Medical treatment currently consists of hormones such as danazol or gonadotropin-releasing hormone analogues that suppress cyclical hemorrhage.[2] Suppression of ovarian function for 6 months reduces endometriosis-associated pain. The hormonal drugs are equally effective, but their side-effect profiles and costs vary.[31] Nonsteroidal, anti-inflammatory drugs are used to treat the symptoms of endometriosis if the diagnosis has not been definitely established.[12,21] A combined medical and surgical therapy might use medical therapy before, after, or both before and after surgical intervention.[30] Laparoscopy can be used to diagnose and treat endometriosis.[12] Treatment during laparoscopy may include ablation of implants, lyses of adhesions, or removal of endometrioma implants.[12,21] Surgical therapy is appropriate, especially for advanced stages of the disease. Radical surgery is performed only in patients who have severe symptoms when there is no desired fertility potential and especially when other forms of treatment have failed.[30] Total abdominal hysterectomy and

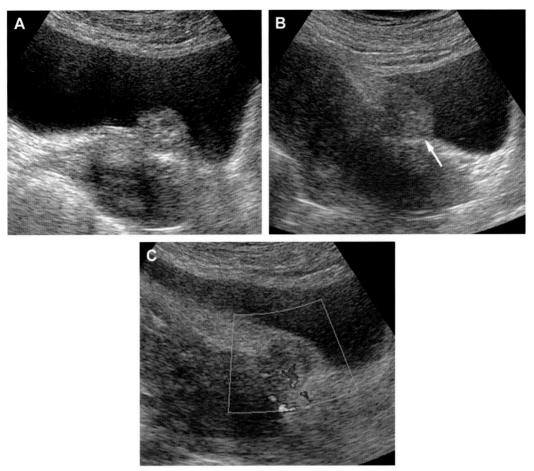

Fig. 19. Bladder endometriosis. The patient had history of surgical removal of endometrioma and right ovarian recurrent endometrioma and now presented with cyclic pelvic pain. (A) Transverse and (B) longitudinal sono-grams of the pelvis through the vesicouterine pouch demonstrate a hypoechoic mass (*arrow*) protruding into the posterior wall of the urinary bladder. (C) Power Doppler sonogram reveals vascularization of the lesion.

bilateral salpingo-oophorectomy are performed with any endometriotic lesions resected as com-pletely as possible.[30]

Medical Treatment

Oral contraceptive pills

Oral contraceptive pills usually are the first line of therapy in adolescents because of their low side-effect profile and their ability to be taken in-definitely.[8] Oral contraceptive pills reduce the endometrial lining and thus reduce the amount of tissue that produces prostaglandins. They also suppress ovulation and the subsequent lu-teal-phase symptoms of endometriosis.[8] This therapy is only suppressive, not curative.

Progestational agents

Progestational agents cause decidualization of ectopic, endometrial tissue and subsequent

atrophy.[8] The relatively low side-effect profile of these agents makes them a good choice in the long-term management of endometriosis in adolescents.[8]

Danazol

Danazol decreases the volume of ectopic endo-metrial tissue by inducing a hyperandrogenic state. The main benefit is pain improvement.[8] Da-nazol diminishes pain symptoms, but irreversible androgenic side effects are substantial.[8]

Gonadotropin-releasing hormone agonists

Gonadotropin-releasing hormone agonists create a hypoestrogenic, hypogonadal situation.[8] A 6-month duration of treatment decreases pain scores.[8] The likelihood of recurrence of symptoms is 10% after 1 year and 50% after 5 years.[8]

Medical therapy only suppresses the disease, and the recurrence rate is 11% each year.[66]

Medical treatment for endometriomas reduces the cyst size by between 40% to 57%, but there is a rapid return to the original size following the cessation of treatment.[67] Recent studies do not support any benefit of medical therapy for endometriosis-associated infertility.[66] In these patients surgery is more appropriate.[66,68]

SURGERY

Laparoscopic fenestration or excision of endometrioma is an effective treatment.[66,68] In some patients operative laparoscopy may be contraindicated because of previous surgery and/or adhesions.[66] Conservative surgery results in a good reproductive outcome.[66] Overall 30% to 70% of patients achieve pregnancy, depending on the severity of the disease.[66] A study comparing endoscopic versus laparoscopic management of endometriomas reported recurrence rates of 11.1% and 19% and pregnancy rates of 42.8% and 46.6%, respectively, following laparoscopy and laparotomy.[69] Excisional surgery of endometriomas seems to be more effective than drainage and ablation in preventing recurrence of the endometriomas.[67] Excisional surgery also is more effective than drainage and ablation in reducing symptoms of dysmenorrhea, dyspareunia, and nonmenstrual pelvic pain.[67] There is a minimal risk of reduced ovarian reserve and early menopause following surgical treatment of endometriosis.[67] Postoperative ovarian suppression would merely delay pregnancy. If the patient is suffering from significant pelvic pain, it would be appropriate to treat areas of deep infiltrating endometriosis.[67] Endometriomas are best treated surgically by capsule stripping, and there is little evidence for the efficacy of adjuvant medical treatment either pre- or postoperatively.[67]

An alternative approach to surgical techniques, ultrasound-guided aspiration of endometrioma (plus 3 months of hormone suppression before or after the procedure) has been performed in infertile patients who had endometrioma to improve their reproductive outcome.[66] A low recurrence rate of 31.8% and successful reproductive outcome in 40.9% of patients has been reported with this therapeutic approach.[66] One problem of aspiration is the possibility of missing the malignancy, because aspiration cytology may not always correlate with histology.[66] Ultrasound-guided aspiration is not an effective treatment for ovarian endometrioma but may be helpful in patients who have had prior surgery and present with a recurrence.[38]

Clinically, there is poor correlation between the size of the lesion and symptoms such as infertility and pelvic pain.[38] Surgery is more effective in alleviating pelvic pain and correcting infertility in severe disease than in mild disease.[38]

SUMMARY

Ultrasound imaging is a useful modality for following up patients who have a known history of endometrioma. The sonographic characteristics of endometriomas are diverse and may overlap with those of other adnexal lesions such as hemorrhagic cysts. The presence of hyperechoic wall foci and low level echoes are very specific for endometriomas. Endometriosis should be considered in the differential diagnosis in any woman of reproductive age who presents with pelvic pain or infertility.

REFERENCES

1. Eskenazi B, Warner ML. Epidemiology of endometriosis. Obstet Gynecol Clin North Am 1997;24: 235–58.
2. Woodward PJ, Sohaey R, Mezzetti TP Jr. Endometriosis: radiologic-pathologic correlation. Radiographics 2001;21:193–216.
3. Rawson JM. Prevalence of endometriosis in asymptomatic women. J Reprod Med 1991;36:513–5.
4. Bhatt S, Kocakoc E, Dogra VS. Endometriosis: sonographic spectrum. Ultrasound Q 2006;22:273–80.
5. Olive DL, Schwartz LB. Endometriosis. N Engl J Med 1993;328:1759–69.
6. Moore J, Copley S, Morris J, et al. A systematic review of the accuracy of ultrasound in the diagnosis of endometriosis. Ultrasound Obstet Gynecol 2002; 20:630–4.
7. Dmowski WP, Lesniewicz R, Rana N, et al. Changing trends in the diagnosis of endometriosis: a comparative study of women with pelvic endometriosis presenting with chronic pelvic pain or infertility. Fertil Steril 1997;67:238–43.
8. Attaran M, Gidwani GP. Adolescent endometriosis. Obstet Gynecol Clin North Am 2003;30:379–90.
9. Huffman JW. Endometriosis in young teen-age girls. Pediatr Ann 1981;10:44–9.
10. Clement PB. Pathology of endometriosis. Pathol Annu 1990;25:245–95.
11. Amer S. Endometriosis. Obstetrics Gynaecology and Reproductive Medicine 2008;18:126–33.
12. Kuligowska E, Deeds L 3rd, Lu K 3rd. Pelvic pain: overlooked and underdiagnosed gynecologic conditions. Radiographics 2005;25:3–20.
13. Arumugam K, Lim JM. Menstrual characteristics associated with endometriosis. Br J Obstet Gynaecol 1997;104:948–50.
14. Sampson JA. Peritoneal endometriosis due to the menstrual dissemination of endometrial tissues into

the peritoneal cavity. Am J Obstet Gynecol 1927;14: 422–69.

15. Oosterlynck DJ, Cornillie FJ, Waer M, et al. Women with endometriosis show a defect in natural killer activity resulting in a decreased cytotoxicity to autologous endometrium. Fertil Steril 1991;56:45–51.

16. Gougoutas CA, Siegelman ES, Hunt J, et al. Pelvic endometriosis: various manifestations and MR imaging findings. AJR Am J Roentgenol 2000;175:353–8.

17. Ghezzi F, Raio L, Cromi A, et al. "Kissing ovaries": a sonographic sign of moderate to severe endometriosis. Fertil Steril 2005;83:143–7.

18. Lebovic DI, Mueller MD, Taylor RN. Immunobiology of endometriosis. Fertil Steril 2001;75:1–10.

19. Wu MY, Ho HN. The role of cytokines in endometriosis. Am J Reprod Immunol 2003;49:285–96.

20. Bis KG, Vrachliotis TG, Agrawal R, et al. Pelvic endometriosis: MR imaging spectrum with laparoscopic correlation and diagnostic pitfalls. Radiographics 1997;17:639–55.

21. Daly S, Outwater E. Endometrioma/endometriosis. Emedicine. Available at: www.emedicine.com. Accessed May, 2005.

22. Jenkins S, Olive DL, Haney AF. Endometriosis: pathogenetic implications of the anatomic distribution. Obstet Gynecol 1986;67:335–8.

23. Clement PB. Disease of the peritoneum. In: Kurman RJ, editor. Blaustein's pathology of the female genital tract. 4th edition. NewYork: Springer-Verlag; 1994. p. 660–80.

24. Brosens I, Puttemans P, Campo R, et al. Diagnosis of endometriosis: pelvic endoscopy and imaging techniques. Best Pract Res Clin Obstet Gynaecol 2004; 18:285–303.

25. Vercellini P, Aimi G, De Giorgi O, et al. Is cystic ovarian endometriosis an asymmetric disease? Br J Obstet Gynaecol 1998;105:1018–21.

26. Chapron C, Dumontier I, Dousset B, et al. Results and role of rectal endoscopic ultrasonography for patients with deep pelvic endometriosis. Hum Reprod 1998;13:2266–70.

27. Chapron C, Vieira M, Chopin N, et al. Accuracy of rectal endoscopic ultrasonography and magnetic resonance imaging in the diagnosis of rectal involvement for patients presenting with deeply infiltrating endometriosis. Ultrasound Obstet Gynecol 2004;24:175–9.

28. Park SB, Kim JK, Cho KS. Sonography of endometriosis in infrequent sites. J Clin Ultrasound 2008;36:91–7.

29. Revised American Society for Reproductive Medicine classification of endometriosis: 1996. Fertil Steril 1997;67:817–21.

30. Kinkel K, Frei KA, Balleyguier C, et al. Diagnosis of endometriosis with imaging: a review. Eur Radiol 2006;16:285–98.

31. Kennedy S, Bergqvist A, Chapron C, et al. ESHRE guideline for the diagnosis and treatment of endometriosis. Hum Reprod 2005;20:2698–704.

32. Kitawaki J, Kusuki I, Koshiba H, et al. Detection of aromatase cytochrome P-450 in endometrial biopsy specimens as a diagnostic test for endometriosis. Fertil Steril 1999;72:1100–6.

33. Harada T, Kubota T, Aso T. Usefulness of CA19-9 versus CA125 for the diagnosis of endometriosis. Fertil Steril 2002;78:733–9.

34. Bedaiwy MA, Falcone T, Sharma RK, et al. Prediction of endometriosis with serum and peritoneal fluid markers: a prospective controlled trial. Hum Reprod 2002;17:426–31.

35. Donnez J, Squifflet J, Casanas-Roux F, et al. Typical and subtle atypical presentations of endometriosis. Obstet Gynecol Clin North Am 2003;30:83–93.

36. Nisolle M, Paindaveine B, Bourdon A, et al. Histologic study of peritoneal endometriosis in infertile women. Fertil Steril 1990;53:984–8.

37. Guerriero S, Mais V, Ajossa S, et al. The role of endovaginal ultrasound in differentiating endometriomas from other ovarian cysts. Clin Exp Obstet Gynecol 1995;22:20–2.

38. Brosens J, Timmerman D, Starzinski-Powitz A, et al. Noninvasive diagnosis of endometriosis: the role of imaging and markers. Obstet Gynecol Clin North Am 2003;30:95–114.

39. Exacoustos C, Zupi E, Carusotti C, et al. Staging of pelvic endometriosis: role of sonographic appearance in determining extension of disease and modulating surgical approach. J Am Assoc Gynecol Laparosc 2003;10:378–82.

40. Webb EM, Green EG, Scoutt LM. Adnexal mass with pelvic pain. Radiol Clin North Am 2004;42:329–48.

41. Clarke L, Edwards A, Pollard K. Acoustic streaming in ovarian cysts. J Ultrasound Med 2005;24:617–21.

42. Seow KM, Lin YH, Hsieh BC, et al. Transvaginal three-dimensional ultrasonography combined with serum CA 125 level for the diagnosis of pelvic adhesions before laparoscopic surgery. J Am Assoc Gynecol Laparosc 2003;10:320–6.

43. Carbognin G, Guarise A, Minelli L, et al. Pelvic endometriosis: US and MRI features. Abdom Imaging 2004;29:609–18.

44. Alcazar JL, Laparte C, Jurado M, et al. The role of transvaginal ultrasonography combined with color velocity imaging and pulsed Doppler in the diagnosis of endometrioma. Fertil Steril 1997;67:487–91.

45. Guerriero S, Ajossa S, Mais V, et al. The diagnosis of endometriomas using colour Doppler energy imaging. Hum Reprod 1998;13:1691–5.

46. Patel MD, Feldstein VA, Chen DC, et al. Endometriomas: diagnostic performance of US. Radiology 1999;210:739–45.

47. Pascual MA, Tresserra F, Lopez-Marin L, et al. Role of color Doppler ultrasonography in the diagnosis of endometriotic cyst. J Ultrasound Med 2000;19: 695–9.

48. Jeong YY, Outwater EK, Kang HK. Imaging evaluation of ovarian masses. Radiographics 2000;20: 1445–70.

49. Brown DL, Frates MC, Muto MG, et al. Small echogenic foci in the ovaries: correlation with histologic findings. J Ultrasound Med 2004;23:307–13.

50. Tamarkin SW, Dogra V. Benign and malignant adnexal lesions. In: Dogra V, Rubens DJ, editors. Ultrasound secrets. Philadelphia: Hanley and Belfus; 2004. p. 97–104.

51. Buy JN, Ghossain MA, Mark AS, et al. Focal hyperdense areas in endometriomas: a characteristic finding on CT. AJR Am J Roentgenol 1992;159:769–71.

52. Togashi K, Nishimura K, Kimura I, et al. Endometrial cysts: diagnosis with MR imaging. Radiology 1991; 180:73–8.

53. Glastonbury CM. The shading sign. Radiology 2002; 224:199–201.

54. Atri M, Nazarnia S, Bret PM, et al. Endovaginal sonographic appearance of benign ovarian masses. Radiographics 1994;14:747–60 [discussion: 761–2].

55. Jain KA. Sonographic spectrum of hemorrhagic ovarian cysts. J Ultrasound Med 2002;21:879–86.

56. Kinkel K, Hricak H, Lu Y, et al. US characterization of ovarian masses: a meta-analysis. Radiology 2000; 217:803–11.

57. Kurjak A, Kupesic S, Anic T, et al. Three-dimensional ultrasound and power Doppler improve the diagnosis of ovarian lesions. Gynecol Oncol 2000;76:28–32.

58. Kim SH, Sim JS, Seong CK. Interface vessels on color/power Doppler US and MRI: a clue to differentiate subserosal uterine myomas from extrauterine tumors. J Comput Assist Tomogr 2001;25:36–42.

59. Taylor AA, Kenny N, Edmonds S, et al. Postmenopausal endometriosis and malignant transformation of endometriosis: a case series. Gynecol Surg 2005;2:135–7.

60. Yoshida S, Onogi A, Shigetomi H, et al. Two cases of pregnant women with ovarian endometrioma mimicking a malignant ovarian tumor. J Clin Ultrasound 2008.10.1002/jcu.20496.

61. Singh M, Sivanesan K, Ghani R, et al. Caesarean scar endometriosis. Arch Gynecol Obstet 2008.10.1007/s00404-008-0672-x.

62. Hensen JH, Van Breda Vriesman AC, Puylaert JB. Abdominal wall endometriosis: clinical presentation and imaging features with emphasis on sonography. AJR Am J Roentgenol 2006;186:616–20.

63. Francica G, Giardiello C, Angelone G, et al. Abdominal wall endometriomas near cesarean delivery scars: sonographic and color Doppler findings in a series of 12 patients. J Ultrasound Med 2003;22: 1041–7.

64. Pastor-Navarro H, Giménez-Bachs JM, Donate-Moreno MJ, et al. Update on the diagnosis and treatment of bladder endometriosis. Int Urogynecol J Pelvic Floor Dysfunct 2007;18:949–54.

65. Stanley KE Jr, Utz DC, Dockerty MB. Clinically significant endometriosis of the urinary tract. Surg Gynecol Obstet 1965;120:491–8.

66. Mittal S, Kumar S, Kumar A, et al. Ultrasound guided aspiration of endometrioma—a new therapeutic modality to improve reproductive outcome. Int J Gynaecol Obstet 1999;65:17–23.

67. Wright JT, Nightingale AL, Ballard KD. Evidence-based gynaecological practice: clinical review 1. Management of ovarian endometriomas. Gynecol Surg 2007;4:275–80.

68. Fayez JA, Vogel MF. Comparison of different treatment methods of endometriomas by laparoscopy. Obstet Gynecol 1991;78:660–5.

69. Daniell JF, Kurtz BR, Gurley LD. Laser laparoscopic management of large endometriomas. Fertil Steril 1991;55:692–5.

Pelvic Congestion Syndrome

Musturay Karcaaltincaba, MD[a],*, Deniz Karcaaltincaba, MD[b],
Vikram S. Dogra, MD[c]

KEYWORDS

- Pelvic congestion syndrome • Pelvic varices
- US • CT • MR imaging • Ovarian venography

Chronic pelvic pain is a significant health problem in women particularly during childbearing age and may account for 10% of outpatient gynecologic visits.[1–4] Etiology of chronic pelvic pain includes irritable bowel syndrome, endometriosis, adenomyosis, pelvic congestion syndrome, atypical menstrual pain, urologic disorders, and psychosocial issues.[2,3] Pelvic congestion syndrome is defined as a syndrome characterized by visible congestion of the pelvic veins on selective ovarian venography in multiparous, premenopausal women with a history of chronic pelvic pain for at least 6 months and was first described by Richet in 1857.[1–5] Pelvic congestion syndrome can present with nonspecific pelvic pain, dyspareunia, and persistent genital arousal.[2–7] In the era of cross-sectional imaging, this entity is increasingly recognized by ultrasound (US), CT, and MR imaging. Presence of dilated pelvic veins and pelvic varices is a frequent finding on transabdominal and transvaginal ultrasound (TVUS) examinations and can be found in approximately half of the women with chronic pelvic pain.[1–4,8,9] Pelvic varices can be seen in 10% of women in the general population[10] and up to 60% of patients with pelvic varices may develop pelvic congestion syndrome.[5] Pelvic congestion syndrome appears to be a multifactorial disease. Mechanical and hormonal factors may contribute to its pathogenesis. Pelvic congestion can occur in premenstrual syndrome, intermenstrual syndrome, and chronic pelvic congestion syndrome.[11] Premenstrual and intermenstrual syndromes are cyclical and can

easily be differentiated from chronic pelvic congestion syndrome by clinical findings, but radiologic findings may overlap. On physical examination, varices can be seen in the vulva, buttocks, and legs.[2–4,12,13]

Pelvic congestion syndrome occurs mostly because of ovarian vein reflux, but can also occur because of the obstruction of ovarian vein outflow resulting in reversed flow. Reversed flow can be attributable to left renal vein stenosis and left ovarian vein stenosis and coexistence of nutcracker and pelvic congestion syndrome has been described.[14–16] The term "midline congestion" has been used by Scholbach[17] to denote that pelvic congestion syndrome may have a common causative factor (congestion of left renal vein) with other pathologies such as migraine, back pain, and headache. Also, pelvic vein kinking owing to uterine malposition may lead to venous stasis.[1] Pelvic varices may be associated with left and right renal vein anomalies including retroaortic and circumaortic left renal veins,[18,19] and anomalous drainage of right ovarian vein into right renal vein.[20] Pelvic congestion can rarely be caused by aorto-left renal vein fistula and inferior vena cava reflux.[21,22]

EVALUATION OF PELVIC CONGESTION SYNDROME
Ultrasound

Ultrasonography is the initial diagnostic modality for the diagnosis of pelvic congestion syndrome.[1–3,9] Current randomized controlled trials

[a] Department of Radiology, Hacettepe University School of Medicine, Sihhiye, Ankara 06100, Turkey
[b] Etlik Women's Hospital Etlik, Ankara, Turkey
[c] Department of Radiology, University of Rochester School of Medicine and Dentistry, 601 Elmwood Avenue, Box 648, Rochester, NY 14642, USA
* Corresponding author.
E-mail address: musturayk@yahoo.com (M. Karcaaltincaba).

Ultrasound Clin 3 (2008) 415–425
doi:10.1016/j.cult.2008.08.002

provide some support for the use of US scanning as an aid to counseling and reassurance for pelvic congestion syndrome.[3] TVUS should be preferred for the demonstration of pelvic varices and to rule out other causes of pelvic pain including endometriosis, adenomyosis, and ovarian cysts.[23] Combination of gray-scale and color flow Doppler (CFD) examination allow accurate diagnosis of pelvic varices (**Fig. 1**). Diagnostic criteria include tortuous pelvic veins with a diameter of greater than 5 to 6 mm, slow (around 3 cm/s) or reversed flow, dilated arcuate veins in myometrium being in communication with pelvic varicose veins, and sonographic detection of polycystic changes in the ovaries.[1,4,20,24–30] The reason for polycystic appearance is not known and there is wide variation in the number of cysts that can be seen in half of the patients.[1,28] Crossing uterine veins in the myometrium (known as arcuate veins) can be seen on transvaginal and transabdominal ultrasonography and CT (**Fig. 2**). They correspond to large crossing veins on selective ovarian venography that allows contralateral filling of contrast

media. Transabdominal pelvic US is useful for the demonstration of size and flow direction of the left ovarian vein (**Fig. 3**). Park and colleagues[1] suggested that demonstration of reversed flow in the distal left ovarian vein was highly accurate for the diagnosis of pelvic congestion syndrome and correlated with the presence of reflux on selective ovarian venography. However, Doppler signal from the ovarian vein may not be obtained in all patients and reversed flow can be seen in healthy patients.[1,8,9]

CFD can also be used in patients who underwent ebolization to demonstrate variceal thrombosis.[31] Pelvic varices can also be caused by increased pressure in the intra-abdominal venous system such as portal hypertension and congestive heart failure and radiologic findings can allow differentiation of these entities from pelvic varices of pelvic congestion syndrome (**Fig. 4**). Pelvic varices are seen as multiple and dilated veins around the ovary and uterus with a venous waveform measuring more than 5 mm in diameter.[1,24–26,28,32] Mayer and Machan[33] suggested that initial

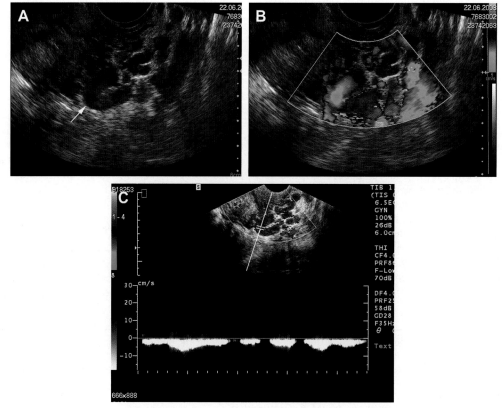

Fig. 1. US findings of pelvic congestion syndrome. Transvaginal gray-scale (*A*) and CFD (*B, C*) US images show multiple pelvic varices (*arrow*).

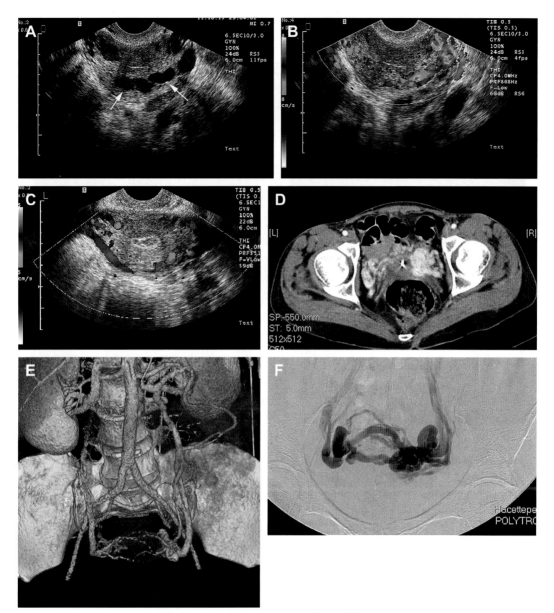

Fig. 2. Gray-scale (*A*) and CFD (*B, C*) US images show arcuate veins (*arrow*) (*arrow* in *A* and *B* are in the same location) within the uterus in two different patients (*arrows*). Note arcuate veins on CT (*C, D*) and ovarian venography (*E*).

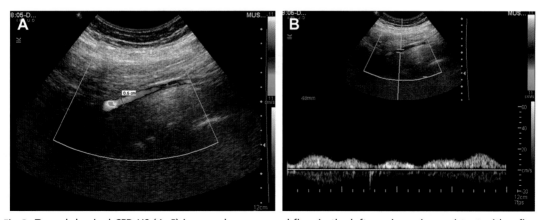

Fig. 3. Transabdominal CFD US (*A, B*) images show reversed flow in the left ovarian vein consistent with reflux.

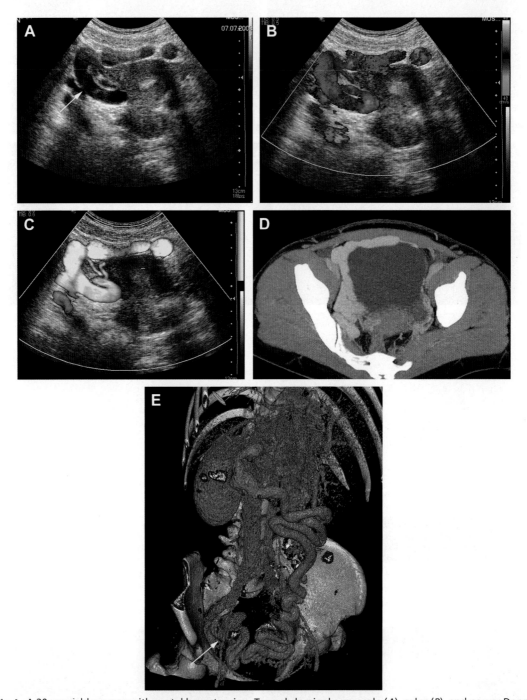

Fig. 4. A 20-year-old woman with portal hypertension. Transabdominal gray-scale (*A*), color (*B*), and power Doppler (*C*) US images show right-sided pelvic varices (*arrow*) with corresponding CT image (*D*). Note that pelvic varices (*arrow*) communicate with dilated paraumbilical vein through abdominal wall varices on CT portography (*E*).

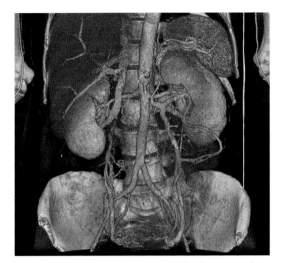

Fig. 5. Volume-rendered MDCT angiography images show retrograde filling of left and right ovarian vein consistent with reflux in a woman with pelvic congestion syndrome.

accentuation in a pelvic varicocele during the Valsalva maneuver was an important Doppler sonographic finding for diagnosing pelvic congestion syndrome, similar to the method of diagnosing scrotal varicoceles in men. However, similar consistent results were not obtained by Park and colleagues[1] and the authors thought that variable Doppler signal on Valsalva maneuver may be attributable to intraperitoneal location of pelvic varices.

Computed Tomography

Multidetector CT (MDCT) allows rapid acquisition (in less than 10 seconds) of submillimeter slices, which enables multiplanar reformation with isotropic resolution. Ovarian veins are well visualized by curved planar reformatted images and pelvic congestion syndrome can be diagnosed by CT.[8,9,34–36] The major disadvantage of CT is its inability to demonstrate flow direction. However,

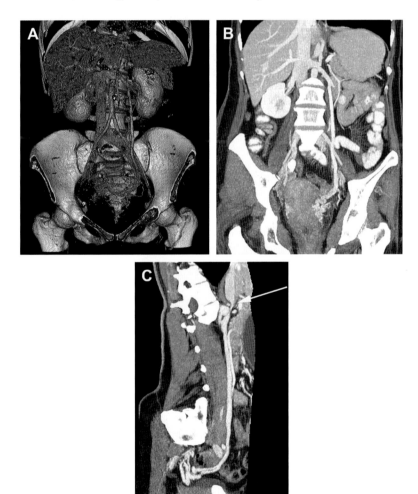

Fig. 6. Coronal volume-rendered MDCT and curved planar reformatted images (*A, B*) show dilatation of left ovarian vein attributable to nutcracker syndrome. Note narrowing of left renal vein (*arrow*) between aorta and superior mesenteric artery (*C*).

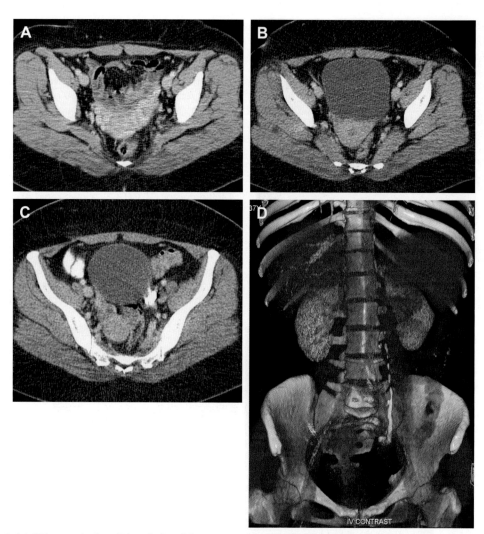

Fig. 7. Axial CT images before (*A*) and after (*B*) treatment show interval resolution of pelvic varices. Axial (*C*) and volume-rendered CT images (*D*) show coils in the left ovarian vein.

reflux can be demonstrated by retrograde filling of ovarian veins in the arterial phase MDCT images (**Fig. 5**).[35] Moreover, stenosis and collaterals can be diagnosed, which are difficult to diagnose by ultrasonography.

Recent studies performed by CT suggest association between pelvic varices and left renal vein variations.[18,19] MDCT allows visualization of pelvic varices, ovarian vein dilatation, and nutcracker syndrome (**Fig. 6**). MDCT can also be used for assessing treatment results and to rule out possible recanalization (**Fig. 7**).

Magnetic Resonance Imaging

MR imaging is becoming widely used for abdominal and pelvic imaging due to improvements in sequences, scanners and parallel imaging.[37] Major advantage of MR IMAGING is lack of radiation when compared with MDCT. Therefore dynamic multiphasic images can be acquired which can allow studying ovarian vein dynamics and acquisition of MR venographic images (**Fig. 8**). Moreover velocity encoded phase contrast images can be used to demonstrate ovarian vein velocity and flow direction. On T1-weighted images, pelvic varices can appear as signal void areas and on gradient-echo MR images, the varices may have high signal intensity. On T2-weighted MR images, they usually appear as an area of low signal intensity; however, hyperintensity or mixed signal intensity may also be noted, possibly because of the relatively slow flow through the vessels.[38] Nascimento and

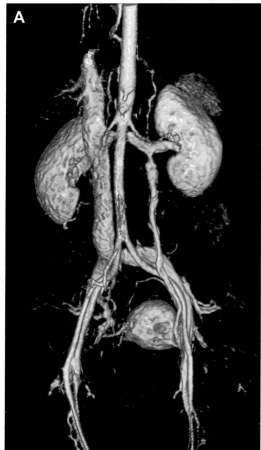

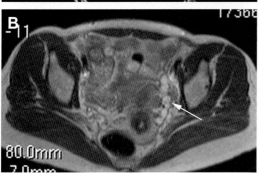

Fig. 8. Volume-rendered MR angiography image (*A*) shows dilated left ovarian vein. Note hyperintense varices on axial T2-weighted image (*arrow*) (*B*).

colleagues[37] reported presence of passive reflux and ovarian vein dilatation (mean size of 6.4 mm) in asymptomatic patients who underwent MR angiography for renal transplant donor evaluation and suggested that MR imaging findings should be correlated with clinical findings. Artifacts from metallic embolization coils also limit follow-up of treated patients with MR imaging.[38] MR imaging can also be used for the diagnosis

of endometriosis and adenomyosis in patients with equivocal findings on ultrasonography in patients with pelvic pain.[5]

Angiography

Selective ovarian venography has been accepted as the gold standard technique for the diagnosis of pelvic congestion syndrome.[13,29,30,39] This technique was first described by Tavernier and Lange[40] in 1965. Ovarian venography should be performed on a tilting table.[39] Ovarian veins can be accessed via a jugular or femoral vein approach. First, left renal vein injection should be performed so as not to miss nutcracker syndrome. Then the left ovarian vein should be catheterized. Also, the right ovarian vein can be catheterized if necessary. Venographic findings include presence of reflux, dilatation of ovarian vein (greater than 8 to 10 mm), pelvic varices, uterine venous engorgement, congestion of the ovarian plexus, and filling of the contralateral pelvic veins through the arcuate veins and/or filling of vulvovaginal and thigh varicosities (**Fig. 9**).[39–47] However, ovarian venography is an invasive technique compared with cross-sectional imaging methods and should be reserved for patients who will undergo treatment. Imaging findings are summarized in **Box 1**.

MANAGEMENT

Pelvic congestion syndrome can be treated by medical, interventional, and surgical treatments. Current evidence from randomized controlled trials provides some support for progestogen (medroxyprogesterone acetate) or goserelin for pelvic congestion and a multidisciplinary approach to assessment and treatment.[3] Medical treatment is noninvasive and progestogen, goserelin, and daflon can be given for symptomatic relief.[48–50] In patients refractory to medical treatment, interventional treatment is a minimally invasive treatment compared with surgical methods.[39–47] The major advantage of interventional techniques is diagnosis and treatment of pelvic congestion syndrome in a single session by ovarian vein occlusion using various embolic agents. Additionally, internal iliac veins can be embolized. Moreover, stents can be placed to treat coexisting nutcracker and pelvic congestion syndrome attributable to left renal vein stenosis.[14–16] The results of endovascular treatment are at least equivalent to those of surgery and better than conventional medical therapy.[39–47] Coils can protrude into the common femoral vein after treatment and rarely pelvic pain can increase after the procedure as complications.[1,51] Surgical methods should be used when interventional methods fail. Surgical alternatives include ligation

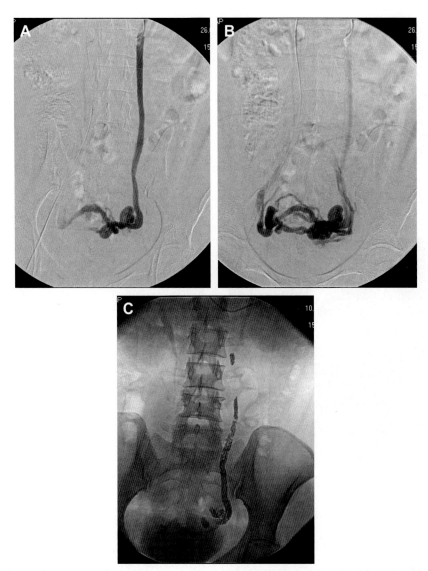

Fig. 9. Selective ovarian venography images show reflux in left ovarian vein (*A*) and pelvic varices (*B*). Subsequent embolization of left ovarian vein (*C*) resulted in treatment of pelvic varices. (*Courtesy of* Barbaros Cil, MD, Ankara, Turkey.)

<table>
<tr><td>Box 1
Summary of findings in pelvic congestion syndrome</td></tr>
</table>

US and CFD

> Pelvic varices (>5 mm) with slow flow
>
> Dilated arcuate veins in myometrium
>
> Polycystic changes in ovaries
>
> Dilated left ovarian vein and reversed flow
>
> Left renal vein stenosis (in patients with accompanying nutcracker syndrome)

CT

> Filling of ovarian veins on arterial phase images
>
> Dilated ovarian vein and pelvic varices
>
> Left renal vein stenosis (in patients with accompanying nutcracker syndrome)

MR imaging

> Filling of ovarian veins on MR angiography images
>
> Pelvic varices appearing
>
> > Signal void on T1-weighted images
> >
> > Hyperintense on gradient-echo images
> >
> > Hypointense, hyperintense, or mixed signal intensity on T2-weighted images

Venography

> Demonstration of reflux into ovarian vein
>
> Dilatation of ovarian vein >8–10 mm
>
> Dilated pelvic veins
>
> Filling of contralateral pelvic varices and extrapelvic varices

---

of ovarian veins and internal iliac veins by open or laparascopic surgery.[52–55]

SUMMARY

Pelvic congestion syndrome has characteristic radiologic findings that include pelvic varices, ovarian cysts, dilated ovarian and arcuate veins, and reversed flow in the ovarian vein. Ultrasonography and CFD should be the initial step in suspect patients. CT and MR imaging can be used as adjunct modalities. Ovarian vein venography is invasive and reserved for patients who will undergo treatment. Embolotherapy of pelvic congestion syndrome and stenting in patients with nutcracker syndrome play a major role in minimally invasive treatment of pelvic congestion syndrome.

REFERENCES

1. Park SJ, Lim JW, Ko TY, et al. Diagnosis of pelvic congestion syndrome using transabdominal and transvaginal sonography. AJR Am J Roentgenol 2004;182:683–8.
2. Liddle AD, Davies AH. Pelvic congestion syndrome: chronic pelvic pain caused by ovarian and internal iliac varices. Phlebology 2007;22(3):100–4.
3. Cheong Y, William Stones R. Chronic pelvic pain: aetiology and therapy. Best Pract Res Clin Obstet Gynaecol 2006;20(5):695–711.
4. Beard RW, Pearce S, Highmanm JH, et al. Diagnosis of pelvic varicosities in women with chronic pelvic pain. Lancet 1984;2:946–9.
5. Kuligowska E, Deeds L 3rd, Lu K 3rd. Pelvic pain: overlooked and underdiagnosed gynecologic conditions. Radiographics 2005;25(1):3–20.
6. Thorne C, Stuckey B. Pelvic congestion syndrome presenting as persistent genital arousal: a case report. J Sex Med 2008;5:504–8.
7. Reiter RC. A profile of women with chronic pelvic pain. Clin Obstet Gynecol 1990;33:130–6.
8. Rozenblit AM, Ricci ZJ, Tuvia J, et al. Incompetent and dilated ovarian veins: a common CT finding in asymptomatic parous women. AJR Am J Roentgenol 2001;176(1):119–22.
9. Belenky A, Bartal G, Atar E, et al. Ovarian varices in healthy female kidney donors: incidence, morbidity, and clinical outcome. AJR Am J Roentgenol 2002; 179:625–7.
10. Mathias SD, Kuppermann M, Liberman RF, et al. Chronic pelvic pain: prevalence, health-related quality of life, and economic correlates. Obstet Gynecol 1996;87:321–7.
11. Charles G. Congestive pelvic syndromes. Rev Fr Gynecol Obstet 1995;90(2):84–90.
12. Bell D, Kane PB, Liang S, et al. Vulvar varices: an uncommon entity in surgical pathology. Int J Gynecol Pathol 2007;26:99–101.
13. Ganeshan A, Upponi S, Hon LQ, et al. Chronic pelvic pain due to pelvic congestion syndrome: the role of diagnostic and interventional radiology. Cardiovasc Intervent Radiol 2007;30:1105–11.
14. Hartung O, Grisoli D, Boufi M, et al. Endovascular stenting in the treatment of pelvic vein congestion caused by nutcracker syndrome: lessons learned from the first five cases. J Vasc Surg 2005;42: 275–80.
15. d'Archambeau O, Maes M, De Schepper AM. The pelvic congestion syndrome: role of the "nutcracker phenomenon" and results of endovascular treatment. JBR-BTR 2004;87:1–8.

16. Scultetus AH, Villavicencio JL, Gillespie DL. The nutcracker syndrome: its role in the pelvic venous disorders. J Vasc Surg 2001;34:812–9.

17. Scholbach T. From the nutcracker-phenomenon of the left renal vein to the midline congestion syndrome as a cause of migraine, headache, back and abdominal pain and functional disorders of pelvic organs. Med Hypotheses 2007;68:1318–27.

18. Koc Z, Ulusan S, Oguzkurt L. Association of left renal vein variations and pelvic varices in abdominal MDCT. Eur Radiol 2007;17:1267–74.

19. Koc Z, Ulusan S, Tokmak N, et al. Double retroaortic left renal veins as a possible cause of pelvic congestion syndrome: imaging findings in two patients. Br J Radiol 2006;79:e152–5.

20. Giacchetto C, Cotroneo GB, Marincolo F, et al. Ovarian varicocele: ultrasonic and phlebographic evaluation. J Clin Ultrasound 1990;18:551–5.

21. Fassiadis N, Macqueen Buchanan E, et al. Retroaortic left renal vein fistula masquerading as pelvic congestion syndrome: Case report. Int J Surg 2007 Apr 10 [e-publication PMID: 17512266].

22. Sugaya K, Miyazato T, Koyama Y, et al. Pelvic congestion syndrome caused by inferior vena cava reflux. Int J Urol 2000;7:157–9.

23. Bhatt S, Kocakoc E, Dogra VS. Endometriosis: sonographic spectrum. Ultrasound Q 2006;22(4):273–80.

24. Adams J, Reginald PW, Franks S, et al. Uterine size and endometrial thickness and the significance of cystic ovaries in women with pelvic pain due to congestion. Br J Obstet Gynaecol 1990;97(7):583–7.

25. Stones RW. Pelvic vascular congestion—half a century later. Clin Obstet Gynecol 2003;46:831–6.

26. Hodgson TJ, Reed MW, Peck RJ, et al. Case report: the ultrasound and Doppler appearances of pelvic varices. Clin Radiol 1991;44:208–9.

27. Saxton DW, Farquhar CM, Rae T, et al. Accuracy of ultrasound measurements of female pelvic organs. Br J Obstet Gynaecol 1990;97:695–9.

28. Juhász B, Kurjak A, Lampé LG. Pelvic varices simulating bilateral adnexal masses: differential diagnosis by transvaginal color Doppler. J Clin Ultrasound 1992;20(1):81–4.

29. Hobbs JT. The pelvic congestion syndrome. Br J Hosp Med 1990;43:200–6.

30. Kennedy A, Hemingway A. Radiology of ovarian varices. Br J Hosp Med 1990;44(1):38–43.

31. Capasso P, Simons C, Trotteur G, et al. Treatment of symptomatic pelvic varices by ovarian vein embolization. Cardiovasc Intervent Radiol 1997;20:107–11.

32. Maleux G, Stockx L, Wilms G, et al. Ovarian vein embolization for the treatment of pelvic congestion syndrome: long-term technical and clinical results. J Vasc Interv Radiol 2000;11:859–64.

33. Mayer AL, Machan LS. Correlation of ultrasound and venographic findings in pelvic congestion syndrome. J Vasc Interv Radiol 2000;11(Suppl):221.

34. Karaosmanoglu D, Karcaaltincaba M, Karcaaltincaba D, et al. MDCT findings of ovarian vein: normal anatomy and pathology. Am J Roentgenol, in press.

35. Desimpelaere JH, Seynaeve PC, Hagers YM, et al. Pelvic congestion syndrome: demonstration and diagnosis by helical CT. Abdom Imaging 1999;24:100–2.

36. Siddall KA, Rubens DJ. Multidetector CT of the female pelvis. Radiol Clin North Am 2005;43:1097–118.

37. Nascimento AB, Mitchell DG, Holland G. Ovarian veins: magnetic resonance imaging findings in an asymptomatic population. J Magn Reson Imaging 2002;15:551–6.

38. Coakley FV, Varghese SL, Hricak H. CT and MRI of pelvic varices in women. J Comput Assist Tomogr 1999;23:429–34.

39. Nicholson T, Basile A. Pelvic congestion syndrome, who should we treat and how? Tech Vasc Interv Radiol 2006;9:19–23.

40. Tavernier J, Lange D. La phlébographie utéro-ovarienne gauche. Presse Med 1965;73:863–6.

41. Stones RW, Mountfield J. Interventions for treating chronic pelvic pain in women. Cochrane Database Syst Rev. 2000;(4):CD000387.

42. Tarazov PG, Prozorovskij KV, Ryzhkov VK. Pelvic pain syndrome caused by ovarian varices. Treatment by transcatheter embolization. Acta Radiol 1997;38:1023–5.

43. Chung MH, Huh CY. Comparison of treatments for pelvic congestion syndrome. Tohoku J Exp Med 2003;201:131–8.

44. Cordts PR, Eclavea A, Buckley PJ, et al. Pelvic congestion syndrome: early clinical results after transcatheter ovarian vein embolization. J Vasc Surg 1998;28:862–8.

45. Venbrux AC, Chang AH, Kim HS, et al. Pelvic congestion syndrome (pelvic venous incompetence): impact of ovarian and internal iliac vein embolotherapy on menstrual cycle and chronic pelvic pain. J Vasc Interv Radiol 2002;13:171–8.

46. Kim HS, Malhotra AD, Rowe PC, et al. Embolotherapy for pelvic congestion syndrome: long-term results. J Vasc Interv Radiol 2006;17:289–97.

47. Sichlau MJ, Yao JS, Vogelzang RL. Transcatheter embolotherapy for the treatment of pelvic congestion syndrome. Obstet Gynecol 1994;83(5 Pt 2):892–6.

48. Soysal ME, Soysal S, Vicdan K, et al. A randomized controlled trial of goserelin and medroxyprogesterone acetate in the treatment of pelvic congestion. Humanit Rep 2001;16:931–9.

49. Taskin O, Uryan II, Buhur A, et al. The effects of daflon on pelvic pain in women with Taylor syndrome. J Am Assoc Gynecol Laparosc 1996;3:S49.

50. Simsek M, Burak F, Taskin O. Effects of micronized purified flavonoid fraction (Daflon) on pelvic pain in women with laparoscopically diagnosed pelvic congestion syndrome: a randomized crossover trial. Clin Exp Obstet Gynecol 2007;34:96–8.

51. Marsh P, Holdstock JM, Bacon JL, et al. Coil protruding into the common femoral vein following pelvic venous embolization. Cardiovasc Intervent Radiol 2008;31:435–8.
52. Schraibman IG. Pelvic congestion syndrome and ligation of ovarian veins. Br J Hosp Med 1990;44:14.
53. Takeuchi K, Mochizuki M, Kitagaki S. Laparoscopic varicocele ligation for pelvic congestion syndrome. Int J Gynaecol Obstet 1996;55:177–8.
54. Rogers A, Beech A, Braithwaite B. Transperitoneal laparoscopic left gonadal vein ligation can be the right treatment option for pelvic congestion symptoms secondary to nutcracker syndrome. Vascular 2007;15:238–40.
55. Gargiulo T, Mais V, Brokaj L, et al. Bilateral laparoscopic transperitoneal ligation of ovarian veins for treatment of pelvic congestion syndrome. J Am Assoc Gynecol Laparosc 2003;10:501–4.

Sonohysterography: Technique and Clinical Applications

Phyllis Glanc, MD[a],[*], Carrie Betel, MD, FRCP(C)[a],
Anna Lev-Toaff, MD, FACR[b]

KEYWORDS

- Sonohysterography • Saline infusion sonohysterography
- Ultrasound • Uterus • Endometrium • Mullerian duct

Sonohysterography (SHG) is a technique used to improve visualization of the endometrial cavity and its relationship to the uterus. A catheter is placed within the endometrial cavity or endocervical canal and an agent, typically saline, is instilled to achieve separation of the walls of the endometrial cavity during continuous transvaginal (TV) ultrasound (US) assessment. In 1993, Parsons and colleagues[1] termed this technique "sonohysterography." Alternate nomenclatures include hysterosonography or saline infused sonohysterography.

SHG is more accurate than TV US and less invasive than hysteroscopy for the detection of endometrial abnormalities.[2–5] SHG can accurately distinguish global versus focal endometrial pathology, endometrial versus subendometrial conditions, and provide a precise description of submucosal fibroids, thus permitting the clinician to determine the optimal therapeutic approach. SHG with the addition of three-dimensional (3D) US is an excellent technique for the evaluation of mullerian duct anomalies (MDA).[6,7] In the authors' experience, SHG can also be helpful in distinguishing between pseudo-endometrial thickening and true endometrial abnormalities in patients with adenomyosis.

TECHNIQUE
Scheduling Patients

SHG should be performed within the first 10 days after spontaneous or progestin induced menstrual flow, preferably between days four and seven. This time period is when the endometrium is thinnest and is before ovulation. Day 10 is the last recommended day to avoid the possibility of aborting an early pregnancy and to avoid the thicker secretory endometrium of the second half of the menstrual cycle. The thicker secretory endometrium may appear mildly "wrinkled" which can result in a false-positive endometrial pathology diagnosis.[1,8] If the menstrual cycle is irregular, the examination may be performed after a negative pregnancy test. Perimenopausal patients SHGs are scheduled similarly to those who are premenopausal, as an unexpected pregnancy may occur. Postmenopausal patients' on cyclical hormonal therapy should be scheduled similarly to a patient who is naturally cycling. Patients on continuous hormone replacement therapy with unopposed estrogen may undergo the procedure at any time.

Bleeding is not a contraindication to the procedure but should be avoided in order to limit the likelihood of a false-positive endometrial

[a] Department of Medical Imaging, University of Toronto, Sunnybrook Hospital, Room AG280, 2075 Bayview Avenue, Toronto, Ontario, Canada M4N 3 M5
[b] Department of Radiology, University of Pennsylvania, Hospital of the University of Pennsylvania 3400 Spruce Street Founders 1, Philadelphia, PA 19104-4283, USA
* Corresponding author. Department Medical Imaging, Women's College Hospital, 76 Grenville Street, Toronto, Ontario, Canada M5S 1 B2.
E-mail address: phyllis.glanc@wchospital.ca (P. Glanc).

Ultrasound Clin 3 (2008) 427–449
doi:10.1016/j.cult.2008.09.001

pathology diagnosis (due to the presence of blood clots). In the patient with irregular bleeding or prolonged menses, optimal scheduling may not be an option; however, gentle catheter manipulation and saline flushing during real-time sonography will diminish the likelihood of mistaking an adherent true lesion from a free-floating blood clot.[9]

Indications

The most common indication is abnormal uterine bleeding in premenopausal and postmenopausal women. Additional indications include the evaluation of infertility and recurrent abortions, congenital or acquired uterine abnormalities, detailed evaluation of the uterine cavity (for leiomyomas, polyps, or synechiae), abnormalities noted on TV US, or a suboptimally-visualized endometrium on TV US.[10]

Contraindications

Contraindications include pregnancy or active pelvic disease. The presence of an intrauterine device is considered a relative contraindication.[8] Women with known bilateral tubal occlusion may be placed on prophylactic antibiotics or monitored postprocedure. Active bleeding is not a contraindication and may, in fact, be the indication for the examination. However, it may make interpretation more challenging.

Preprocedure Medications and Consent

The most common complication is discomfort or mild pain during the procedure. We instruct our patients to take a nonsteroidal anti-inflammatory drug approximately 30 to 60 minutes before the procedure. As a general recommendation, we advise the patient to take whatever she normally uses for menstrual cramping. If asked for a specific drug we recommend ibuprofen, 200 to 400 mg.[8,11]

If the patient's history or physical examination is consistent with active pelvic inflammatory disease (PID), we usually delay the examination until after a course of antibiotics to minimize the risk of exacerbating the infection. If the patient has nontender hydrosalpinges, we will perform the examination after discussing the need for prophylactic or periprocedural antibiotics with the referring physician. Many physicians will watch and wait for symptoms before administering antibiotics in patients with obstructed or distended fallopian tubes because the risk of infection is felt to be low (approximately 1%).[12] Some of the authors advocate prophylactic antibiotics, in particular for infertile patients.[13] The evaluation of patients at risk for systemic bacterial endocarditis is a complex issue for which the

authors recommend referring to the American Heart Association's guidelines.[14]

We obtain written informed consent after discussing the risks of pain similar to menstrual cramping, the possibility of infection, and answering any questions the patient may have. The patient is advised to self-monitor postprocedure for abnormal bleeding or symptoms of infection (such as fever, pelvic pain, or foul smelling vaginal discharge) in which case she should contact her physician. Uterine perforation is an extremely unlikely complication; therefore, we do not include it in our informed consent process.[15] Some physicians will recommend the avoidance of intercourse for several days postprocedure to minimize the risk of infection.[9]

Psychologic Component

Many patients are anxious about undergoing a SHG for a variety of reasons including "fear of the unknown," prior painful gynecologic examination, or concern about their diagnosis. We have found it helpful to encourage patient involvement by requesting she become part of the team and immediately inform us of any discomfort, which results in stopping that component of the examination. We feel this technique of "patient empowerment" has resulted in diminished anxiety and improved cooperation in our patient population. We prefer the patient to be in a slightly upright position, approximately 45 degrees, to enable operator-patient eye contact. Slightly indenting the drapes centrally facilitates eye contact. We communicate to the patient regarding features provided for her comfort; including a locked door environment, adequate draping to ensure physical privacy, a "heating pad" on the lower abdomen to provide a comfort point to focus on, a prewarmed speculum, and a female in attendance.

At the end of the examination, a review of what the patient may expect, such as minimal spotting, and providing a sanitary napkin will provide a positive ending to the examination. The patient will often ask the results of the examination. When possible, informing her of the results, particularly if normal, is helpful.

Examination Technique

The patient is placed in a semi-upright lithotomy position with her thighs flexed and abducted, feet resting in padded stirrups, and buttocks extending slightly over the edge of a gynecologic examination table for ease of probe manipulation. If such a table is unavailable, a specially designed firm, angled pad with a cutout for probe maneuverability can be purchased. Preliminary routine TV

US is performed. Preprocedural knowledge of uterine flexion and version can be useful in directing speculum and catheter placement.

In patients who have undergone childbirth, we begin with a medium Miller speculum with biconcave wide blades and an open side hinge through which the catheter can easily be removed before speculum withdrawal. The Graves speculum is similar but without the open side hinge. For a sexually active but nulliparous female, a medium Pederson with its narrower and straight blades may be chosen. A small (pediatric) Pederson speculum is useful in patients with a small introitus or atrophic vaginal mucosa. Application of gel to the speculum may be helpful to ease insertion. In pelvic floor prolapse, vaginal wall laxity, or obese patients, a large Graves speculum may help with optimal visualization. With extremely lax vaginal walls, a condom or glove with the tip cut open can be placed over the speculum or lateral vaginal sidewall retractors may be used. Disposable, internally illuminated plastic speculums can be used but tend to have thinner blades than the Graves or Miller models.

The metal speculum is always prewarmed in sterile water for patient comfort and ease of insertion. This is usually achieved by placing the unopened container of saline in a basin of hot tap water, although a microwave can also be used. The closed speculum is slowly inserted at a 45-degree angle downward toward the posterior vaginal wall and then rotated into a horizontal position. The blades are opened and the speculum maneuvered until the cervix comes into full view, the speculum is then secured open by tightening the thumbscrew.

The external cervical os is cleansed and a catheter inserted into the endocervical canal or uterine cavity. Simple maneuvers such as using the other hand to press down on the abdomen or repositioning the speculum may modify the uterine angle to achieve success. If difficulty persists, additional options include an outer introducer sheath placed into the external cervical os, a guide wire to stiffen the catheter, or a larger (thus stiffer) catheter.[12,15] Occasionally a tenaculum is required to provide traction to straighten the cervix, in particular in the case of a very soft cervix, or an acutely anteflexed or retroflexed cervix. The tenaculum is placed on the anterior cervical lip at the 12 o'clock position with minimum ratcheting to decrease pressure on the cervical tissue. The 3 and 9 o'clock positions are avoided to minimize bleeding from paracervical vessels. Cervical dilators may be required in the setting of cervical stenosis.

If a balloon catheter is used, it is slowly inflated with approximately 1 mL of sterile normal saline. Then cautious mild traction is applied to ensure stable placement. If the catheter has been advanced too far so that it touches the uterine fundus, it may elicit a vasovagal response or cramping.[9,11] Prior knowledge of the cervix length and visual marking of the catheter will enable approximate placement of the catheter. Subsequently the speculum can be removed and the TV US probe introduced.

Slow instillation of 3 to 10 mL of prewarmed sterile saline, with accompanying gradual distension of the endometrial cavity, will diminish the likelihood of precipitating cramping. The saline acts as a negative contrast agent against the more echogenic endometrial lining. Positive contrast media has been used, more commonly, for evaluation of tubal patency. Exalto and colleagues[16] performed a study using a sterile gel preparation of hydroxyethylcellulose and glycerol containing lidocaine where an average volume of 4 mL provided stable distension of the uterine cavity for several minutes due to lower leakage velocity through the fallopian tubes and cervix. This preliminary work suggests this may be an attractive alternative that will provide stable uterine cavity distension. A limitation of this gel technique is that saline flushing, as an aid to distinguish blood clots from polyps, cannot readily be performed.[16]

Catheter choices vary widely and are a matter of operator preference. A popular option is a balloon tip catheter that can be inflated to minimize saline reflux or catheter dislodgement, particularly for patients with a patulous or incompetent cervix. The catheter should be flushed with water and the balloon filled with water to avoid obscuration of structures by gas. A simple thin pediatric feeding catheter or slightly stiffer insemination catheters are inexpensive options. Foley catheters, although inexpensive, are soft and flexible, increasing the difficulty of the procedure from the physician's perspective. A catheter equipped with a stopper affixed to the external cervical os, such as the Goldstein catheter or ZUI-2.0 catheter, is better tolerated by patients. However, a balloon catheter ensures a better seal requiring less fluid instillation.[17] Speldoch and colleagues[11] published a prospective randomized trial comparing cervical versus uterine placement of a balloon catheter. After initial inflation, there was significantly less pain with intracervical placement and a smaller volume of saline instillation was required for adequate visualization. They speculated that the different innervation of the cervix and its relative lack of smooth muscle compared with the uterus may minimize pain stimulation and perception.

Examination Documentation

Once adequate distension of the uterine cavity has been achieved, we acquire a sagittal sweep from cornua to cornua, followed by an axial sweep from fundus to external cervical os. If a balloon catheter has been inflated in the lower uterine segment, it is now deflated with a second series of images obtained of the lower uterine segment and cervix as the catheter is withdrawn. If 3D imaging software is available, then 3D volumes are obtained initially from the midline sagittal plane and then from the midpoint of the uterus in an axial plane. At the end of the examination, we briefly evaluate the presence of free fluid. When present, it indicates at least one fallopian tube is patent. If there is no free fluid, we advise the patient that her risk of potential PID may be increased and review the self-monitoring instructions for potential infection.

Potential Pitfalls

Potential pitfalls resulting in false-positive diagnosis may occur due to blood clots, mucus plugs, or endometrial shearing by the catheter. Blood clots may be identified by motion during saline flushing or catheter manipulation; whereas fixed or adherent endometrial lesions cannot be flushed from their location.[18] If color flow is demonstrated, a blood clot can be excluded. Soft-tip catheters minimize inadvertent endometrial shearing. Endocervical catheter placement of a balloon catheter or use of the Goldstein-type catheter will avoid endometrial shearing. However, saline flushing and catheter manipulation with respect to a suspected clot will not be available. The balloon catheter may obscure local pathology and should be deflated before ending the examination (**Fig. 1**A, B). Overdistension of the endometrial

cavity may result in underestimation of the degree of pathology. Obstruction to catheter placement past the internal cervical os may indicate cervical pathology such as a mass or adhesions. This knowledge is particularly relevant to women undergoing assisted-reproduction techniques and may require pre-procedural cervical lesion resection or dilation.

Role of Three-Dimensional Sonohysterography

The addition of 3D SHG to conventional two-dimensional (2D) SHG involves a rapid acquisition of data volumes which is then stored for subsequent analysis. At the time of acquisition, a rapid review ensures adequate coverage has been obtained. A second volume may be required to complete coverage of the uterus and cervix. The addition of 3D US is relatively rapid with no concerns about image degradation by motion as in obstetric imaging.[19] The advantages include the digital storage of entire data volume sets, rapid simultaneous correlation of three orthogonal planes (**Fig. 2**), and decreased time required to maintain uterine cavity distension. Although the coronal multiplanar reformatted (MPR) view obtained from the 3D volume is inherently lower in resolution than an image acquired in-plane, the addition of a coronal view may add significant diagnostic information in as many as 30.8% of patients.[20–22] This includes evaluation of the external uterine contour,[23] detection of adhesions,[24] and identification of focal pathology.[20] Benacerraf and colleagues[24] found an improvement in diagnostic information and examiner confidence in approximately 24% of cases. Rendered 3D images provide a sense of depth and spatial relationships (**Fig. 3**). The volume of data can be sliced

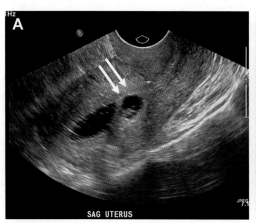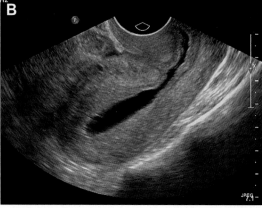

Fig. 1. Normal SHG: (*A*) Technical artifact in the lower-uterine segment due to shadowing from minimal amount of air in the balloon of the SHG catheter (*arrows*). (*B*) Post-balloon deflation and pullout of catheter while injecting saline demonstrates normal lower-uterine segment and cervical canal.

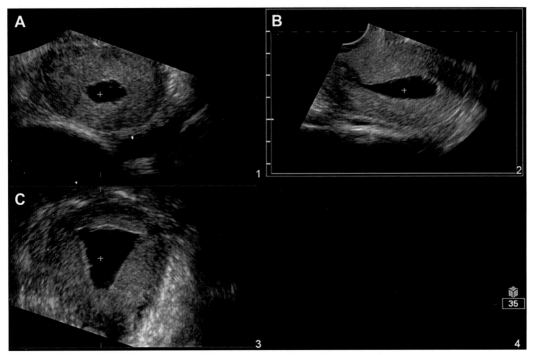

Fig. 2. Normal uterus and uterine cavity demonstrated on multiplanar display of 3D sonohysterogram. (A) Transverse. (B) Sagittal. (C) Coronal reconstructed view.

into sequential images at a prescribed thickness and interval (Fig. 4).The most common artifact encountered is the "enhancement artifact" in which the echogenic endometrium appears to extend beyond the endometrial–myometrial interface.[25]

CLINICAL APPLICATIONS

Histology remains the definitive diagnosis in all women with abnormal uterine bleeding unresponsive to medical or hormonal therapy.[26] The role of imaging is to: (1) determine if endometrial pathology is global or focal, (2) guide the type of histologic sampling technique, (3) document and guide the method of resection of submucosal or intracavitary fibroids, and (4) define mural (rather than endometrial) abnormalities such as fibroids or adenomyosis. The driving force behind histologic sampling is that in postmenopausal women (PMW) abnormal bleeding is the presenting sign in 80% to 85% of endometrial cancers; thus offering an opportunity for early-stage resection. Alternatively, endometrial cancer accounts for only 10% of postmenopausal bleeding, whereas postmenopausal atrophy accounts for 40% to 50%.[27] In premenopausal women, abnormal bleeding is proportionately less often due to endometrial cancer, although 5% to 10% of endometrial cancers occur in women less than age 40.[5,26,27] When

a patient presents with bleeding per the vagina, there is a long differential to consider; including lesions anywhere along the genital tract, medical conditions, and iatrogenic causes.

What is the Role of Sonohysterography in Abnormal Uterine Bleeding?

TV US provides good screening for abnormal uterine bleeding in that it is widely accessible, well tolerated, relatively inexpensive, and has a high sensitivity (96%) in the detection of endometrial

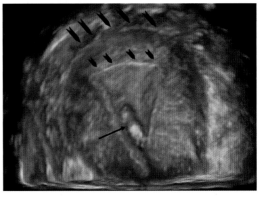

Fig. 3. Normal uterus and uterine cavity on rendered coronal view obtained from 3D SHG. Note outer convex contour (long arrowheads); convex fundal contour (short arrowheads), triangular endometrial cavity, and catheter in lower uterus (arrow).

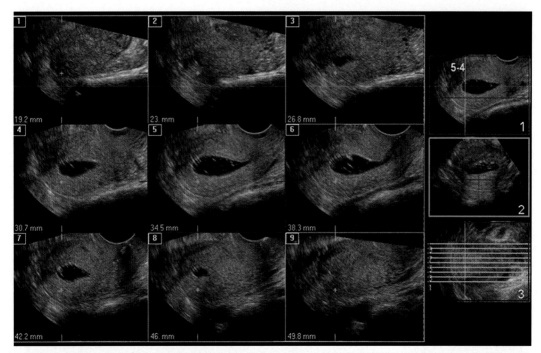

Fig. 4. Normal uterus and uterine cavity seen in a multiple sagittal slices format, obtained by means of 3D volume SHG. This so-called "iscan format" displays a series of images in a selected view (sagittal, axial, or coronal) obtained from the volume data set at a prescribed thickness and interval.

cancer in postmenopausal women at a cutoff of greater than 5 mm[28–30] compared with SHG (89%), nondirected endometrial biopsy (87%), and hysteroscopy (86%).[29,31,32] In premenopausal women, the sensitivity of TV US in detection of endometrial pathology is much lower: 67% at a cutoff of 16 mm.[33] SHG and hysteroscopy demonstrate similar performance characteristics with sensitivities and specificities of 95% and 88%, respectively, for SHG[34] and 96% and 90% for hysteroscopy.[3] The key advantage of hysteroscopy is its ability to provide histologic sampling. SHG is less invasive, less expensive, well tolerated without a need for sedation, and has no major complications. SHG can provide a guide for focal hysteroscopic resection, decrease the rate of negative hysteroscopy, and redirect the approximately one third of women for whom hysteroscopy is not the appropriate therapy.[4] This includes cases such as: normal endometrium, global endometrial pathology, subendometrial pathology as in fibroids or adenomyosis, or as a problem solver when the results of the TV US and the biopsy are discordant. SHG plays an important role in the significant percentage of patients in whom TV US does not optimally visualize the endometrium; typically quoted as 5% to 10%, but ranging as high as 18%.[10,35] Suboptimal endometrial visualization is commonly due to an angulated uterus limiting the ability of the probe to image perpendicular to the long axis of the uterus, co-existing pathology (such as fibroids), or an indistinct endometrial–myometrial interface. Many of these challenges can be overcome by the incorporation of 3D US into the 3D SHG.

Endometrial Thickness Measurements

How much endometrial thickness should be considered abnormal remains a controversial topic. Nonetheless, endometrial thickness is a good indicator of absence or presence of proliferation; limiting the need for biopsy of symptomatic women to those in whom the bilayer measurements (two basalis layers and the central specular reflection of the lumen) is greater than 4 to 5 mm.[36–38] Endometrial cancer is rare with a negative predictive of value of 96% when the endometrium is less than 5 mm, regardless of whether the woman was on hormone replacement therapy.[37] Smith-Bindman and colleagues'[36] meta-analysis suggests that the endometrial cancer risk in symptomatic PMW is less than 0.07% if the endometrium is less than or equal to 5 mm, and 7.3% if the endometrium is greater than 5 mm. In the asymptomatic PMW, the risk of endometrial cancer is 0.002% if the endometrium is less than or equal to 11 mm, and 6.7% when the endometrium measures greater than 11 mm. They concluded that biopsy is unnecessary in the asymptomatic

PMW with an endometrial measurement less than or equal to 11 mm. Approximately 5% of PMW will have an endometrial measurement between 5 and 11 mm.[39] The risk of cancer or atypical hyperplasia in the 5 to 11 mm range is not zero.[37,38,40,41] Also, no consensus has been reached on the usefulness of screening by TV US or on which cut-off between 5 and 11 mm should trigger further investigations.[42] The Society for Radiologists in Ultrasound Consensus Conference[43] determined that with an endometrium less than or equal to 5 mm the risk of endometrial cancer is low at approximately 1%, achieving a sensitivity similar to endometrial blind biopsy whether the patient was on hormone replacement therapy or not. They also concluded that there is no known acceptable upper limit of normal for any patient and that further evaluation is warranted in symptomatic patients with an endometrial thickness measurement greater than 5 mm. A paper published by Bree and colleagues[18] reported that almost one third of patients with an endometrial thickness less than or equal to 5 mm had an abnormality; leaving unanswered the question of the importance of finding benign disease. There are well established norms in the premenopausal endometrium reported as measuring 2 to 4 mm in the early proliferative phase after cessation of menses, in the periovulatory phase measuring 8 to 10 mm with a layered appearance, and in the postovulation secretory phase appearing uniformly echogenic measuring up to 16 mm.[44]

Endometrial Polyps

Endometrial polyps are a source of bleeding in both premenopausal and postmenopausal women. They are associated with infertility and account for 30% of bleeding in PMW. The majority of polyps are benign. However, as US cannot reliably distinguish between benign and malignant polyps, they are all resected for histologic evaluation. The incidence of malignancy in polyps ranges from 0.5% to 1.5%.[45] The prevalence of uterine polyps is approximately 10% in asymptomatic women versus 33% in symptomatic women.[46]

Endometrial polyps are generally isoechoic relative to the endometrium and echogenic to the myometrium. They may be pedunculated on a stalk or sessile, but the underlying endometrial–myometrial interface is preserved. The margins are usually smooth (**Figs. 5** and **6**). [47,48] Use of color Doppler ultrasound to identify a single central-feeder vessel may have a positive predictive value up to 81.3%,[48] potentially providing an alternative to SHG (**Fig. 7**). Submucosal or pedunculated fibroids show either no vascular pedicle or an arborizing pattern.[18,49] Cystic change within polyps

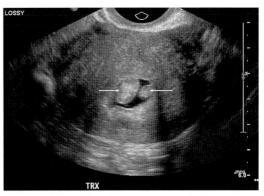

Fig. 5. Endometrial polyps: Transverse image from sonohysterogram demonstrates two endometrial polyps (*arrows*) which are homogenous and smoothly marginated with preserved underlying endometrial–myometrial interface.

is relatively common and may be due to hemorrhage, infarction, inflammation, dilated glands, or mucinous metaplasia as in tamoxifen-associated polyps (**Fig. 8**). Atypical polyps may contain larger cystic spaces, are multiple, broad-based, hypoechoic, or heterogenous. Endometrial hyperplasia is similarly echogenic and may contain cystic spaces so that TV US alone cannot reliably distinguish between these two entities. The addition of saline to separate the endometrial walls will permit distinction of a focal, versus a diffuse, endometrial abnormality, thus directing management. In a patient who has recently undergone a dilation and curettage (D&C) or is postpartum with an endometrial polypoid lesion, a placental polyp originating from chronic retained placental fragments should be considered. These polyps may be vascular, resulting in bleeding and persistent mild elevation of beta-human chorionic gonadotropin.

Cervical polyps have a low incidence of malignancy (0.3%); however, they are often removed as they tend to cause bleeding.[50,51] Perhaps of greater significance is their association with endometrial polyps in 26.7% of patients, more specifically in all PMW on tamoxifen and 40.8% of PMW (**Fig. 9**).[51]

Endometrial Hyperplasia

Endometrial hyperplasia results from unopposed estrogenic stimulation of the endometrium, causing PMB in roughly 4% to 8% of cases.[8] Simple hyperplasia rarely progresses to endometrial carcinoma; whereas in atypical hyperplasia, approximately 23% will progress to endometrial cancer.[52] As US cannot distinguish between these two subtypes of endometrial hyperplasia, histopathological correlation is recommended in all cases.[53]

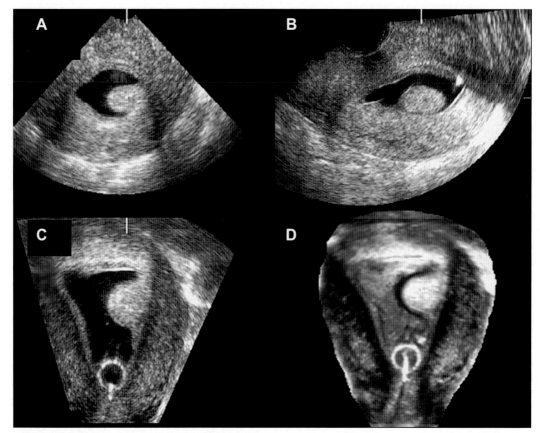

Fig. 6. Multiplanar display with rendered coronal view obtained during SHG using 3D volume sonography demonstrates single endometrial polyp. (*A*) Transverse. (*B*) Sagittal. (*C*) Coronal reconstructed view. (*D*) Rendered coronal view.

Endometrial hyperplasia generally appears as a diffuse thickening of the endometrium; however, it may be focal, may contain cysts in approximately 50%, and concomitant polyps are present in approximately 25% (**Fig. 10**).[54] The US appearance can mimic the normal endometrial thickening of the secretory phase, underscoring the importance of performing SHG in the early proliferative phase.

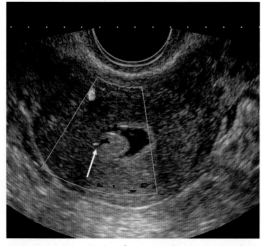

Fig. 7. Transverse image from sonohysterogram demonstrates broad-based polyp with single vascular pedicle (*arrow*).

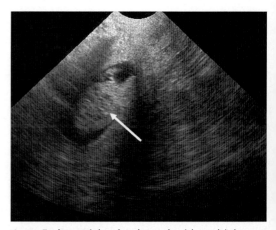

Fig. 8. Endometrial polyp (*arrow*) with multiple cysts on sonohysterogram.

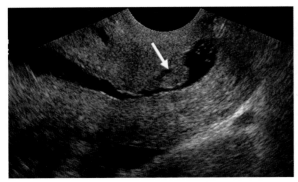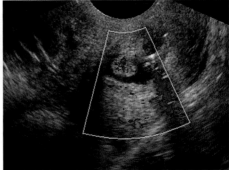

Fig. 9. Cervical polyp on SHG demonstrated by slow removal of the SHG catheter while instilling additional saline at the end of the procedure. (*A*) Sagittal image with polyp (*arrow*). (*B*) Transverse image with color Doppler sonography (CDS) demonstrates flow within polyp.

Endometrial Cancer

The peak of endometrial cancer occurs at age 55, 75% of patients are PMW, and 5% to 10% are less than age 40.[5,26,27] Although endometrial cancer is the fourth most common cancer in women in the United States, and the most common invasive gynecologic malignancy, it is not a leading cause of death due to early detection and treatment. Endometrial cancer, as in endometrial hyperplasia, is related to unopposed estrogen stimulation. The most important single risk factor is age followed by obesity (secondary to increased estrogen production and bioavailability as weight increases.) Other risk factors include nulliparity, early menarche, late menopause, hypertension, diabetes,

and polycystic ovarian syndrome. Approximately 85% to 90% are well-differentiated adenocarcinomas with a good prognosis. Less common are adenosquamous, clear cell or papillary serous carincomas, and sarcomatous variants with more aggressive patterns and poorer prognosis.[29]

Endometrial cancer is typically a diffuse process but will occasionally present as a polypoid or focal mass.[47,55] The US features are nonspecific so that endometrial cancer is difficult to distinguish from hyperplasia or polyps, resulting in a recommendation for histologic correlation in any of these findings, especially in PMW. Color Doppler has not been proven to reliably distinguish a benign from malignant process. MR imaging is also limited in the distinction of endometrial carcinoma from

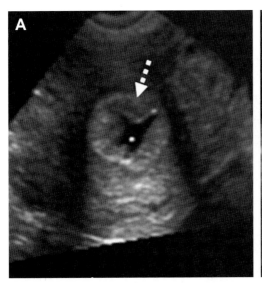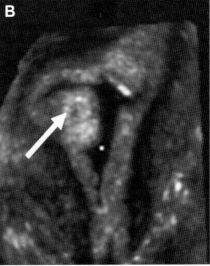

Fig. 10. Multiplanar display obtained during sonohysterography using 3D volume sonography demonstrates diffuse mild endometrial thickening and polyps. Pathology confirmed benign endometrial hyperplasia and polyps. (*A*) Transverse view: Benign endometrial hyperplasia (*perforated arrow*). (*B*) Reconstructed Coronal view: Fundal polyp (*arrow*) clearly delineated from surrounding endometrial hyperplasia.

hyperplasia, but is helpful for staging the depth of myometrial invasion.[44] Suspicious ultrasound features include: heterogeneity, irregular or ill-defined margins, loss of underlying endometrial–myometrial interface of concern for invasion, and lack of uterine cavity distensibility (**Fig. 11**).[47]

Although theoretic concerns have been raised about the risk of flushing malignant cells into the peritoneal cavity during an SHG, several small prospective studies have demonstrated it is doubtful that viable malignant cells are disseminated.[56,57] Until further research is available it may be prudent to use low volumes to minimize potential transtubal dissemination of viable cancer cells.

Tamoxifen Induced Endometrial Changes

Tamoxifen is an adjunct therapy for breast cancer in PMW. It has an antiestrogenic effect in breast tissue, but a weakly estrogenic effect on the endometrium resulting in a 2.2 fold increased risk of endometrial cancer.[58] Subsequent studies by Tepper and colleagues[59] and Fong and colleagues[60] demonstrated a high incidence of endometrial abnormalities ranging from 32% to 40% in patients treated with tamoxifen, but no cases of atypical endometrial hyperplasia or endometrial cancer. The consensus statement from the Society of Radiologists in Ultrasound[43] concluded that routine screening in asymptomatic patients on tamoxifen therapy is warranted. Cystic changes are commonly found in endometrial polyps, hyperplasia, or carcinoma, in addition to areas of glandular cystic atrophy or within the subendometrial myometrium. It is believed that tamoxifen causes reactivation of adenomyosis in the inner layer of the myometrium resulting in an apparent thickening of the endometrium on TV US. SHG can reliably distinguish the subgroup

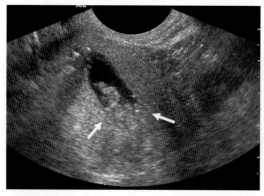

Fig. 11. Endometrial cancer: Transverse image from sonohysterogram demonstrates an irregular polypoid mass with loss of endometrial–myometrial interface (*between the arrows*).

of patients on Tamoxifen (~8%) who develop sub-endometrial cystic changes which require no further intervention from those with endometrial pathology.[61]

Postmenopausal Endometrial Atrophy

Women with PMB but a thin endometrium less than or equal to 5 mm presumably have a senile endometritis, prone to superficial ulcerations and bleeding. Senile hyperplasia or cystic atrophy of the endometrium represents dilated but nonproliferative glands occurring in up to 8% of asymptomatic PMW.[62]

Approach to the Patient with Bleeding

In the setting of postmenopausal bleeding or premenopausal bleeding unresponsive to hormonal or medical therapy, further evaluation with a TV US is appropriate. If the endometrium appears normal ($\leq$5 mm in PMW or $\leq$16 mm in premenopausal patient), the recommended choice is a clinical evaluation; although some clinicians may recommend a SHG[28] for the reassurance a negative result confers. If the TV US demonstrates thick, abnormal, or suboptimally visualized endometrium, then SHG or hysteroscopy may be performed. If the SHG demonstrates a focal lesion then hysteroscopic resection is appropriate. If there is global endometrial pathology, then endometrial sampling by D&C or blind biopsy is recommended. There are a number of alternate approaches which may begin with blind endometrial biopsy (EMB) or blind EMB after transvaginal ultrasound with any abnormality. Further work needs to be done to optimize the best algorithm on a cost-effective basis.

Benign Uterine Pathology

Uterine leiomyomas or fibroids

Uterine leiomyomas or fibroids are the most common gynecologic tumors occurring in 20% to 40% of women, of which 25% will present with symptoms of bleeding, pain, or infertility.[63–65] Fibroids account for approximately 10% of PMB.[55] They are benign smooth muscle tumors typically surrounded by a pseudocapsule. The classic fibroid is a well-defined hypoechoic (relative to the myometrium) lesion associated with posterior attenuation of sound, edge shadows, recurrent refractive shadowing, and a diffuse arborizing pattern of vascularity.[63,65] Fibroids may have a variable appearance, particularly as they enlarge and outstrip their vascular supply which can result in areas of cystic, myxoid, calcific, or hemorrhagic degeneration. Occasionally a fibroid has a high lipomatous content and appears echogenic. Leiomyosarcoma is difficult to distinguish from leiomyoma unless there is local invasion or distant metastases. Rapid growth, especially in PMW, should raise the possibility of sarcomatous transformation. SHG has proven clinically useful in the diagnosis and classification of submucosal fibroids. Submucosal fibroids are broad based, continuous with the underlying myometrium with a similar echogenicity, well defined, and with obtuse angles to the underlying endometrium unless they are almost completely intracavitary. A smooth echogenic endometrial lining should cover the surface of the relatively hypoechoic fibroid, although erosions are not infrequent.[55] Occasionally the overlying endometrium is thick and irregular suggesting chronic inflammation or edema.[55] The number, size, location, and depth of myometrial involvement or protrusion into the endometrial cavity should be documented. Larger mural fibroids may also distort the endometrial cavity but their epicenter is within the

myometrium. For potential hysteroscopic resection of larger submucosal fibroids, it is important to document the remaining peripheral rim of myometrium as less than or greater than 1 cm.[64] The location of a submucous fibroid with respect to the uterine cavity may be classified according to the European Society of Hysteroscopy system in which Type 0 are entirely intracavitary, Type 1 are greater than 50% intracavitary, and Type 2 are less than or equal to 50% intracavitary (**Figs. 12–14**).[66]

Adenomyosis

Adenomyosis is a common gynecologic condition affecting menstruating women. It is characterized by migration of endometrial glands and stroma into the myometrium, associated with surrounding smooth muscle hypertrophy.[67] Patients present with non-specific symptoms such as dysmenorrhea, uterine tenderness, menorrhagia, and

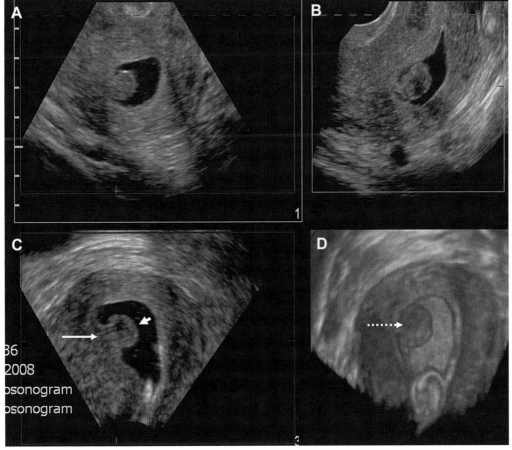

Fig. 12. Intracavitary submucous fibroid, Type 0. Multiplanar display with rendered coronal view obtained during SHG using 3D volume sonography. (*A*) Transverse image. (*B*) Sagittal image. (*C*) Coronal reconstructed view demonstrates continuity with the underlying myometrium (*arrow*) and the surface covered by a thin layer of endometrium (*arrowhead*). The fibroid is isoechoic with the myometrium. (*D*) Rendered coronal view provides depth perception and depicts the spatial relationship of the fibroid within the uterine cavity (*perforated arrow*).

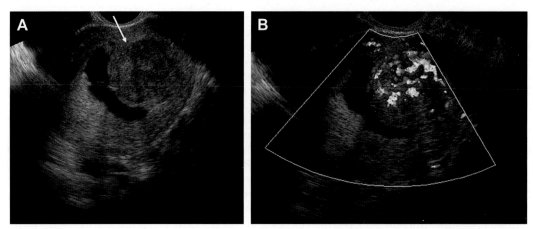

Fig.13. SHG demonstrates a Type 2 submucous fibroid with less than 50% protruding intracavitary. (*A*) Transverse image of fibroid (*arrow*) demonstrates refractive shadowing and overlying echogenic line of endometrium. (*B*) Transverse image of fibroid with CDS demonstrates an arborizing pattern of flow.

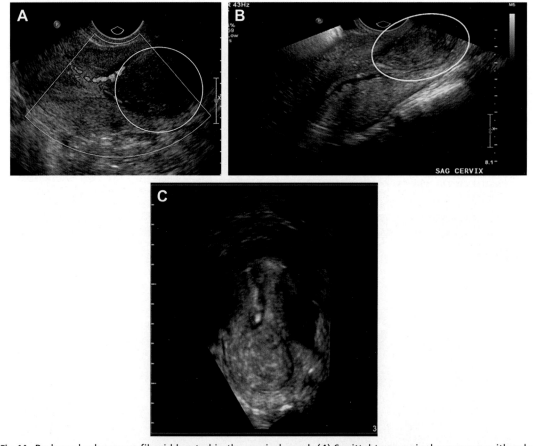

Fig.14. Prolapsed submucous fibroid located in the cervical canal. (*A*) Sagittal transvaginal sonogram with color Doppler demonstrates hypoechoic mass in region of the lower uterine segment and cervix with vessels coursing toward it. (*B*) Sagittal view from 3D volume sonohysterogram shows minimal fluid above cervical lesion. The vascularized stalk of the prolapsing myoma was seen on another sagittal plane. (*C*) Reconstructed coronal plane from 3D volume sonohysterogram obtained with minimal fluid demonstrates otherwise normal endometrial cavity and expanded cervical canal due to prolapsing fibroid.

uterine enlargement. Although they commonly co-exist with fibroids, their distinction is important as their treatments are different. Fibroids can be surgically resected, whereas adenomyosis is treated medically with agents such as gonadotropin-releasing hormone inhibitors, oral contraceptives, nonsteroidal inflammatory agents, or endometrial ablation or resection.[68]

There is a spectrum of sonographic appearances including: subendometrial or myometrial cysts, indistinct endometrial–myometrial interface, subendometrial islands of echogenic nodules or linear striations surrounded by the relatively hypoechoic myometrium, an undulating appearance of the outer margin of the endometrium, asymmetric myometrial thickening, or a globular uterus (**Fig. 15**). The myometrium has abnormal echotexture typically hypoechoic or heterogenous with multiple-edge shadows but relatively little mass effect. In contrast, fibroids are well defined with mass effect. Both fibroids and adenomyosis may demonstrate edge shadows, refractive shadowing, and arborizing vascular patterns; although the vascularity may be more peripheral in fibroids. Less common appearances include localized mass or focal adenomyosis, or a larger adenomyotic cyst (presumably due bleeding into the ectopic endometrium). Adenomyosis may present with pseudoendometrial thickening, which can be distinguished from true endometrial abnormality using SHG.

Adhesions

The majority of adhesions are related to uterine trauma, typically a curettage performed in a recently gravid uterus, with the risk increasing as the number of procedures increases.[69,70] Clinical presentation may include menstrual disturbances (hypomenorrhea, amenorrhea, or cyclic pelvic pain), infertility, and recurrent pregnancy losses. Approximately 50% of women with intrauterine adhesions will suffer from a degree of infertility.[13,70] Despite the presence of extensive synechiae, TV US may appear normal, whereas after saline distension of the endometrial cavity adhesions are readily identified.[13] The sensitivity of SHG in the diagnosis of adhesions is 75%, the specificity is 93%,[8] and the positive predictive value is 43%.[69] The high false-positive rate implies that this examination is best used for screening, rather than diagnosis,[69] and should be followed by a definitive hysterocopic diagnosis and therapy as appropriate.

Adhesions are seen as bridging bands of tissue with no associated mass. They may be thin and mobile or thick and adherent bands which constrict or obliterate the endometrial cavity as in Asherman's syndrome (**Figs. 16** and **17**).[13,55] Lysis of adhesions is chosen for patients with infertility, recurrent pregnancy losses, or pain. After lysis of adhesions, SHG may be helpful to determine the adequacy of the procedure and evaluate for recurrence.[13]

True uterine arteriovenous malformations
True uterine arteriovenous malformations are rare. They may be congenital or acquired. Patients may present with uterine bleeding. The sonographic appearance is nonspecific with a tangle of tubular anechoic spaces in the myometrium containing abundant high-velocity turbulent flow and low-resistance pattern. Angiography confirms the diagnosis by demonstrating early venous filling.[71] The US appearance may overlap with entities such as trophoblastic disease, retained products of conception, or abnormal placentation. This distinction is important as treatment by D&C of a true arteriovenous malformation may increase the risk for bleeding.

Retained products of conception
In general, retained products of conception (RPOC) are diagnosed based on clinical and routine TV US findings. Immediately postpartum, the inner myometrium may be increased in echogenicity so that it is difficult to determine the endometrium–myometrium interface, limiting measurement accuracy. By six to eight weeks the uterus should be normal in size and appearance.[72] The endometrial measurements for diagnosis are arbitrary, with cut off values ranging from 5 to 20 mm.[44] Hertzberg and colleagues[73] suggest that with an endometrial thickness less than 15 mm RPOC is unlikely. RPOC on US is nonspecific, but a focal echogenic mass or mass with punctate hyperechoic foci associated with abundant flow and adherent to the uterine wall is highly

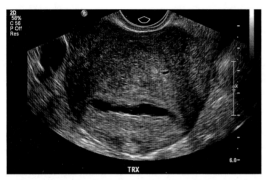

Fig. 15. Adenomyosis: Transverse image from sonohysterogram demonstrates asymmetric thickening of the anterior myometrium with heterogenous echotexture and scattered small cysts.

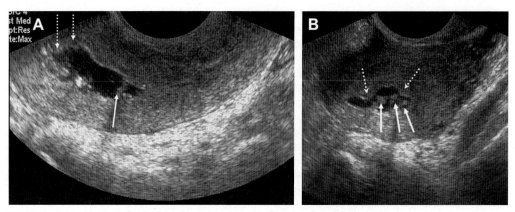

Fig. 16. SHG demonstrates multiple adhesions (*arrows*) with localized restriction of distention of the uterine cavity (*perforated arrows*). The patient has a history of prior D&C. (*A*) Sagittal. (*B*) Transverse.

suggestive.[47,73–75] The presence of color Doppler flow in a region of suspected RPOC is generally deemed supportive evidence; however, the reliability of this finding has conflicting published values and remains unknown.

After a term delivery or abortion, there may also be subinvolution of the placental bed or nonregression of trophoblastic tissue with abundant subendometrial and myometrial turbulent vascular flow with velocities as high as 90 to 100 cm per second. If there is no clear evidence of retained products or placental tissue within the endometrial cavity itself, conservative therapy awaiting spontaneous regression is generally

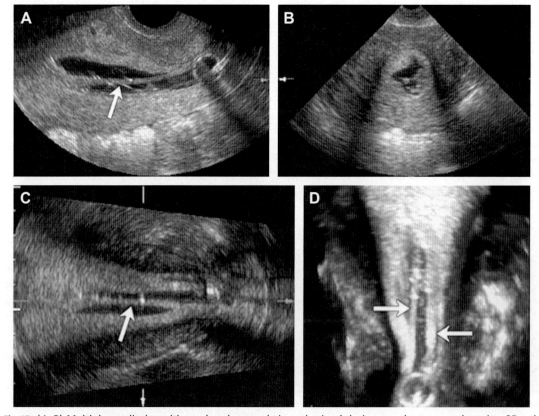

Fig. 17. (*A–D*) Multiplanar display with rendered coronal view obtained during sonohysterography using 3D volume sonography demonstrates thick adhesions (*arrows*) traversing the uterine cavity with minimal restriction in distension of the endometrial cavity. The patient has a history of D&C.

appropriate. However, the subset with higher peak systolic velocities, at least greater than 80 cm per second, may be at increased risk of significant bleeding and should be stratified into a group for careful monitoring and consideration of uterine artery embolization.[71,75] The group with peak systolic velocities under 40 cm per second appear to do well with conservative therapy alone.[71,75] SHG may play a role by confirming an intracavitary component suggesting RPOC in association with nonregression of trophoblastic tissue rather than a vascular malformation. SHG is useful when there are persistent clinical symptoms despite a negative TV US, or when symptoms persist after D&C. In these cases, SHG may be able to detect and localize a small amount of residual tissue for directed hysteroscopic resection.[55] SHG may also be useful to distinguish RPOC from a blood clot because if a directed saline flush or catheter manipulation cannot move the lesion it implies an adherent lesion more likely to represent RPOC (**Fig. 18**).[72]

Cesarean section niche
In virtually all patients who have undergone a cesarean delivery, the SHG will reveal triangular outpouching in the anterior lower uterine segment, with an average depth of 6 mm.[76] This defect, or cesarean section niche, occurs within the scar and is likely related to scar tissue retraction (**Fig. 19**). A larger defect may retain menstrual blood and be a cause for intermenstrual bleeding.

Intrauterine fluid
A small amount of intrauterine fluid is considered normal, but a significant amount requires careful evaluation with consideration of both endometrial and cervical pathology. This "natural SHG" is an opportunity to assess the endometrium, rather

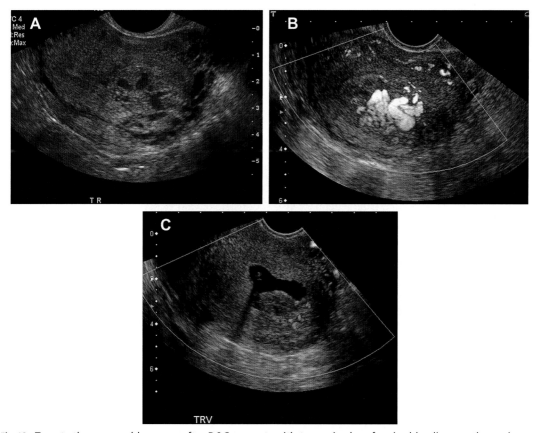

Fig. 18. Twenty-three year old woman after D&C presents with two episodes of major bleeding per the vagina requiring blood transfusions. Initial TV US demonstrated vascularized mass of heterogeneous echotexture located centrally in the upper uterus with peak systolic velocity as high as 150 cm per second. Initial treatment was angiographic embolization. Patient continued to bleed and therapeutic D&C was performed with no complications and evacuation of trophoblastic tissue. (*A*) TV US sagittal image demonstrates heterogeneous mass with tubular anechoic spaces. (*B*) TV US transverse image demonstrates a tangle of large blood vessels. (*C*) Transverse image from sonohysterogram demonstrates a small intracavitary component. The majority of the flow is in the myometrium consistent with subinvolution of trophoblastic tissue and RPOC.

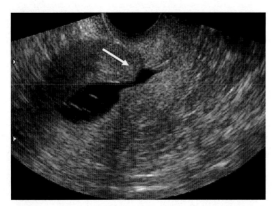

Fig. 19. Sagittal view from SHG demonstrates small tri-angular-shaped cesarean section defect (*arrow*).

than the fluid itself. In the premenopausal patient, early pregnancy, menstruation, or the pseudoges-tational sac of an ectopic pregnancy are consider-ations. Benign causes of obstruction and fluid production include polyps, infection, and submu-cosal fibroids. In the postmenopausal patient, the most commonly associated benign condition is a degree of cervical stenosis.

Intraoperative SHG may provide guidance for vi-sualization of focal pathology in the saline dis-tended uterine cavity, direct retrieval of sponges or foreign bodies, monitor the extent of removal of intrauterine synechiae, directed resections, or placement of intracavitary radiation seeds.[77]

Infertility

SHG is an important screening examination for in-fertility patients. It provides similar diagnostic results to office hysteroscopy, but uses a less in-vasive and less expensive technique.[78] Both MR imaging and SHG with MPR capabilities provide a noninvasive technique for Mullerian duct and ac-quired uterine anomaly evaluation. They demon-strate the relationship of the uterine cavity to the uterus and the external uterine contour, and have similar diagnostic accuracies.[6] High sensitivities and specificities approaching 100% can be achieved in the diagnosis of normal, arcuate, and major uterine MDA such as septate or bicornuate uterus with 3D SHG.[6,79]

The Mullerian ducts develop into the uterus, cer-vix, upper four-fifth of the vagina, and the fallopian tubes. In the normal population, MDA has an inci-dence of approximately 1%; whereas congenital or acquired uterine pathology may be present in up to 10% of infertile women, and in as much as 15% to 55% of patients with recurrent pregnancy losses.[6,7] The correct diagnosis is important to tri-age patients for whom interventional therapy such

as hysteroscopic resection (septate uterus) or abdominal metroplasty (bicornuate uterus) is appropriate.

The most widely used classification for MDA is from the American Fertility Society (AFA),[80] which is based on embryologic etiology (with the excep-tion of Class VII, which is reserved for embryologic abnormalities secondary to in utero exposure to diethylstilbestrol). This classification is limited be-cause it does not account for complex MDAs crossing categories or for vaginal anomalies such as septums; and, perhaps most important, be-cause it provides no measurements to help distin-guish whether a uterus is bicornuate, septate, or arcuate. Therefore, a detailed description of the findings are important. Salim and colleagues[81] modified the AFA classification system by adding observations and measurements which are ob-tained from the coronal view. The external uterine fundal contour should be convex, flat, or with an indentation less than1 cm.[75,81] Another method is to determine the distance from the external con-tour to a line drawn between the two interstial components of the fallopian tube: the interostial line. When the fundal indentation is less than or equal to 5 mm above the interostial line the uterus is considered to be either bicornuate or didelphic. In a septate uterus, the fundal indentation should be greater than 5 mm above the interostial line. If a line is drawn perpendicular to the midpoint of the interostial line to bisect the endometrial cavity and the angle at this central point is obtuse (greater than 105°), it is consistent with a bicornu-ate uterus. An acute angle of less than 75 to 90° is consistent with a septate uterus. Unfortunately, the majority of angles of divergence fall between these two numbers (**Table 1**).

The normal uterus has a single triangular uterine cavity and the external uterine fundal contour is either flat or convex outward. A mild concave in-dentation up to 1 cm may be within normal limits. Similarly, the uterine fundal contour (superior fun-dal contour of the uterine cavity) should be convex or flat; a concave contour would be considered abnormal (**Fig. 20**).[81]

AFA Class 1 MDA is associated with variable degrees of Mullerian agenesis and hypoplasia. Mayer-Rokitansky-Kuster-Hauser syndrome is the most common manifestation with complete vaginal agenesis and 90% association with uterine agenesis.

AFA Class II MDA anomaly is a unicornuate uterus (~20% of all MDA), with a single uterine cavity which may be associated with a rudimentary communicating or noncommunicating horn. Renal abnormalities are present in up to 40%, typically ipsilateral to the rudimentary horn, with ipsilateral

Table 1
Mullerian duct anomalies: distinguishing features on sonohysterography

	External Contour	Fundal Contour (Uterine Cavity)	Separation of Uterine Horns	Cervix
Normal	Convex, flat, or <1 cm fundal cleft	Convex or flat	Single triangular cavity	Single
Unicornuate	Convex or flat	Convex or flat Single cornual ostia on SHG	Single banana-shaped cavity	Single
Didelphys	Two well-formed uterine cornua, convex or flat	Two well formed uterine cornua with convex fundal contour in each with no communication	2 horns widely divergent, obtuse angle at the central point	Double
Bicornuate	Fundal cleft >1 cm	Two well-formed symmetric uterine cornua with convex fundal contour in each, fused caudally, communicate	2 horns widely divergent, obtuse angle at the central point	Single or double
Septate	Convex, flat, or <1 cm fundal cleft	Two well-formed symmetric uterine cornua, communicate	2 horns close, acute angle at the central point	Single or double (rare)
Subseptate	Convex, flat, or <1 cm fundal cleft	Two well-formed symmetric uterine cornua fused caudally, communicate	2 horns close, acute angle at the central point	Single
Arcuate	Convex, flat, or <1 cm fundal cleft	Single cavity with a broad shallow indentation	Obtuse angle at the central point (>105)	Single

Abbreviation: SHG, sonohysterography.

renal agenesis the most common finding. The unicornuate uterus has an elongated curved "banana" like configuration with overall reduction of uterine volume, smaller and deviated from the midline. The addition of MPR 3D US coronal view permits the demonstration of only one cornual angle confirming the diagnosis.

AFA Class III didelphys uterus (~5%) results from almost complete failure of fusion of the Mullerian ducts which results in two separate uterocervical cavities. The horns may vary from rudimentary to fully developed, but are always widely separated; therefore they may be difficult to image on a single 2D plane. There are separate but adjacent cervical canals. A longitudinal vaginal septum is present in up to 75%. When a transverse vaginal septum is present, women may present early due to hematometrocolpos.

AFA Class IV bicornuate uterus (~10%) results from incomplete fusion of the superior fundal aspect of the two Mullerian ducts. This results in an abnormal external fundal uterine contour which is concave with a fundal cleft greater than 1 cm. Imoaka and colleagues[82] suggest, based on MRI studies, that bicornuate uterus has an intercornual distance greater than 4 cm, fundal cleft depth greater than 1 cm, and widely divergent uterine horns with a large fundal cleft obtuse angle greater than 105 degrees. The cornua are typically symmetric and fused more caudally, resulting in a communicating cavity unlike the didelphic uterus. These rarely require surgery although surgical union of the two horns may be performed in selected patients with recurrent second and third trimester losses.[83] The cervix may be single or double.

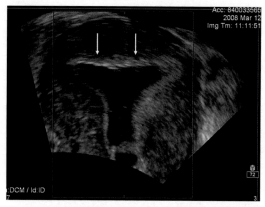

Fig. 20. Coronal reconstructed view from an SHG obtained with volume sonography shows a normal external fundal contour as well as a normal flat contour to the myometrium facing the fundal aspect of the uterine cavity (*arrows*).

AFA Class V septate uterus results from a failure of resorption of the uterovaginal septum after the Mullerian ducts have undergone complete fusion. The septate uterus is the most common Mullerian duct anomaly (55%) associated with both recurrent pregnancy losses and the worst obstetric outcomes of the MDAs. The outcomes may improve if the septum is resected. The septum arises in the fundus and extends caudally as far as the upper vagina. The septum is considered complete if it extends to the external cervical os. Extension into the upper vagina occurs in 25%. Typically the upper septum is myometrial tissue and the lower septum fibrous tissue (relatively hypoechoic to the myometrium). The external uterine contour is unremarkable and the endometrial cavities are close; the horns have an acute angle of divergence of less than 75° (**Fig. 21**).[7] If the septum does not

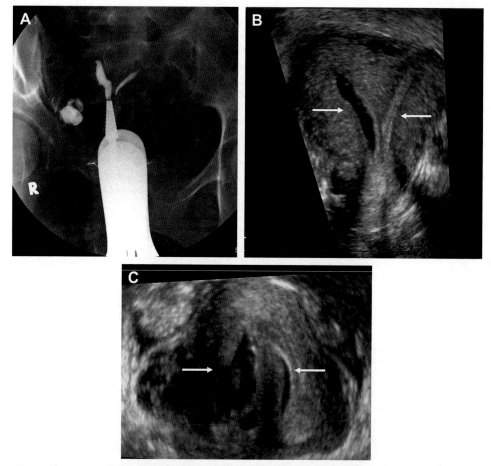

Fig. 21. Twenty-three year old female with history of resection of transverse vaginal septum and two first-trimester pregnancy losses. (*A*) Hysterosalpingogram demonstrates two separate uterine cavities, slighty more capacious on the right. (*B*) SHG coronal view after cannulation of the right cervical os demonstrates two separate endometrial cavities (*arrows*) with a narrow angle of divergence, and a normal external contour consistent with a septate uterus. There was no communication between the right and left hemicavities. (*C*) SHG coronal view demonstrates two separate cervical canals (*arrows*), indicating a septate uterus with septate cervix.

extend to the uterine isthmus it is termed a subseptate uterus (**Fig. 22**).

AFA Class VI arcuate uterus has a normal external uterine contour. There may be mild thickening of the midline fundal myometrium such that it measures greater than 1.5 cm depth, resulting in a myometrial fundal cavity indentation that is smooth and broad but less than 1 cm. The definition of an arcuate uterus with respect to the degree of fundal indentation remains controversial. However, it is generally accepted as a broad shallow fundal indentation with an obtuse angle at the central point, and a normal external contour. Controversy persists whether this represents a true anomaly or a normal anatomic variant. The literature reports both good and poor outcomes; however, it is generally considered compatible with normal term gestation. The true prevalence is unknown as this is a subtle abnormality easily missed on TV US, although readily identified on 3D SHG or MRI (**Fig. 23**).

AFA Class VII anomalies are sequelae of in utero diethystilbestrol exposure, most commonly resulting in a T-shaped uterine cavity; this drug was discontinued in 1971. Other findings include hypoplastic uterus, constriction, and associated abnormalities of the cervix and fallopian tubes.

Sonosalpingography or Fallopian Tube Evaluation

Positive contrast agents are widely available in Europe, but no longer commercially available in North America. Sonosalpingography (SSG) is best performed after saline SHG has initially evaluated the endometrial cavity because the positive contrast agent will mask the presence of endometrial pathology. There is additional advantage if the saline spills into the adnexae because it provides a hypoechoic background in which to better visualize the echogenic positive contrast agent spilling from a patent fallopian tube. Before injecting positive contrast agent, any negative contrast fluid should be aspirated from the uterine cavity. Agitated saline, echogenic due to multiple dispersed gas bubbles, may be used however it appears less successful than positive contrast agents. Campbell and colleagues demonstrated that sonosalpingography is as accurate for tubal patency as HSG. Campbell and colleagues[84] demonstrated that SSG (with Levovist) is as accurate for tubal patency as HSG. Diagnosis is based on contrast spill distally with free flow for at least 10 seconds without formation of a hydrosalpinx. Proximal obstruction is diagnosed by lack of interstial flow, failure to form a hydrosalpinx, or intraperitoneal fluid accumulation. Distal obstruction is diagnosed by hydrosalpinx formation. Tubal spasm may mimic proximal obstruction. A balloon catheter is useful to minimize or stop contrast spill via the cervical lumen.

FUTURE DIRECTIONS

As three-dimensional software becomes more readily available and user friendly, the standard will likely be rapid volumetric acquisitions providing shorter examination duration while improving accuracy and reproducibility. Dubinsky and colleagues[85] published a preliminary study in which directed biopsy was performed at the time of SHG. As technical difficulties are overcome, this

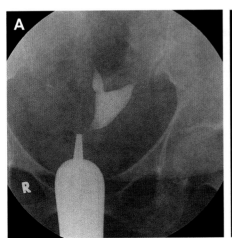
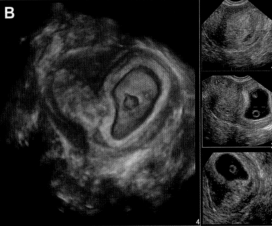

Fig. 22. (*A*) Hysterosalpingogram demonstrates asymmetric separation of the upper endometrial cavity. The differential diagnosis includes bicornuate or subseptate uterus. (*B*) Subsequent pregnancy with "natural SHG" due to presence of amniotic fluid demonstrates left-sided implantation of the pregnancy in a subseptate uterus.

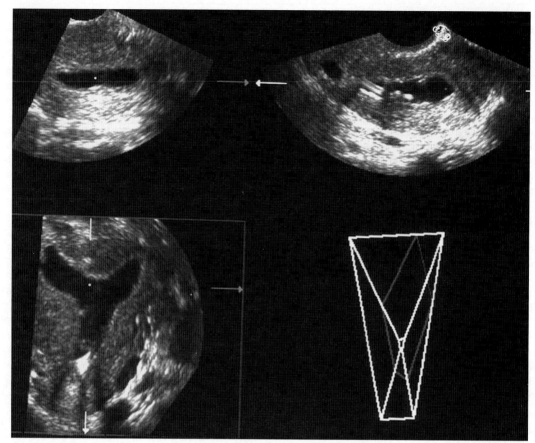

Fig. 23. Multiplanar display obtained during SHG using 3D volume sonography demonstrates an arcuate uterus with broad shallow indentation of the fundal contour, convex toward the lumen.

technique may become a standard of care, potentially reducing the need for hysteroscopic evaluation.

SUMMARY

SHG is an elegant extension of the TV US examination in providing detailed information on the separated endometrial walls as well as of the endometrium, and for evaluation of congenital anomalies, endometrial, and subendometrial conditions. It is well tolerated with few complications. The improved anatomic resolution increases diagnostic confidence and helps direct the patient to appropriate therapeutic options, potentially decreasing the need for more costly or invasive examinations. The addition of 3D US to SHG has made the examination quicker and expanded the utility of the procedure in particular in the area of congenital uterine anomalies and the evaluation of potentially resectable submucosal fibroids. The authors suspect it will continue to play a growing role in the evaluation of common gynecologic problems and in defining uterine pathology.

REFERENCES

1. Parsons AK, Lense JJ. Sonohysterography for endometrial abnormalities: preliminary results. J Clin Ultrasound 1993;21:87–95.
2. De Kroon CD, de Bock GH, Dieben SW, et al. Saline contrast hysterosonography in abnormal uterine bleeding; a systematic review and meta-analysis. Br J Obstet Gynaecol 2003;110:947–88.
3. van Dongen H, de Kroon C, Jacobi CE, et al. Diagnostic hysteroscopy in abnormal uterine bleeding: a systematic review and meta-analysis. Br J Obstet Gynaecol 2007;114:664–75.
4. Erdem M, Bilgin U, Bozkurt N, et al. Comparison of transvaginal ultrasonography and saline infusion sonohysterography in evaluating the endometrial cavity pre- and post menopausal patients with abnormal uterine bleeding. Menopause 2007;14:846–52.

5. Lindheim S, Morales A. Comparison of sonohyster-ography and hysteroscopy: lessons learned and avoiding pitfalls. J Am Assoc Gynecol Laparosc 2002;9(2):223–31.

6. Deutch TD, Abuhamad AZ. The role of 3-dimensional ultrasonography and magnetic resonance imaging in the diagnosis of mullerian duct anomalies: a review of the literature. J Ultrasound Med 2008;27:413–23.

7. Troiano RN, McCarthy SM. Mullerian duct anomalies: imaging and clinical issues. Radiology 2004;233:19–34.

8. Berridge D, Winter T. Saline infusion sonohysterography: technique, indications, and imaging findings. J Ultrasound Med 2004;23:97–112.

9. Lindheim S, Sprague C, Winter T. Hysterosalpingography and sonohysterography: lessons in technique. AJR Am J Roentgenol 2006;186:24–9.

10. American Institute of Ultrasound in Medicine. AIUM practice guideline for the performance of sonohysterography. Revised February 15, 2007. Published in conjunction with ACR, ACOG. Available at: http://www.aium.org/publications/clinical/sonohysterography.pdf. Accessed July 1, 2008.

11. Spieldoch R, Winter T, Schouweiler C, et al. Optimal catheter placement during sonohysterography. Obstet Gynecol 2008;111(1):15–22.

12. Bonnamy L, Marret H, Perrotin F, et al. Sonohysterography: a prospective survey of results and complications in 81 patients. Eur J Obstet Gynecol Reprod Biol 2002;102:41–7.

13. Cullinan J, Fleischer A, Kepple D, et al. Sonohysterography: a technique for endometrial evaluation. Radiographics 1995;15(3):501–14.

14. Dajani AS, Taubert KA, Wilson W, et al. Prevention of bacterial endocarditis; recommendations by the American Heart Association. Circulation 1997;96:358–66. Available at: http://circ.ahajournals.org/cgi/content/full/96/1/358.

15. Lindheim S, Adsuar N, Kushner D, et al. Sonohysterography: a valuable tool in evaluating the female pelvis. Obstet Gynecol Surv 2003;58(11):770–82.

16. Exalto N, Stappers C, van Laamsdonk LA, et al. Gel instillation hysterosonography: first experience with a new technique. Fertil Steril 2007;87:152–5.

17. Dessole S, Farina M, Capobianco G, et al. Determining the best catheter for sonohysterography. Fertil Steril 2001;76:605–9.

18. Bree R, Bowerman R, Bohm-Velez M, et al. US evaluation of the uterus in patients with postmenopausal bleeding: a positive effect on diagnostic decision-making. Radiology 2000;216(1):260–4.

19. Abuhamad AZ, Singleton S, Zhao Y, et al. The Z technique: an easy approach to the display of the midcoronal plane of the uterus in volume sonography. J Ultrasound Med 2006;25:607–12.

20. Andreotti RF, Fleischer AC, Mason LE Jr. Three-dimensional sonography of the endometrium and adjacent myometrium; preliminary observations. J Ultrasound Med 2006;25:1313–9.

21. Jurkovic D. Three-dimensional ultrasound in gynecology: a critical evaluation. Ultrasound Obstet Gynecol 2002;19:109–17.

22. Bega G, Lev-Toaff AS, O'Kane P, et al. Three-dimensional ultrasonography in gynecology: technical aspects and clinical applications. J Ultrasound Med 2003;22:1249–69.

23. Ghate S, Crockett M, Boyd B, et al. Sonohysterography: do 3D reconstructed images provide additional value? AJR Am J Roentgenol 2008;190:W227–33.

24. Benacerraf BR, Shipp TD, Bromley B. Which patients benefit from a 3D reconstructed coronal view of the uterus added to standard routine 2D pelvic sonography. AJR Am J Roentgenol 2008;190:626–9.

25. Nelson TR, Pretorius DH, Hull A, et al. Sources and impact of artifacts on clinical three-dimensional ultrasound imaging. Ultrasound Obstet Gynecol 1984;149:285–90.

26. Lee SI. An imaging algorithm for evaluation of abnormal uterine bleeding: does sonohysterography play a role? Menopause 2007;14:823–5.

27. Medverd JR, Dubinsky TJ. Cost analysis model: US versus endometrial biopsy in evaluation of peri- and postmenopausal abnormal vaginal bleeding. Radiology 2002;222:619–27.

28. Bree RL, Carlos RC. US for postmenopausal bleeding: consensus development and patient-centered outcomes. Radiology 2002;222:595–8.

29. National Cancer Institute. Cancer topics. Available at: http://www.cancer.gov/cancertopics/types/endometrial. AccessedJuly 4, 2008.

30. Smith-Bindman R, Kerlikowske K, Feldstein VA. Endovaginal ultrasound to exclude endometrial cancer and other endometrial abnormalities. JAMA 1998;280:1510–7.

31. Clark TJ, Voi D, Gupta JK, et al. Accuracy of hysteroscopy in the diagnosis of endometrial cancer and hyperplasia: a systematic quantitative review. JAMA 2002;288:1610–21.

32. Critchley HO, Warner P, Lee AJ, et al. Evaluation of abnormal uterine bleeding: comparison of three outpatient procedures within cohorts defined by age and menopausal status. Health Technol Assess 2004;8:1–139.

33. Smith P, Bakos O, Heimer G, et al. Transvaginal ultrasound for identifying endometrial abnormality. Acta Obstet Gynecol Scand 1991;70:591–4.

34. de Kroon CD, de Bock GH, Dieben SW, et al. Saline contrast hysterosonography in abnormal uterine bleeding: a systematic review and meta-analysis. BJOG 2003;110(10):938–47.

35. Bredella MA, Felstein VA, Filly RA, et al. Measurement of endometrial thickness at US in multicenter drug trials: value of central quality assurance reading. Radiology 2000;217:516–20.

36. Smith-Bindman R, Weiss E, Felstein V. How thick is too thick? When endometrial thickness should prompt biopsy in postmenopausal women without vaginal bleeding. Ultrasound Obstet Gynecol 2004; 24:558–65.

37. Karlsson B, Granberg S, Wikland M, et al. Transvaginal ultrasonography of the endometrium in women with postmenopausal bleeding – Nordic multi-center study. Am J Obstet Gynecol 1995;172:1488–94.

38. Ferrazzi E, Torri V, Trio D, et al. Sonographic endometrial thickness: a useful test to predict atrophy in patients with postmenopausal bleeding. An Italian multicentric study. Ultrasound Obstet Gynecol 1996;7:315–22.

39. Parsons A. Opinion: resetting endometrial thresholds: we should avoid double standards. Ultrasound Obstet Gynecol 2004;24:495–9.

40. Deckardt R, Lueken RP, Gallinat A, et al. Comparison of transvaginal ultrasound, hysteroscopy and dilation and curettage in the diagnosis of abnormal vaginal bleeding and intrauterine pathology in perimenopausal and postmenopausal women. J Am Assoc Gynecol Laparosc 2002;9:277–82.

41. Gupta JK, Chien PF, Voit D, et al. Ultrasonographic endometrial thickness for diagnosing endometrial pathology in women with postmenopausal bleeding: a meta-analysis. Acta Obstet Gynecol Scand 2002; 81:799–816.

42. Jurkovic D, Alfirevic Z. DISQ 2: endometrial thickness in asymptomatic women. Ultrasound Obstet Gynecol 2005;26:203.

43. Goldstein RB, Bree RL, Benson CB, et al. Evaluation of the woman with postmenopausal bleeding: Society of Radiologists in Ultrasound-sponsored consensus conference statement. J Ultrasound Med 2001; 20:1025–36.

44. Nalaboff K, Pellerito J, Ben-Levi E. Imaging the endometrium: disease and normal variants. Radiographics 2001;21(6):1409–24.

45. Anastasiadis PG, Koutlaki NG, Skaphida PG, et al. Endometrial polyps: prevalence, detection, and malignant potential in women with abnormal uterine bleeding. Eur J Gynaecol Oncol 2000;21:180–3.

46. Clevenger-Hoeft M, Syrop CH, Stovall DW, et al. Sonohysterography in premenopausal women with and without abnormal bleeding. Obstet Gynecol 1999;94:516–20.

47. Laifer-Narin S, Ragavendra N, Lu D, et al. Transvaginal saline hysterosonography: characteristics distinguishing malignant and various benign conditions. AJR Am J Roentgenol 1999;172:1513–20.

48. Lev-Toaff AS, Toaff ME, Liu JB, et al. Value of sonohysterography in the diagnosis and management of abnormal uterine bleeding. Radiology 1996;201: 179–84.

49. Timmerman D, Verguts J, Konstantinovic MI, et al. The pedicle artery sign based on sonography with color Doppler imaging can replace second-stage tests in women with abnormal vaginal bleeding. Ultrasound Obstet Gynecol 2003;22:166–71.

50. Bossselmann K, Schwarz H. Cervical and endometrial polyps and carcinoma of the genital tract. Geburtshilfe Frauenheilkd 1972;32:687–90.

51. Coeman D, Van Belle Y, Vanderick G, et al. Hysteroscopic findings in patients with a cervical polyp. Am J Obstet Gynecol 1993;169:1563–5.

52. Kurman RJ, Kaminski PF, Norris HG. The behaviour of endometrial hyperplasia: a long-term study of "untreated" hyperplasia in 170 patients. Cancer 1985; 56:403–12.

53. Fleischer AC, Shappell HW. Color Doppler sonohysterography of endometrial polyps and submucosal fibroids. J Ultrasound Med 2003;22:601–4.

54. Jorizzo JR, Chen MY, Martin D, et al. Spectrum of endometrial hyperplasia and its mimics on saline hysterosonography. AJR Am J Roentgenol 2002; 179:385–9.

55. Davis P, O'Neill M, Yoder I, et al. Sonohysterographic findings of endometrial and subendometrial conditions. Radiographics 2002;22(4):803–16.

56. Berry E, Lindheim SR, Connor JP, et al. Sonohysterography and endometrial cancer: incidence and functional viability of disseminated malignant cells. Am J Obstet Gynecol 2008 [Epub ahead of print].

57. Alcazar JL, Errasti R, Zornoza A. Saline infusion sonohysterography in endometrial cancer: assessment of malignant cells dissemination risk. Acta Obstet Gynecol Scand 2000;321(79):321–2.

58. Fisher B, Costantino JP, Redmond CK, et al. Endometrial cancer in tamoxifen-treated cancer patients: findings from the national surgical adjuvant breast and bowel project (NSABP) B14. J Natl Cancer Inst 1994;86:527–37.

59. Tepper R, Beyth Y, Altaras MM, et al. Value of sonohysterography in asymptomatic postmenopausal tamoxifen-treated patients. Gynecol Oncol 1997; 64:386–91.

60. Fong K, Kung R, Lytwyn A, et al. Endometrial evaluation with transvaginal US and hysterosonography in asymptomatic postmenopausal women with breast cancer receiving tamoxifen. Radiology 2001;220: 765–73.

61. Hann LE, Giess CS, Bach AM, et al. Endometrial thickness in tamoxifen-treated patients: correlation with clinical and pathological findings. Am J Roentgenol 1997;168:657–61.

62. Weigle M, Friese K, Strittmatter HG, et al. Measuring the thickness is that all we have to do for sonographic assessment of endometrium in

postmenopausal women? Ultrasound Obstet Gynecol 1995;6:97–102.

63. Caoili EM, Hertzberg BS, Kliewer MA, et al. Refractory shadowing from pelvic masses on sonography: a useful diagnostic sign for uterine leiomyomas. Am J Roentgenol 2000;174:97–101.

64. Becker E Jr, Lev-Toaff AS, Kaufman EP, et al. The added value of transvaginal sonohysterography over transvaginal sonography alone in women with known or suspected leiomyoma. J Ultrasound Med 2002;21:237–47.

65. Stewart EA. Uterine fibroids. Lancet 2001;357:293–8.

66. Cohen LS, Valle RF. Role of vaginal sonography and hysterosonography in the endoscopic treatment of uterine myomas. Fertil Steril 2000;73:197–204.

67. Atri M, Reinhold C, Mehio AR, et al. Adenomyosis: US features with histological correlation in an in vitro study. Radiology 2000;215:783–90.

68. Andreotti RF. The sonographic diagnosis of adenomyosis. Ultrasound Q 2005;213:167–70.

69. Kodaman P, Arici A. Intra-uterine adhesions and fertility outcome: how to optimize success? Curr Opin Obstet Gynecol 2007;19:207–14.

70. Schenker JG. Etiology and therapeutic approach to synechia uteri. Eur J Obstet Gynecol Reprod Biol 1996;65:109–13.

71. Timmerman D, Wauters J, Van Calenbergh S, et al. Color Doppler imaging is a valuable tool for the diagnosis and management of uterine vascular malformations. Ultrasound Obstet Gynecol 2003;21:570–7.

72. Zalel Y, Cohen S, Oren M, et al. Sonohysterography for the diagnosis of residual trophoblastic tissue. J Ultrasound Med 2001;20:877–81.

73. Hertzberg BS, Bowie JD. Ultrasound of the postpartum uterus. Prediction of retained placental tissue. J Ultrasound Med 1991;10:451–60.

74. Wolman I, Gordon D, Yaron Y, et al. Transvaginal sonohysterography for the evaluation and treatment of retained products of conception. Gynecol Obstet Invest 2000;50:73–6.

75. Van Den Bosch T, Van Schoubroeck D, Lu C, et al. Color Doppler and gray-scale ultrasound evaluation of the postpartum uterus. Ultrasound Obstet Gynecol 2002;20:586–91.

76. Monteagudo A, Carreno C. Saline infusion sonohysterography in nonpregnant women with previous cesarean delivery: the "niche" in the scar. J Ultrasound Med 2001;20:1105–15.

77. Lindheim SR, Kavic S, Sauer MV. Intraoperative applications of saline infusion ultrasonography. J Assist Reprod Genet 1999;16:390–4.

78. Kim AH, McKay H, Keltz MD, et al. Sonohysterographic screening before in vitro fertilization. Fertil Steril 1998;69:841–4.

79. Kupesic S, Kurjak A. Ultrasound and Doppler assessment of uterine anomalies. In: Kupesic S, de Ziegler D, editors. Ultrasound and infertility. Pearl River (NY): Parthenon; 2000. p. 147–53.

80. The American Fertility Society. The American Fertility Society classifications of adnexal adhesions, distal tubal occlusion, tubal occlusion secondary to tubal ligation, tubal pregnancies, mullerian anomalies, and intrauterine adhesions. Fertil Steril 1988;49:944–55.

81. Salim R, Woelfer B, Backos M, et al. Reproducibility of three-dimensional ultrasound diagnosis of congenital uterine anomalies. Ultrasound Obstet Gynecol 2003;21:578–82.

82. Imaoka I, Wada A, Matsuo M, et al. MRI imaging of disorders associated with female infertility: use in diagnosis, treatment, and management. Radiographics 2003;23:1401–21.

83. Strassman EO. Fertility and unification of the double uterus. Fertil Steril 1996;17:165–76.

84. Campbell S, Bourne TH, Tan SL, et al. Hysterosalpingocontrast sonography (HyCoSy) and its future role within the investigation of infertility in Europe. Ultrasound Obstet Gynecol 1994;4:245–53.

85. Dubinsky TJ, Reed S, Mao C, et al. Hysterosonographical guided endometrial biopsy: technical feasibility. Am J Roentgenol 2000;174:1589–91.

Ovarian Torsion and Its Mimics

Deniz Akata, MD

KEYWORDS

- Ovarian torsion • Adnexal masses
- Color Doppler sonography • Ultrasongraphy

During routine clinical practice, radiologists often must evaluate a wide range of cases with acute abdominal and pelvic pain. Although ultrasound (US) is the primary imaging modality of choice for the evaluation of pelvic pain in the female patient, MR imaging has proven to be a valuable adjunct to characterize the adnexal mass. Computed tomography (CT) is mostly performed if US findings are equivocal or if the abnormality extends beyond the field of view achievable with the endovaginal probe.

Adnexal torsion is an uncommon but serious cause of lower abdominal pain in women, found in less than 3% of cases presenting with acute pelvic pain.[1,2] It can mimic other conditions, such as ovarian cyst rupture, ectopic pregnancy, pelvic inflammatory diseases (PID), and even acute appendicitis.[3]

This article reviews the radiologic evaluation of ovarian torsion and its mimics. The complementary roles of US, CT, and MR imaging in the evaluation of various acute pelvic disorders is also discussed.

OVARIAN TORSION
Clinical Findings

Adnexal torsion is the fifth most common gynecologic emergency, with a reported prevalence of 3% in some series.[1,2] It primarily affects women of reproductive age or younger. Ovarian torsion most commonly occurs in premenapausal age. In premenapausal adults, there is usually a concurrent benign ovarian cyst or mass.[4,5] Adnexal torsion is accompanied with pregnancy in 20% of the cases (**Fig 1**), with the right ovary being the most commonly affected. In the postmenapausal

period, it is almost always seen with ovarian neoplasm. Ovarian torsion may occur in the absence of ovarian disease, usually in children, and has been attributed to excessive mobility of the adnexa.[6–8] In 10% of the cases, the contra lateral ovary is also torsed.

The diagnosis is complicated by its vague clinical presentation. In most cases, ovaries are frequently difficult to palpate, so physical examination findings often do not suggest the diagnosis.[6] It is the most difficult diagnosis that can be predicted preoperatively in patients with acute pelvic pain.[9] Because of the variable pain characteristics and frequent lack of definitive clinical findings, the diagnosis of ovarian torsion is often delayed, thereby limiting the possibility of ovarian salvage. In a study,[9] it has been shown that in 100 nonpregnant patients who went through emergent laparotomy or laparoscopy, ovarian torsion was the preoperative diagnosis in 66 cases; however, only 29 of them (44%) were confirmed surgically.

The only consistent symptom cited in most studies is abdominal pain, usually localized to lower quadrant.[10,11] Unfortunately, the differential considerations for abdominal pain in female patients include many etiologies, such as appendicitis, cholecystitis, PID, urinary collecting system calculi, and ruptured benign adnexal cysts. It has been reported by Shadinger and colleagues,[6] that all of the 39 patients with pathologically proven ovarian torsion had presented with abdominal pain: 33 (85%) reported vomiting, 22 (56%) had leukocytosis, and 7 (18%) had a documented elevated temperature.

In the setting of acute pelvic pain, ovarian torsion is often a leading diagnostic consideration.

Department of Radiology, Hacettepe University Medical School, Sıhhiye 06100 Ankara, Turkey
E-mail address: dakata@hacettepe.edu.tr

Ultrasound Clin 3 (2008) 451–460
doi:10.1016/j.cult.2008.07.002

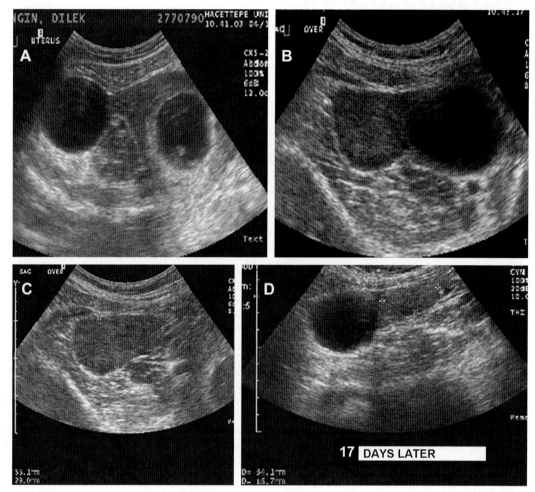

Fig. 1. Spontaneous detorsion. An 8-week-pregnant patient presents with right lower quadrant pain, suspicious for acute appendicitis. (A) Transabdominal sonogram in the transverse plane demonstrates intrauterine gestational sac with embryonic pole. There is an adnexal cyst, 60 mm × 42 mm in size, on the right. (B) A cyst is attached to the ovary. (C) The ovary is also significantly enlarged, measuring 53 mm × 33 mm in size. No follicles are seen within the ovarian stroma secondary to edema. Sonographic diagnosis was ovarian torsion; however, the patient was managed conservatively. (D) US scan of the pelvis after 17 days shows that ovary is normal in size, measuring 34 mm × 16 mm. Also, the cyst, which was previously located medially, has moved to the lateral of the ovary.

Gray scale US combined with Doppler US is the method of choice for imaging of lower abdominal and pelvic pain in female patients. Major advantages of US are that it is radiation-free, cost-effective, and has easy availability. US offers high-resolution anatomic detail of the uterus and adnexa; however, CT or MR imaging can be performed when alternative diagnoses are considered, particularly if torsion is subacute or intermittent. CT plays a particularly important role in (a) the evaluation of patients with suspected pelvic abscess or hematoma, postpartum complications, or complications related to pelvic inflammatory disease, and (b) the exclusion of bowel disease and (c) renal stones.

Imaging Findings

Sonographic findings in ovarian torsion are variable and include an enlarged ovary with peripherally distributed follicles (small peripheral cystic structures), an associated cyst or mass, and lack of vascularity (**Fig. 2**). The presence of enlarged ovary is the most common finding and has been documented in all patients in the majority of the studies.[5,6,12] Free fluid in the cul-de-sac is also frequently observed but it is a nonspecific finding seen in many physiologic and pathologic conditions. If torsion is associated with a cyst or mass, it is usually a complex one with septations and debris caused by ischemic necrosis and

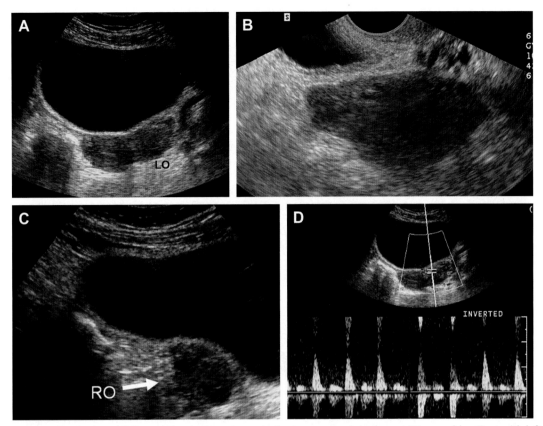

Fig. 2. Ovarian torsion. (*A*) Transabdominal sonogram in the transverse plane from a 13-year-old patient with left lower quadrant pain shows an enlarged ovary next to the uterus. (*B*) Focused view of the left ovary delineates hypoechoic, enlarged ovary without any conspicuous follicles. (*C*) Right ovary (RO, *white arrow*) is normal in size with normal follicles. (*D*) Color flow Doppler sonography of the left ovary demonstrates presence of arterial blood flow in the periphery. Patient underwent exploratory laparatomy. The left ovary was found to be necrotic from torsion and was resected.

hemorrhage.[13] Additional findings suggestive of torsion include deviation of the uterus to the twisted side and engorged blood vessels on the twisted side.

The most common mass associated with ovarian torsion is mature cystic teratoma . Torsed mature cystic teratomas are relatively larger, with a mean diameter of 11 cm, than the average 6-cm teratoma. This enlargement could be the result of the torsion rather than the cause of it.[4] Torsion of a teratoma, even in chronic cases, does not eradicate the fatty elements.

Because ovarian enlargement is the most consistent sonographic finding, the normal size of the ovaries from newborn age to the postmenapausal period should be well kept in mind. The ovarian volume can be assessed by the volume ellipsoid formula: volume = 1/2 length $\times$ width $\times$ height. The upper limit of normal for ovarian volume in adults is generally accepted as 15 cm^3. Previously established pediatric ovarian

size guidelines state that the mean volumes are 1 cm^3 or less in girls of 6 years and younger, 1.2 cm^3 to 2.3 cm^3 in girls of 6 to 10 years, and 2 cm^3 to 4 cm^3 in girls of 11 to 12 years. However, because of the effect of maternal hormones, the ovarian volume can reach to 3.6 cm^3 in the first 3 months and even in the first year of life. The mean volume in postmenopausal women is 8 cm^3. In torsion, the ovaries or—when the ovary and mass could not be differentiated—the ovary/mass complexes, are uniformly enlarged, ranging from 24 cm^3 in a 3-year-old patient to 957 cm^3 in an adult.[6] Comparison with the morphologic appearance and flow patterns of the contra lateral ovary will aid in diagnosis. In the author's experience, a torsed ovary is almost always associated with abnormal morphologic appearance.

Color flow Doppler (CFD) sonography plays an important role in diagnosing ovarian torsion. CFD findings in ovarian torsion are variable. Complete absence of arterial and venous flow in a morphologically abnormal ovary is the sine qua non of ovarian torsion; however, presence of blood flow does not exclude ovarian torsion. Ben-Ami and colleagues[14] reported that the positive predictive value for torsion in the absence of venous flow was 94%, and torsion was very unlikely when Doppler interrogation revealed venous flow (**Fig. 3**). To the contrary, several case reports and retrospective studies of adnexal torsion have described an abnormal appearance of the ovary with ovarian torsion in the presence of arterial and venous Doppler signals.[15,16] Penna and colleagues reported that CFD findings were normal in 60% (6 of 10), and abnormal (decreased or absent) in 40% of cases, suggestive of ovarian torsion. In cases involving ovulation induction, Doppler sonography findings were normal in 25% of the cases.[16] Dual arterial blood supply of the ovary is proposed as the major justification of this finding. Presence of blood flow in an ovary predicts its viability in the presence of ovarian torsion. Fleischer and colleagues and Lee and colleagues have shown that the presence of arterial and venous flow within ovaries that are found to be torsed is predictive of their viability. Absence of blood flow within the twisted vascular pedicle is highly predictive for necrotic ovaries.[17,18]

Albayram and Hamper[19] have shown that the duration of pain did not show a statistically significant relationship with the presence or absence of ovarian arterial flow. However, the relationship between the duration of pain and the absence of venous flow was significant and unexpectedly inverse.

CT and MR imaging are helpful in difficult cases as problem solving modalities. CT findings in ovarian torsion have been described previously[15,20] and include deviation of the uterus to the twisted side, ascites, obliteration of fat planes, and an enlarged ovary or adnexal mass displaced from its normal location in the adnexa or to the contralateral side of the pelvis (**Fig. 4**). Intravenous

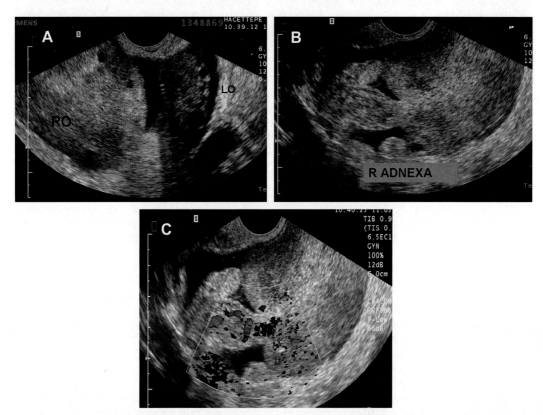

Fig. 3. Complete ovarian torsion. Endovaginal US and CFD study of a 24-year-old patient with right lower quadrant pain and tenderness. (A) The US scan in the transverse plane shows normal size of the left ovary with well-defined follicles. The mass-like structure next to the left ovary is the enlarged right ovary (RO) because of edema. (B) Thickened, right salpinx and twisted right ovary are well seen. Free fluid encircles both ovaries within the pelvis. (C) CFD delineates flow only in the salpinx but not in the ovary. Noise artifacts within the ovary are because of the color gain adjusted for very slow flow. Findings are compatible with complete torsion. The diagnosis confirmed after right salpingoopherectomy.

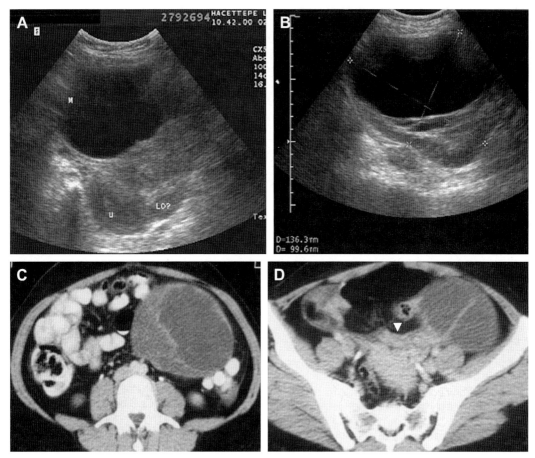

Fig. 4. Twisted vascular pedicle sign on CT. A 17-year-old woman with a history of lower abdominal tenderness and palpable abdominal mass. (*A*) Transabdominal US scan in the transverse plane shows the uterus (U) deviated to the right. There is a large mass (M) with cystic and solid components located anterior and to the left lateral of the uterus. There is a solid structure on the left, probably representing left ovary (LO?). (*B*) No right ovary other than the mass is identified. The mass measures 136 mm × 99 mm in size. The solid component is eccentrically located. (*C*) Contrast-enhanced CT scan shows a large, unilocular cystic mass. Eccentric smooth wall thickening (maximum wall thickness, 15 mm) is noted along the right lateral margin of the mass. (*D*) Contrast-enhanced CT scan obtained caudate to (*C*) shows an amorphous mass like structure (*arrowhead*) connecting the cyst and the uterus. This finding represents a twisted vascular pedicle of a right ovarian cyst with hemorrhagic infarction.

contrast-enhanced CT or MR imaging may reveal surrounding enhancing blood vessels, a finding that is consistent with congestion.[6,20] In lesions with hemorrhagic infarction, a beaked or serpentine protrusion at the periphery of the twisted ovary, lack of enhancement, hematoma, or gas[3,21] may be observed. This can best be appreciated on sequential scans obtained before and after torsion.

There is growing evidence that untwisting the involved adnexa to observe for tissue reperfusion and viability is safe. However, significant delay in diagnosis and surgical intervention may result in irreversible tissue necrosis, rendering the adnexa unsalvageable.

Diagnosis of adnexal torsion is still a diagnostic challenge and because of that, patients are most commonly treated with adnexal resection.[22]

OVARIAN TORSION MIMICS

In the evaluation of acute pelvic pain in a nonpregnant female patient, hemorrhagic ovarian cyst, ovarian hyperstimulation syndrome, endometriosis, PID, endometritis, adhesions, and acute appendicitis should also be considered in the differential diagnosis. Ectopic pregnancy is a common cause of acute pelvic pain in patients with positive pregnancy test and is described in detail in this issue by Gurel and Akata. Endometriosis

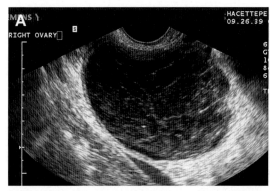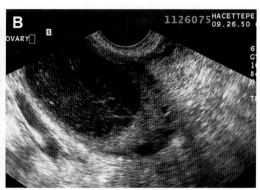

Fig. 5. Hemorrhagic cyst with "fishnet appearance." A 25-year-old patient with right lower quadrant pain. (A) There is a complex cyst in the right ovary measuring 4 cm × 3.5 cm in size. (B) The cyst has reticular pattern consistent with "fishnet appearance" of hemorrhagic cyst.

results in chronic pain rather than acute pain in the majority of the cases. Additional pain in endometriosis need not be cyclical.

Hemorrhagic Ovarian Cyst

Significant hemorrhage in an ovarian cyst often presents with sudden onset of pelvic pain. It is the most straightforward diagnosis that can be predicted preoperatively in patients with acute pelvic pain.[9] There may be hemorrhage into a corpus luteal cyst or follicular cyst (Fig. 5). If there is cyst rupture, it is associated with hemoperitoneum. Although hemoperitoneum is untreated in most cases, it can be a life-threatening condition, especially in patients who are undergoing anticoagulation therapy (Fig. 6).[23] At US, hemorrhagic ovarian cysts can mimic a variety of solid and mixed solid-cystic masses. Its classical appearance is described as a "fishnet appearance." In essence, its appearance corresponds to evolution of hemorrhage or clot. Patients with hemorrhagic cysts are usually followed at an interval of 6 to 8 weeks to demonstrate their resolution or decrease in size to exclude the possibility of an ovarian tumor presenting with hemorrhage. Contrast-enhanced CT may delineate the cyst wall, and delayed CT may be useful in demonstrating the site of pooling of contrast-enhanced blood in the pelvis.[6] CT is also helpful in excluding other intra-abdominal diseases, such as acute appendicitis and urinary calculi that can lead to acute pelvic pain.

A ruptured ectopic pregnancy could manifest with a similar clinical picture, and correlation with β-HCG levels before imaging to exclude this possibility is essential. If the disease is correctly diagnosed, patients with hemorrhagic ovarian cysts often do well with conservative treatment and supportive therapy.

Ovarian Hyperstimulation Disease and Polycystic Ovary Syndrome

Ovarian hyperstimulation disease (OHD) is usually secondary to ovarian stimulant drug therapy for infertility[24] but may occur as a spontaneous event in pregnancy. Enlargement of the ovaries are quite different than the ovaries that are torsed. The ovaries in OHS are enlarged secondary to distended, usually peripherally located corpora lutea cysts of varying sizes. The imaging findings are similar at US, CT, and MR imaging[24–26] and described as having a "wheel spoke" appearance (Fig. 7). Extravascular accumulation of exudates leading to weight gain, ascites, pleural effusions,

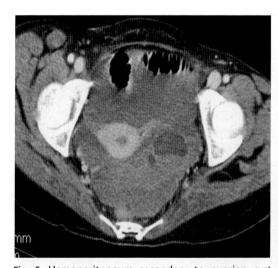

Fig. 6. Hemoperitoneum secondary to ovarian cyst rupture. Patient on anticoagulation therapy presents with pelvic pain and hypotension. Free-fluid levels within the left ovarian cyst and high-density free-fluid accumulation within the pelvis are present. Findings are compatible with hemorrhagic ovarian cyst rupture and hemoperitoneum.

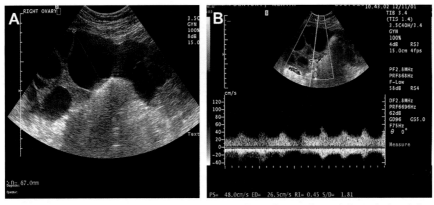

Fig. 7. Ovarian hyperstimulation syndrome. Both ovaries are enlarged secondary to distended peripherally located follicle cysts of varying sizes. (*A*) The largest cyst measures 6 cm to 7 cm in size. The greatest dimension of the right ovary is 13 cm. (*B*) Because of hyper stimulation, low resistant flow is detected around the wall of the cysts.

intravascular volume depletion with hemoconcentration, and oliguria in varying degrees are the dominating features of this syndrome. Pain, abdominal distention, nausea, and vomiting are also frequently seen. Familiarity with ovarian hyperstimulation syndrome and the appropriate clinical setting should help avoid the incorrect diagnosis of an ovarian cystic neoplasm or ovarian torsion.

Polycystic ovary syndrome (POS) is a painless condition presenting as an endocrine disorder, amenorrhea, hirsutism, irregular bleeding, and infertility. There are multiple cysts at the periphery of the ovaries with stromal increased echogenicity. The US criteria for diagnosing POS includes demonstration of 12 or more 2-mm to 9-mm follicles in the ovary on transvaginal US examination. The ovaries are bilaterally enlarged and round in shape. Although it is not a diagnostic problem, because of this enlargement (ovarian volume greater than 10 cm^3) they are prone to torsion (**Fig. 8**).

Pelvic Inflammatory Disease

PID is one of the most common causes of acute pelvic pain in women, and imaging findings vary with the severity of the disease. US is the primary imaging modality. CT can be a helpful in determining the extent of disease and identifying associated complications, Clinical findings of fever, leukocytosis, and cervical motion tenderness are very important in suggesting this diagnosis. In mild cases, US and CT findings are most often normal or demonstrate a small amount of fluid in the cul-de-sac. With progression to tubo-ovarian abscess, CT findings include bilateral thick-walled,

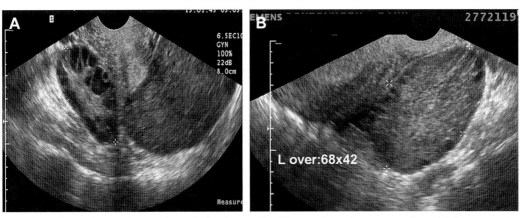

Fig. 8. POS with ovarian torsion. Endovaginal US scan of a 22-year-old patient presenting with lower quadrant pain. (*A*) Right ovary is 50 mm × 30 mm in size with hyperechoic stroma and peripherally located follicles. (*B*) Left ovary is significantly enlarged, measuring 68 mm × 42 mm in size. Follicles are also peripherally located but the stroma is significantly hypoechoic and edematous. Findings are consistent with left ovarian torsion of the polycystic ovarian syndrome. Patient had left salpingo-oopherectomy and the diagnosis was confirmed.

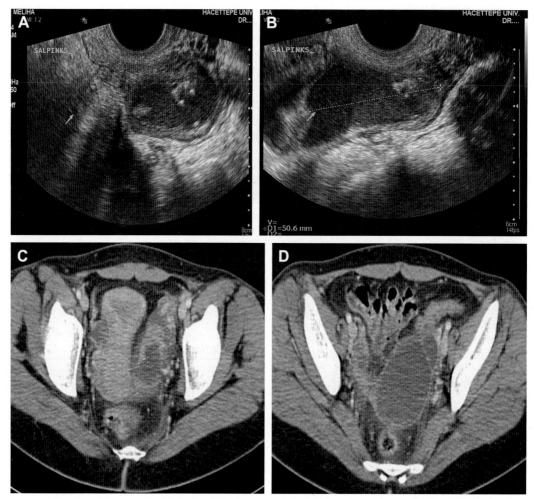

Fig. 9. Tubo-ovarian abscess. Left adnexal cystic mass in a patient with pelvic pain and fever. (*A*) US scan in transverse and (*B*) in sagittal plane delineates a fusiform cystic mass with thickened wall, debris, and thick fluid. These findings are consistent with tubo-ovarian abscess. (*C*) CT scan shows contrast enhanced left complex adnexal mass. (*D*) Although fluid density is high, the inhomogenity of the fluid is better appreciated by US.

low-attenuation adnexal masses with thick septations and debris corresponding to a dilated, pus-filled fallopian tube (**Fig 9**). CFD shows increased vascularity in the adnexa secondary to inflammation. The tubular nature of the mass may also help distinguish a tubo-ovarian abscess from other complex cystic masses.[2–5] Associated findings include thickening of the uterosacral ligaments, increased attenuation of the presacral fat secondary to edema, hydronephrosis, and indistinct margins of adjacent bowel loops. The inflammatory process may extend to involve the appendix or colon and greater omentum. Anterior displacement of a thickened broad ligament and loss of definition of the uterine border are suggestive of an adnexal origin for the inflammatory process and help distinguish a tubo-ovarian abscess from other causes of pelvic abscess, such as

diverticulitis.[27] Patients with an intrauterine device are prone to infection with *Actinomyces israelii*, an invasive organism, which leads to chronic suppurative infection.[27,28] It can often be difficult to differentiate infection with this organism from pelvic neoplasm with carcinomatosis (**Fig 10**).

SUMMARY

Abnormal flow detected by Doppler sonography is highly predictive of adnexal torsion and is useful in the diagnosis of ovarian torsion. However, when normal flow is detected by Doppler sonography, it does not necessarily exclude an ovarian torsion and may indicate its viability. Ovarian torsion should be suspected in the presence of abnormal morphology despite the presence of arterial and venous blood flow on CFD. Mature cystic teratoma

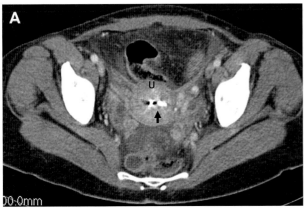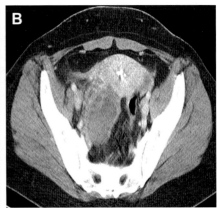

Fig. 10. (A) PID with *Actinomyces israelii* infection. Patient with an intrauterine device (IUD) (*arrow*) in place. There is fluid around the uterus (U), uterine ligaments are thickened. (B) Accompanying right cystic mass with thickened wall and septi is compatible with tuba ovarian abscess.

is the most common ovarian mass associated with ovarian torsion. Mimics of the ovarian torsion include hemorrhagic cyst, endometrioma, and PID. Non-gynecologic emergencies, such as acute appendicitis or renal stone disease, can also mimic ovarian torsion.

US and CFD are the primary imaging modality in assessing patients with ovarian torsion. However, advances in technology and improved availability have led to increased use of CT and MR imaging as adjunct problem solving modalities in ambiguous cases.

REFERENCES

1. Hibbard LT. Adnexal torsion. Am J Obstet Gynecol 1985;152(4):456–61.
2. Burnett LS. Gynecological causes of the acute abdomen. Surg Clin North Am 1988;68(2):385–98.
3. Rha SE, Byun JY, Jung SE, et al. CT and MR imaging features of adnexal torsion. Radiographics 2002; 22(2):283–94.
4. Outwater EK, Siegelman ES, Hunt JL. Ovarian teratomas: tumor types and imaging characteristics. Radiographics 2001;21(2):475–90.
5. Bennett GL, Slywotzky CM, Giovanniello G. Gynecologic causes of acute pelvic pain: spectrum of CT findings. Radiographics 2002;22(4):785–801.
6. Shadinger LL, Andreotti RF, Kurian RL. Preoperative sonographic and clinical characteristics as predictors of ovarian torsion. J Ultrasound Med 2008; 27(1):7–13.
7. Graif M, Shalev J, Strauss S, et al. Torsion of the ovary: sonographic features. Am J Roentgenol 1984;143(6):1331–4.
8. Stark JE, Siegel MJ. Ovarian torsion in prepubertal and pubertal girls: sonographic findings. Am J Roentgenol 1994;163(6):1479–82.
9. Cohen SB, Weisz B, Seidman DS, et al. Accuracy of the preoperative diagnosis in 100 emergency laparoscopies performed due to acute abdomen in nonpregnant women. J Am Assoc Gynecol Laparosc 2001;8(1):92–4.
10. Lee CH, Raman S, Sivanesaratnam V. Torsion of ovarian tumors: a clinicopathological study. Int J Gynecol Obstet 1989;28(1):21–5.
11. Nichols DH, Julian PT. Torsion of the adnexa. Clin Obstet Gynecol 1985;28:375–80.
12. Servaes S, Zurakowski D, Laufer MR, et al. Sonographic findings of ovarian torsion in children. Pediatr Radiol 2007;37(5):446–51.
13. Graif M, Itzchak Y. Sonographic evaluation of ovarian torsion in childhood and adolescence. Am J Roentgenol 1988;150(3):647–9.
14. Ben-Ami M, Perlitz Y, Haddad S. The effectiveness of spectral and color Doppler in predicting ovarian torsion: a prospective study. Eur J Obstet Gynecol Reprod Biol 2002;104:64–6.
15. Hurh PJ, Meyer JS, Shaaban A. Ultrasound of a torsed ovary: characteristic gray scale appearance despite normal arterial and venous flow on Doppler. Pediatr Radiol 2002;32(8):586–8.
16. Pena JE, Ufberg D, Cooney N, et al. Usefulness of Doppler sonography in the diagnosis of ovarian torsion. Fertil Steril 2000;73(5):1047–50.
17. Fleischer A, Stein S, Cullinan J, et al. Color Doppler sonography of adnexal torsion. J Ultrasound Med 1995;14:523–8.
18. Lee EJ, Kwon HC, Joo M, et al. Diagnosis of ovarian torsion with color Doppler sonography: depiction of twisted vascular pedicle. J Ultrasound Med 1998; 17:83–9.
19. Albayram F, Hamper U. Ovarian and adnexal torsion: spectrum of sonographic findings with pathologic correlation. J Ultrasound Med 2001;20(10): 1083–9.

20. Villalba ML, Huynh B, So M, et al. An ovary with a twist: a case of interesting sonographic findings of ovarian torsion. J Emerg Med 2005;29(4):443–6.
21. Anders JF, Powell EC. Urgency of evaluation and outcome of acute ovarian torsion in pediatric patients. Arch Pedtr Adolesc Med 2005;159(6):532–5.
22. Bayer AI, Wiskind AK. Adnexal torsion: can the adnexa be saved? Am J Obstet Gynecol 1994; 171(6):1506–10.
23. Garel L, Dubois J, Grignon A. Ultrasound of the pediatric female pelvis: a clinical perspective. Radiographics 2001;21(6):1393–407.
24. Schenker JG, Polishuk WZ. Ovarian hyperstimulation syndrome. Obstet Gynecol 1975;46(1): 23–8.
25. Kim IY, Lee BH. Ovarian hyperstimulation syndrome US and CT appearances. Clin Imaging 1997;21(4): 284–6.
26. Jung BG, Kim H. Severe ovarian hyperstimulation syndrome with MR findings. J Comput Assist Tomogr 2001;25(2):215–7.
27. Hochsztein JG, Koenigsberg M, Green DA. US case of the day: actinomycotic pelvic abscess secondary to an IUD with involvement of the bladder, sigmoid colon, left ureter, liver and upper abdominal wall. RadioGraphics 1996;16(3):713–6.
28. Maenpaa J, Taina E, Gronroos M, et al. Abdomino-pelvic actinomycosis associated with intrauterine devices: two case reports. Arch Gynecol Obstet 1988;243(4):237–41.

Color Flow Doppler Evaluation of Uterus and Ovaries and Its Optimization Techniques

Mustafa Secil, MD[a], Vikram S. Dogra, MD[b],*

KEYWORDS

• Doppler ultrasound • Uterus • Ovary • Optimization

Color flow Doppler (CFD) imaging provides valuable information about the vascularity of tissue, organs, or systems. CFD imaging is commonly used during the evaluation of uterus and ovaries in addition to gray-scale imaging[1] and is a helpful imaging modality in the diagnosis of various pathologic conditions in gynecology and obstetrics.[2–12] The main limitation of CFD imaging is its user dependency that may lead to misdiagnosis owing to the artifacts or pitfalls derived from improper technique, incorrect use of imaging parameters, and unawareness of physical properties of the modality by the user. This article summarizes the CFD imaging technique, the optimization of imaging parameters, and the useful findings in the evaluation of uterus and ovaries.

VASCULAR ANATOMY
Uterus

The arterial blood supply of the uterus is provided by the uterine arteries originating from the anterior branch of internal iliac artery on each side. Uterine arteries ascend on the lateral surfaces of the uterus, up to the hilum of the ovary, and join to the ovarian arteries. Branches arise from the main uterine arteries and penetrate the outer myometrium, forming a spoke wheel configuration of arcuate arteries.[1,2,13] The radial branches of the uterine artery traverse the myometrium and

form the basal and spiral arterioles, which supply the endometrium. The uterine plexus of veins accompanies the arcuate arteries and is larger than the associated arterial channels.

Uterine arteries on each side can be detected by color Doppler sonography at the level of the corporocervical junction (**Fig. 1**). The arcuate arteries can be depicted on their course in the outer myometrium with the descending cervical and ascending uterine branches.[1] The depiction of further uterine artery branches depends on several factors, including the sensitivity of the scanner and the age and parity of the patient.[2] In nonmedically suppressed women of childbearing age, myometrial vessels can be seen as well as spiral vessels within the endometrium in the luteal phase. Vessels within the basal layer can be seen as straighter vessels than those that course within the basal layers, whereas spiral vessels are more tortuous and scattered within the luteal phase endometrium. Postmenopausal women typically have relatively hypovascular myometrium and endometrium.

Doppler waveforms of uterine artery flow typically have a high-velocity, high-resistance pattern with an identifiable dicrotic notch.[14] The Doppler spectrum of basal and spiral arterioles varies depending on the time of menstruation cycle, gestation, or postmenopausal status (**Fig. 2**). Uterine artery branches haves high-resistance

[a] Department of Radiology, Dokuz Eylul University, 35350, Izmir, Turkey
[b] Department of Radiology, University of Rochester School of Medicine and Dentistry, 601 Elmwood Avenue, Box 648, Rochester, NY 14642, USA
* Corresponding author.
E-mail address: vikram_dogra@URMC.Rochester.edu (V.S. Dogra).

Ultrasound Clin 3 (2008) 461–482
doi:10.1016/j.cult.2008.07.004

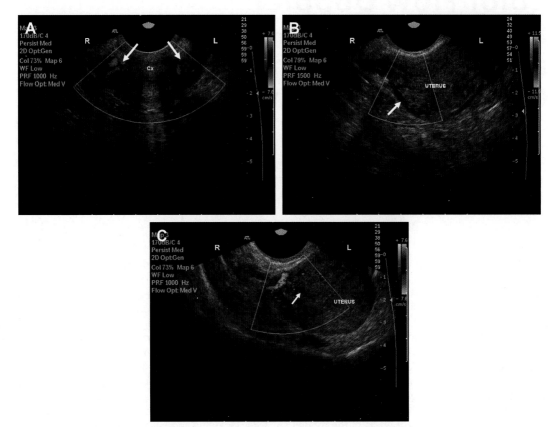

Fig. 1. Normal uterine vessels. (*A*) Transverse transvaginal Doppler image demonstrates the main uterine arteries (*red*) and veins (*blue*) at the corporocervical junction (*arrows*). Cx denotes the cervix uteri. (*B*) The right arcuate artery is seen on the lateral surface of the uterus (*arrow*). (*C*) The radial artery penetrating the myometrium (*arrow*).

flow with resistive index values around 0.7 in premenopausal, nonpregnant women.[15] In the postmenopausal period the same values are 0.93 plus or minus 0.09.[16] During gestation, the flow characteristically gains low-resistance pattern, the resistive and pulsatility indices in uterine artery branches decrease gradually with increasing gestational week.[17,18]

Ovaries

The ovaries have dual arterial blood supply through the ovarian artery and the adnexal branches of the uterine artery.[1,13,19] Ovarian arteries originate from the aorta inferior to the renal arteries on each side. They cross the external iliac arteries and veins at the pelvic brim and course medially within the suspensory ligament of the ovary and then pass posteriorly in the meso-ovarium.[13] Adnexal branches of the uterine artery anastomose with the ovarian artery at the ovarian hilum (**Fig. 3**). The venous system roughly parallels the arterial system, having a pampiniform plexus that directly connects to gonadal veins. The ovarian veins drain into the inferior vena cava on the right and the renal vein on the left.

Doppler imaging findings of the ovary depend on the phase of the menstruation cycle (**Fig. 4**). After the development of a corpus luteum, a vascular arcade is created within the wall of a functioning corpus luteum, seen as vascular ring on color or power Doppler sonography.[1,19] On spectral imaging, in the dominant ovary where the follicle develops, the arterioles show low-resistance flow.[19] This pattern coincides with the luteinizing hormone surge that increases through the periovulatory period and remains at this level for 4 to 5 days after ovulation into the luteal phase of the cycle.[1] Ovarian arterial blood flow then gradually returns to a high-resistance pattern during the menstrual period.[14,15,19] The dormant ovary shows high-impedance arterial flow throughout the menstrual cycle.[1] In the postmenopausal period the ovaries have low vascularity on color Doppler and the spectrum of arterial waveforms are in a high-resistance pattern. The ovarian veins have a continuous waveform with minimal phasic variations.

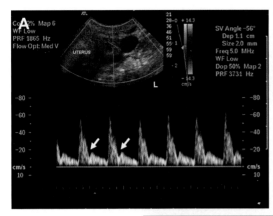
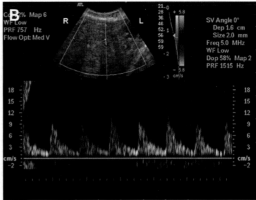
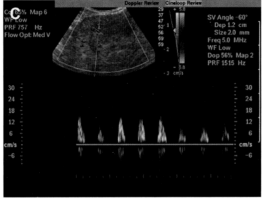

Fig. 2. Normal waveform of uterine artery and its branches. (*A*) Spectral Doppler analysis of uterine artery at the corporocervical junction level reveals high-resistance waveform with typical dicrotic notch (*arrows*). (*B*) The spectrum of a uterine artery branch in the myometrium in a premenopausal woman; high-resistance waveform, RI value is around 0.7. (*C*) High-resistance waveform uterine artery with RI value 1.0, in a postmenopausal woman.

COLOR FLOW DOPPLER EVALUATION TECHNIQUE OF UTERUS AND OVARIES
Transducers

Sonographic evaluation of the uterus and ovaries is commonly performed by transabdominal or transvaginal approach. Transrectal and transperineal approach are rarely used methods in very specific conditions. Transabdominal imaging provides a global anatomic survey, whereas transvaginal imaging provides improved texture determination and characterization of the internal architecture of the uterus, ovary, vascular anatomy, and adnexal area.[7] Transrectal ultrasound is performed whenever there is a contraindication to transvaginal scan, such as in the evaluation of the pediatric pelvis or in women who have never been sexually active.[7] Transperineal scans also have a role to play in determining the origin and extent of some tumors.

Transabdominal transducers are in the low-frequency range with wide field of view and high sound penetrability, whereas transvaginal transducers are in medium to high frequencies with a limited field of view and low sound penetration. Transvaginal approach is the preferred method in suitable patients as it provides better gray-scale resolution owing to the higher frequencies than the transabdominal transducers. The high-frequency property of transvaginal transducers has an additional advantage of better detection of Doppler signals.[20] Higher frequency transducers are more sensitive to Doppler shifts because the intensity of the scattered sound varies in proportion to the fourth power the Doppler frequency.[21] The main limitation of high-frequency transducers is the attenuation of sound and loss of beam penetration for both gray-scale and Doppler imaging.

Sonographic Examination Steps of Uterus and Ovaries

Gray-scale imaging

A complete and proper gray-scale evaluation of uterus and ovaries is essential before further examination by CFD imaging. Gray-scale imaging not only provides morphologic information and

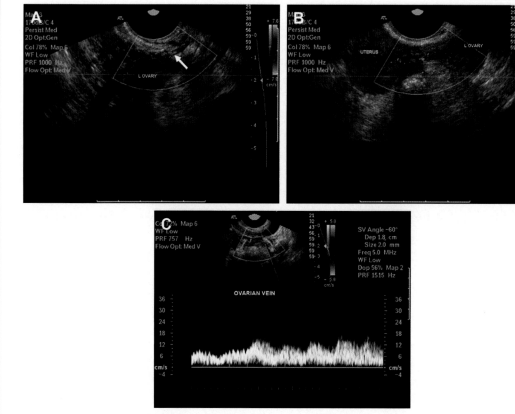

Fig. 3. Normal ovarian vascularization. (*A*) Ovarian artery and (*B*) adnexal branches of uterine artery constitutes the dual arterial supply of ovary. (*C*) Normal venous waveform of the ovarian vein. The flow is continuous character with minimal phasic variations.

initial orientation to pelvic structures, but also affect the technical quality of Doppler evaluation. As the color-flow Doppler data are superimposed on gray-scale image, basic gray-scale parameters should be optimized first. The presets dedicated to pelvic or gynecologic imaging on the ultrasound scanners for the parameters are satisfactory in most of the conditions. However, parameters such as the gain, location and number of focal zones, depth of field, zoom, and orientation settings are actively set during the examination in every patient. Improper setting of these parameters negatively influences the CFD imaging.[20] High gray-scale gain settings suppress the color information (**Fig. 5**) and contrarily low settings highlight the color on the image. A balance should be maintained between the gray-scale and color priority, based on the imaging findings and the clinical condition of the patient. For the evaluation of suspicion of an ovarian torsion, for example, low-level color is preferable at the beginning of the examination and then is tuned to higher values for detection of ovarian vascularity.[4] Highly vascular pathologies such as uterine arteriovenous malformation or fistula, on the other hand, may cause

color dominance on the image and may obscure the gray-scale findings necessitating the adjustment of the priority to gray-scale. Increasing the depth of view, the number and depth of focal zones, and applying zoom are other important gray-scale parameters for the quality CFD imaging. The main effects of inappropriate use of these parameters are the loss of gray-scale information and the decreased frame rate. The frame rate varies inversely with the depth of field, zoom application, and the number of focal zones.[20]

Color Doppler imaging

The second step of CFD imaging of uterus and ovaries is the application of a "color box" at the area of interest. Color box is the sample volume of color Doppler imaging where the Doppler shifts are detected and displayed on the image as color pixels. The data of color Doppler and gray-scale are obtained by two separately sent and received pulses and are tied to be displayed on the same image. However, the scanner needs some time to detect the Doppler frequency shifts and this time is considerably less than the acquisition time of gray-scale information. As the color box

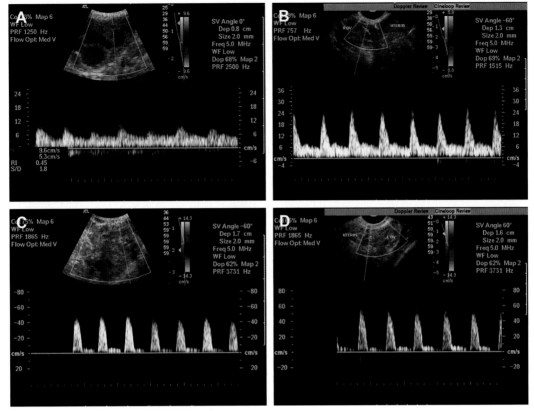

Fig. 4. Normal variation of ovarian arterial flow depending on the menstrual cycle. The dominant ovary of the cycle with the maturing follicle has low-resistance waveform in the ovarian artery branch (*A*) and also in the adnexal branch of uterine artery supplying the ovary (*B*). The dormant site ovary demonstrates high-resistance waveform in the ovary (*C*), and in the adnexal branch of uterine artery (*D*).

covers the area that will be scanned for frequency shifts, the size of the color box is important for the amount of Doppler data that will be collected, determining the frame rate of color box.[20] The time consistency between color and gray-scale display is inversely affected by the size of the color box.

Working with a decreased frame rate causes the loss of synchronization between the gray-scale and color imaging, resulting in image orientation loss. Trying to catch up the time delay on the image is very annoying for the operator and may not be possible in conditions when very wide color

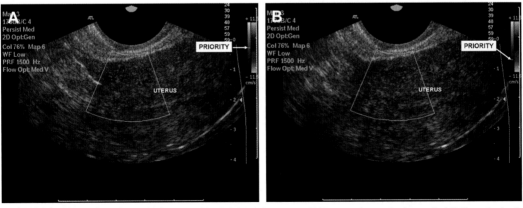

Fig. 5. Gray-scale versus color priority. Priority is denoted as a small line on the scale (*arrow*). (*A*) No priority between the gray-scale and color. (*B*) The selection of priority toward gray-scale instead of color results in a decrease of color encoding.

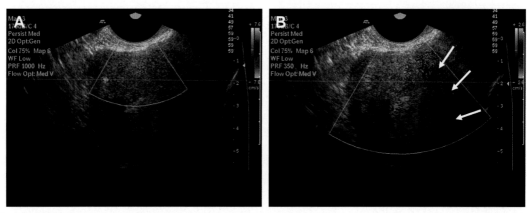

Fig. 6. (*A*) Color box is the sample volume of color Doppler imaging that should be as small as possible to cover only the area of interest. (*B*) For the scanner, a wide color box means more pixels to compute, and also more waiting time to collect data from deep signals. Flash artifact (*arrows*) owing to any small motion become apparent during the computation of data, particularly in low PRF values.

box is used. The other negative effect of a wide color box is the facilitation of the color Doppler artifacts to occur (**Fig. 6**). For optimization, the width and depth size of the color box should be kept small to improve frame rate and obtain better color resolution.[1,20] The box should cover only the area of interest for sampling of vessels of the uterus, ovary, or of a detected mass.

Spectral Doppler imaging

The flow spectrum is obtained by real-time interrogation of a vessel by a cursor, "the spectral gate," positioned on a vessel that is detected either on the color box or on gray-scale image (**Fig. 7**).

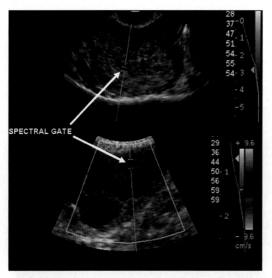

Fig. 7. Spectral gate is the sample volume of spectral Doppler imaging. The gate can be applied either on the gray-scale image if the vessel can be visualized (*upper*) or on the color box (*lower*).

The use of color box as a guide to detect the vessel is the frequently used and preferred method. However, in conditions that decrease the frame rate because of real-time color interrogation, spectral imaging can be performed by applying the cursor on the gray-scale image, if the vessel can be visualized. The obtained spectral waveform depicts the spectrum of frequency shifts of all blood traversing the sampled volume during the period of data acquisition[22] and contains the hemodynamic information describing the velocity and character of the blood flow in the specific vessel being insonated.[20] Besides the characterization of flow, the waveform provides velocity-time information of the sampled vessel, which can be used in quantification of the flow. There are several velocity and velocity-derived, or time and time-derived measurement methods that are being used in CFD imaging of uterus and ovaries (**Box 1**). Owing to the complexity of the imaging parameters, spectral analysis has a high risk of making mistakes, which can lead to false diagnosis because of wrong characterization, or more importantly to incorrect measurement of flow.

COLOR-FLOW DOPPLER PARAMETERS AND OPTIMIZATION

Color flow Doppler examination is probably the most user-dependent imaging modality. There are several imaging parameters that have to be taken into consideration during the evaluations.[20,23] Most of the imaging parameters are preset by the manufacturers of the sonography devices to perform optimum CFD imaging, however there are certain parameters that should be controlled by the user in each patient. Some, on the other hand, should particularly be checked, not to meet with a potential pitfall or artifact that may lead to false diagnosis. The user should be familiar with the basic Doppler physics including the principles of Doppler artifacts, as well as the operational parameters that should be optimized for a proper imaging. Independent of the type or the manufacturer, all Doppler ultrasound scanners display the gray-scale, color, or spectral Doppler operational parameters of the examination on the display monitors. For optimum imaging, the operator should be familiar with the displayed parameters on the monitors. The general concepts for optimization of color Doppler parameters are summarized in **Table 1**, and of spectral Doppler parameters are summarized in **Table 2**.

SAMPLE VOLUME

The Doppler frequency shifts are measured in the sample volume represented by the color box and by the spectral gate in color and spectral Doppler, respectively. The sample volume is a three-dimensional space. The sound beam is not ultimately thin and has the third dimension (the thickness) not displayed on the image.[23,24] Doppler signals collected from the third dimension may be displayed on the image, just similar to the partial volume artifact in CT or MR imaging. The ovaries are located near the internal iliac vessels. An improper Doppler sampling may cause color or spectral encoding inside of the ovary or ovarian mass because of partial volume averaging. If the spectral gate is kept wide during the sampling of uterine or ovarian artery branches, the waveform may detect the nearby iliac artery branches (**Fig. 8**). Wide spectral gate also depicts arterial and venous flow

on the same spectrum because of the close proximity of arterial and vein branches in uterus and ovaries (**Fig. 9**). The ideal spectral gate size for routine survey of a vessel is about two thirds of the vessel width positioned in the center of the vessel,[24] excluding as much of the unwanted clutter from near the vessel walls as possible.[21]

Sample volume displays the detected signals that are focused on the image. However, the sound is not as homogeneous and well-focused as expected and there is always off-focus sound at the side lobes and grating lobes. The image reflections form the side-lobes and may be displayed in the center if the reflections in these areas are high. This is known as the "side lobe artifact," which may also occur in Doppler imaging.[23] The detected Doppler shifts in the side-lobes may be high enough to be encoded in the central beam areas and may mimic flow on color Doppler images. Intestinal gas in the pelvis may behave as a strong reflector for Doppler frequencies in the side-lobe beam and may cause signal encoding inside of the ovary or of an ovarian mass. Spectral imaging shows bizarre signals in those areas and can be used to demonstrate that the color encoding is not attributable to a real flow (**Fig. 10**).

VELOCITY SCALE

The velocity scale is the range of flow velocities that are depicted with either the color (**Figs. 11** and **12**) or spectral Doppler imaging (**Fig. 13**). The scale is controlled by pulse repetition frequency (PRF) of Doppler imaging. The sampling of any frequency is dependent on the Nyquist theory. Nyquist theory denotes that, for correct observation of a periodical motion, the observation frequency must be at least twice of the observed periodical motion. Aliasing occurs when the pulse repetition frequency is less than 2 times the highest frequency of a Doppler frequency shift (Nyquist limit is exceeded).[25–29] Aliasing is seen as ambiguous color encoding in color Doppler and as a "wrapping around" of the waveform in spectral Doppler imaging. Aliasing can be avoided by optimal use of the velocity scale to allow the actual velocity to fall within the selected range. On the other hand, to increase the PRF (hence the velocity scale) much over the Doppler frequency shifts in a vessel restrains the detection of flow in a patent vessel.

DOPPLER GAIN

Gain refers to amplification of the sampled information for purposes of improving the depiction

Table 1
Color Doppler parameters

Parameter	Effects	Optimization
Color box size	Color encoding competes with gray-scale image during the display. Increased size and width necessitates more sampling resulting in decreased frame rate of color display. • Width—more lines to sample • Depth—more lines to sample and increased time for waiting to detect Doppler shifts	Should be kept small, only to cover the area of interest.
Beam steering (angle of color box)	• Doppler shift detection is zero at 90°. • Doppler shifts near 90° result in directional ambiguity artifact; the direction of flow could not be estimated.	Should be adjusted to obtain a satisfactorily small angle (ie, not 90°). Optimum angle can be achieved by probe manipulations.
Color velocity scale	Determines the sampled velocity range and controlled by PRF. • High scale (High PRF)—Doppler frequencies fall out of the sampling ranges; no flow is detected. • Low scale (Low PRF)—Nyquist limit is exceeded, "color aliasing" occurs.	Depends on the area of interest. Low PRF settings for slow flow, higher PRF settings for increased or turbulent flow detection. Proper adjustment of PRF to obtain a color encoding just over the aliasing limit.
Color gain	Amplifies the color information • High gain—Noise of color encoding at nonvascular areas ("color bleed artifact") • Low gain—No visualization of flow	Should be set just below the noise level.
Color priority	Each pixel is encoded either by color or gray-scale information. • Increased color priority—Low intensity signals at the periphery of vessels • Increased gray-scale priority—More gray-scale information, less color encoding	Best to be kept in balance in between. Rarely needed to be changed.
Color wall filter	Filters eliminate high-intensity–low-frequency noise originating from wall motion of the vessels.	Ideally should be kept at 50–100 Hz. Usually presets are adequate, not necessary to change during routine exams.

of acquired data. The amplification should be set to detect the presence of flow in a vessel without causing an artifact or noise (**Fig. 14**). Too high Doppler gain would result in color encoding in nonvascular areas ("color bleed artifact") and noise that may obscure the waveform in spectral imaging (**Fig. 15**).[27,30] Too low Doppler gain will cause

the lack of depiction of a present flow or will underestimate a flow disturbance, both in color and spectral Doppler analyses.

Inappropriate adjustment of color Doppler gain settings during the evaluation of uterus and ovaries may cause mistakes in various conditions. The vascularity of adenomyosis is typically

Table 2
Spectral Doppler parameters

Parameter	Effects	Optimization
Angle	The most important parameter because the velocity measurements of the spectrum are dependent on the angle. • Doppler shift is maximum at 0° (practically unachievable) and zero at 90°. • Linear relation between velocity and Doppler shifts between 30° and 60°. Exponential differences occur between velocity and Doppler shifts out of this angle range causing incorrect velocity measurements.	Should be parallel to the lumen of the vessel and be kept less than 60°.
Sample gate size	• Too large gate—Spectral impurity; contiguous vessels encoded on the same spectrum (venous flow contamination in sampling of an artery, or vice versa). • Too large gate—Erroneous signal detection from adjacent vessels. • Too small gate—Reduced or no flow depiction.	Should be set in correct size, usually two-thirds of the vessel lumen
Spectral velocity scale	Determines the sampled velocity range and controlled by PRF. • High scale (High PRF)—Doppler frequencies fall out of the sampling ranges. Shallow spectrum is displayed limiting measurements of flow or no spectrum obtained at all. • Low scale (Low PRF)—Nyquist limit is exceeded, spectrum is wrapped around ("spectral aliasing").	Depends on the area of interest. Low PRF settings for slow flow, higher PRF settings for increased or turbulent flow detection. Proper adjustment of PRF to obtain a spectrum just over the aliasing limit.
Spectral gain	Amplifies the spectral information • High gain—Noise contaminates or may obscure the spectrum. • Low gain—No spectrum is displayed	Should be set just below the noise level
Spectral baseline	The direction of flow is displayed over or under the baseline. Improper level disrupts the spectrum and the flow is encoded on both sides of the line.	Should be kept at the level to fit the spectrum in the display.
Spectral wall filter	Filters eliminate high-intensity–low-frequency noise originating from wall motion of the vessels.	Ideally should be kept at 50–100 Hz. Usually presets are adequate, not necessary to change during routine exams.

increased in the affected site and has been defined as a "raindrop" appearance of blood flowing through the center of the tissue.[1] Surrounding tissue unaffected by adenomyosis remains mostly hypovascular. High color gain settings may result in overencoding of colors mimicking adenomyosis in a normal myometrium (**Fig. 16**). The ovary with torsion may be observed to have vascularity in high color gain settings or contrarily a normal ovary may be found to be avascular in low settings.[29]

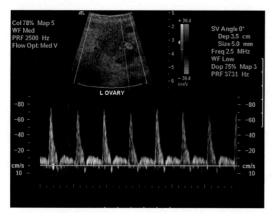

Fig. 8. Incorrect use of location and size of sample gate. Spectral Doppler sampling at the lateral part of the ovary displays the arterial waveform of an internal artery branch inside of the ovary.

Higher level of color gain than normal may cause an image as if there is pelvic inflammatory disease affecting the uterus, adnexa, or ovaries.

Either low or high, improper spectral Doppler gain settings may cause failure in depiction,

characterization, and making correct measurements of the flow in the uterus and ovaries (Fig. 17). Low gain settings cause a faint spectrum or no spectrum at all. High spectral gain results in an unclear spectrum because of the increased display of the background noise.

DOPPLER ANGLE

Doppler angle is the most important parameter of CFD imaging for appropriate sampling and also for correct measurements. Doppler angle parameter includes the two commonly confused terms: "angle of insonation" and "angle correction." The differences between these two terms are important to understand.[20]

The "angle of insonation" is the angle between the transducer and the vessel during the evaluation, which determines the detection of the frequency shifts and acquisition of correct information from the shifts.[20] Angle of insonation is controlled by steering of the beam in the sample volume (color box or spectral gate) by steer button on the ultrasound scanner or by operator manipulations of the probe.

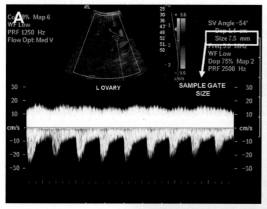

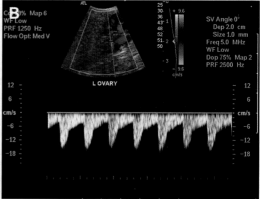

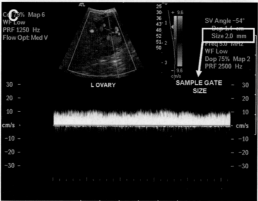

Fig. 9. Incorrect use of size of sample gate. (A) Too-wide sample gate depicts arterial and venous waveforms in the same spectrum of a contiguous artery and vein. Optimum setting of the size and position selectively displays the artery (B) and vein (C).

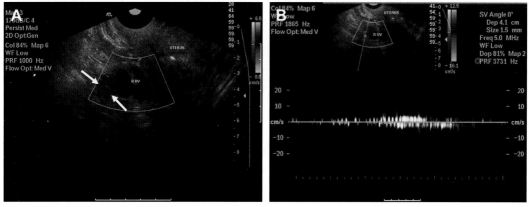

Fig. 10. Side-lobe artifact in Doppler. (*A*) The intestinal gas outside of the color box behaves as a strong reflector for Doppler shifts in the off-focus sound (the "side-lobe" sound). The detected frequency shift is displayed in the focus area as a color artifact (*arrows*). (*B*) Spectral Doppler imaging of that area distinguishes the artifact from a real flow by demonstrating bizarre signals on the spectrum.

The "angle correction" refers to adjustment of the Doppler angle and is used to calibrate the velocity scale to provide the correct angle for the computer to solve the Doppler equation.[20] Angle correction is performed before, during, or after the acquisition of the waveform by proper placing of the angle cursor of spectral gate, parallel to the vessel wall.

Angle of Insonation and Beam Steering

The angle of insonation determines the range of velocities being detected and affects the color or spectral display of the flow. The maximum Doppler shift detection is at 0°, which is practically impossible, and is zero at 90° where no signal is obtained. To detect flow in a vessel, the angle of insonation should be as small as possible. The angle of insonation determines the detected range of frequency shifts, which finally affects the velocity scale and the quality of the obtained spectral waveform (**Fig. 18**). Scanning with extreme angles toward 0° or 90° may result in falsely high or low flow velocities, respectively, owing to the nonlinear relation between velocity and the Doppler shifts in extreme angles.[2] Scanning with angle of

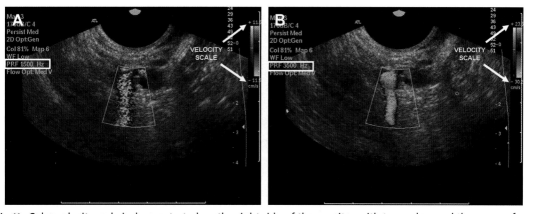

Fig. 11. Color velocity scale is demonstrated on the right side of the monitor with two colors and the range of velocities (*arrows*) determined by the color Doppler PRF (*in rectangles*). The color on the upper side of the color scale depicts the flow toward the transducer and the lower side away from it. (*A*) The encoded color inside of the vessel is speckled and direction of flow cannot be estimated by color. This is known as color "aliasing." (*B*) Optimum PRF correctly depicts the direction of flow that is toward the transducer (*encoded in red*) in this example.

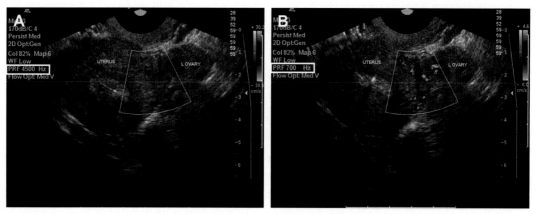

Fig. 12. (*A*) High selection of color velocity scale (too high PRF) underestimates the vascularity in the adnexal area; (*B*) optimum PRF use of the same area depicts the correct amount of vascularity.

insonation near 90° results in another handicap: the "directional ambiguity artifact."[26] This is most common in small vessels, especially those that may be traveling in and out of the imaging

plane.[23] Directional ambiguity is seen as a spectral Doppler waveform displayed with nearly equal amplitude above and below the baseline. Doppler samplings of flow at the parenchymal level vessels

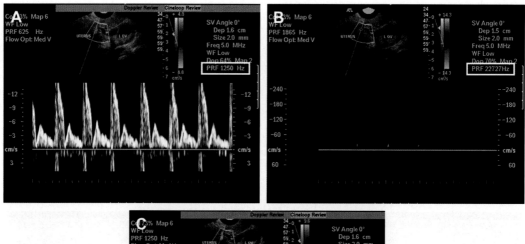

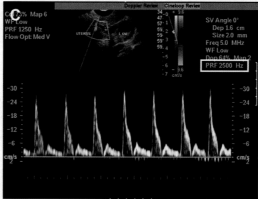

Fig. 13. Spectral velocity scale is determined by spectral PRF (*in rectangles*), which is independent of color PRF. (*A*) Spectral "aliasing" occurs because of too low PRF setting. Some of the Doppler frequency shifts do not fit into the spectrum and the waveform is seen as "wrapped around," and depicted on the other side of the baseline. (*B*) Too high PRF use, resulting in a shallow waveform that is difficult to characterize and perform measurement. Further elevation of PRF would cause total elimination of spectral encoding. (*C*) Optimum PRF and the spectral velocity scale with optimum waveform depiction.

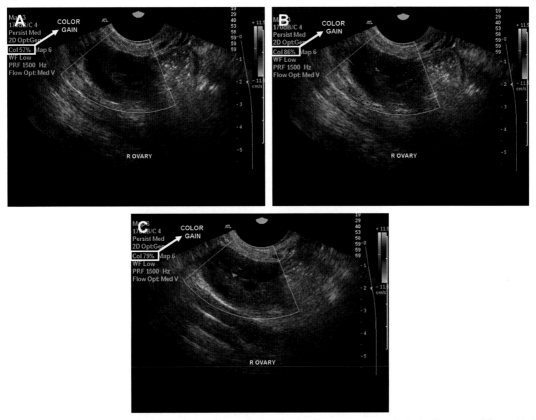

Fig. 14. Color gain setting. (*A*) Too low color gain misses to depict the present vascularity in the ovary. (*B*) Too high color gain causes color noise on the image seen as color encoding in areas other than the vessels of the ovary. (*C*) Optimum color gain detecting the present flow and is just lower than the color noise.

of uterus and ovaries frequently depict directional ambiguity artifact in which the flow direction cannot be determined in these unqualified waveforms (**Fig. 19**). The convex nature of the transducers used for the evaluation of uterus and ovaries limits beam steering on the ultrasound scanner. To obtain a clear spectrum devoid of directional ambiguity artifact, the operator should manipulate the probe to provide an appropriate angle of insonation.

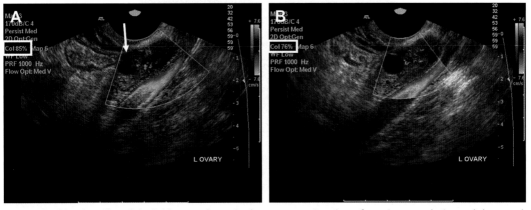

Fig. 15. Color bleed artifact. (*A*) Highly set color gain shows overestimation of ovarian vascularity and shows color encoding in the ovarian cyst. The perivascular color encoding of the iliac vessel is also exaggerated, some color "bleeds" to the ovary from the iliac vessel. (*B*) Optimal color gain of the same area eliminates the color bleed artifact, demonstrates that the cyst is avascular, and depicts the correct vascularity of the ovary.

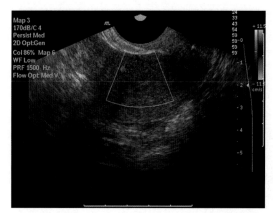

Fig. 16. Over-encoding of color in the normal myometrium because of high color gain setting, which may mimic the "raindrop" color appearance of adenomyosis.

Angle Correction

The frequency shifts are solved by the computer according to the Doppler equation and displayed as a velocity-time spectrum. All velocity measurements on this spectrum are highly dependent on the angle because the computation includes wide range of changes originating from high variations of cosine of the angle. For a correct measurement, the scale of the spectrum should be optimized by correct application of angle cursor of the spectral gate. The angle cursor should always be parallel to the vessel wall. However, angle correction fails in small vessels of the uterus and ovaries in cases where the outline of the vessel could not be accurately determined. Velocity measurements differ in a high range in these conditions (**Fig. 20**). To overcome this limitation, the velocity measurements can be disregarded and only the character of flow can be taken into consideration, or angle-independent parameters such as resistive index, pulsatility index, systole-diastole ratio, and so forth can be used as reference.

WALL FILTERS

Wall filters eliminate the typically low-frequency–high-intensity noise that may arise from vessel

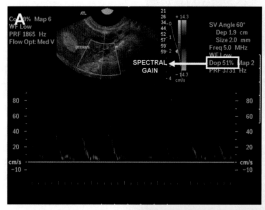
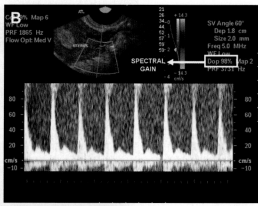
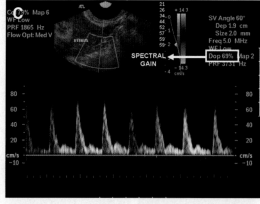

Fig. 17. Spectral gain setting. (A) Too low spectral gain resulting in a faint spectrum. Further decrease would limit the detection of flow in that uterine artery branch. (B) Too high spectral gain causing the contamination of the spectrum by noise. Aliasing and directional ambiguity artifacts are displayed more than normal by high gain settings, which also contribute to the impurity of the spectrum. (C) Optimum spectral gain provides a pure spectrum in the same uterine artery branch.

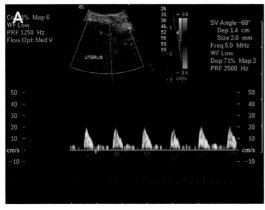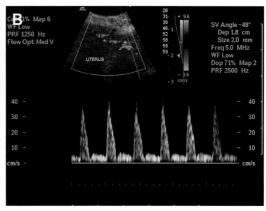

Fig. 18. Angle of insonation is the angle between the transducer and the vessel (the angle between the spectral gate and the vessel that should not be confused with the angle correction denoted as SV angle on the monitor). (A) The spectral gate is in the middle of the color box; the sound reaches to the vessel with approximately 70° to 90°. (B) The gate is located with minimum achievable angle to the trace of the same vessel. The waveform and the detected range of velocities are quite different between (A) and (B).

wall motion (**Fig. 21**).[20,23] Filters are usually preset by the manufacturer, and a high, medium, or low filter setting may be applied separately to spectral, color, and power imaging. To avoid the loss of signal that characterizes slow flow, filter settings should be kept at the lowest possible setting (typically in the 50- to 100-Hz range).[1] Presets of the ultrasound scanners for imaging of uterus and ovaries are generally adequate for a proper evaluation and changes are rarely needed.

USEFUL COLOR FLOW DOPPLER FINDINGS IN UTERINE AND OVARIAN PATHOLOGIES

CFD imaging is a valuable tool in the diagnosis of various pathologic conditions of uterus and ovaries (**Box 2**).

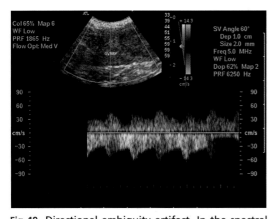

Fig. 19. Directional ambiguity artifact. In the spectral Doppler of the ovary, the spectral gate is just on the midline, the angle of insonation is nearly 90°. The direction of detected frequency shifts could not be correctly displayed and the flow is encoded on both sides of the baseline.

Uterus

Leiomyoma (myoma/fibroid) is the most common tumor of the uterus occurring in 20% to 25% of women older than 30 years.[31] Leiomyomas are classified according to their locations as submucosal, intramural, subserosal. The demonstration of the extent of isoechoic submucosal or intramural leiomyomas may render difficulties, or subserosal leiomyomas growing toward the adnexal area may mimic an adnexal mass. Certain CDF findings are useful in correct diagnosis of these conditions.

Peripheral rim
Depiction of fibroid vascularity by CFD improves the delineation of the size, location, and extent of myometrial involvement.[32] The pseudocapsule of an intramural myoma usually shows an arc of vascularity seen as a "peripheral rim," which helps to identify isoechoic intramural myomas and aids in the diagnosis of subserosal myomas (**Fig. 22**).

Vascular bridging sign
The presence of multiple vessels between the uterus and the presumed adnexal mass is called the "vascular bridging sign" (**Fig. 23**). It is secondary to recruitment of multiple vessels feeding the exophytic uterine fibroid and confirms the origin of the vascular blood supply is from the uterine arteries, implying that the tissue is uterine, not ovarian.[33,34] Color and power Doppler sonography alone have 100% sensitivity and 92% specificity for differentiating subserosal leiomyomas from extrauterine tumors.[34]

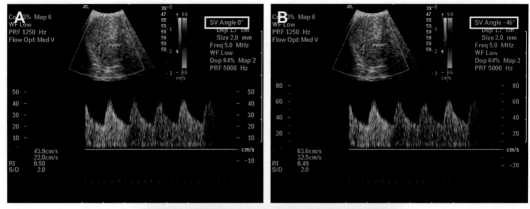

Fig. 20. Angle correction. The same spectrum an ovarian arterial branch with different angle corrections (A–C) demonstrates the considerable variations of flow velocities depending on the angle.

Vascular pedicle sign

A solitary vessel originating from the uterine artery supplying the subserosal leiomyoma is called the "vascular pedicle sign" (**Fig. 24**). The sign shows that the mass and the uterus have a common source of blood supply, which implies that the mass is of uterine origin.[1]

Adenomyosis is a benign condition of the uterus characterized by the presence of endometrial glands and stroma in the myometrium, identified

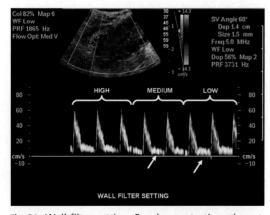

Fig. 21. Wall filter setting. For demonstration, the setting is changed while the spectrum goes by. The effect of lowering the filter is seen as the contamination of the spectrum by low-frequency–high-intensity noise (*arrows*).

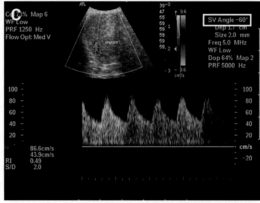

Box 2

Clinical conditions in which CFD is helpful in the evaluation of uterus and ovaries

UTERUS
- Leiomyoma
- Adenomyosis
- Endometrial neoplasms
- Gestational trophoblastic disease
- Abnormal placentation (placenta accreat, increta, percreta; vasa previa)
- Retained products of conception
- Uterine arteriovenous malformations, fistula
- Uterine artery aneurysm

OVARIES
- Torsion
- Ectopic pregnancy
- Ovarian vein thrombosis
- Ovarian malignancy

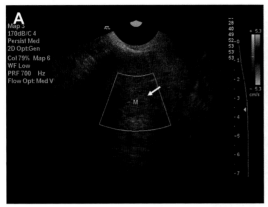
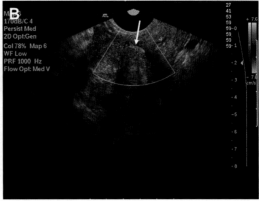

Fig. 22. Peripheral rim of vascularity in intramural (*A*) and subserosal (*B*) leiomyomas. The pseudocapsule of the leiomyoma demonstrates an arc of vascularity seen as a "peripheral rim" (*arrows*), which helps to identify isoechoic intramural myoma (*A*) and aids in the diagnosis of subserosal myomas (*B*).

on imaging by the distortion of the endometrial-myometrial junctional zone and the asymmetry of the uterus.[35,36] Adenomyosis is seen as an ill-defined heterogeneous area in the myometrium in a globularly enlarged uterus. The appearance may mimic an ill-defined leiomyoma and CFD is helpful in discrimination of these two conditions. Unlike leiomyomas, which have a peripheral blood supply, adenomyosis may be distinguished on imaging by its "raindrop" appearance of blood flowing through the center of the tissue and surrounding tissue is hypovascular (**Fig. 25**).[1] On spectral Doppler, RI is usually less than 0.7,[37] the PI of the arteries within or around the adenomyosis tissue is usually greater than 1.17, whereas leiomyomas have a PI of less than or equal to 1.17.[38] The overall sensitivity and specificity of transvaginal US for the diagnosis of adenomyosis is considered to be 80% to 86% and 50% to 96%, respectively.[39]

Endometrial neoplasms include benign hyperplasia, endometrial carcinoma, and endometrial polyps. Sonographically, a considerable overlap exists between the morphologic characteristics of benign and malignant endometrial neoplasms. Also, the studies on the use of CFD imaging in endometrial neoplasms have yielded variable results.[1] The CFD depicts vessels in benign and malignant endometrial lesions (**Fig. 26**). Irregular and randomly dispersed vessels with complex branching in an endometrial lesion favor malignancy.[40] The mean RI in the uterine artery in a normal postmenopausal woman is 0.93 plus or minus 0.09,[16] low-impedance flow with an RI of less than 0.5 and a PI of less than 1.0 have been positively associated with the presence of malignancy.[41] A combination of transvaginal sonography and color

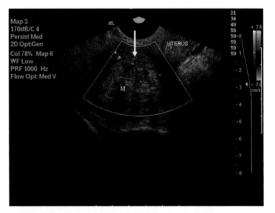

Fig. 24. Vascular pedicle sign of subserosal leiomyoma. The solitary vessel originating from the uterine artery supplying the subserosal leiomyoma (*arrow*). The sign shows that the mass (*M*) and the uterus have common source of blood supply, which implies that the mass is of uterine origin.

Fig. 23. Vascular bridging sign of leiomyoma. The vessels between the uterus and the mass (*M*) confirms the origin of the vascular blood supply is from the uterine arteries, implying that the tissue is uterine, not ovarian.

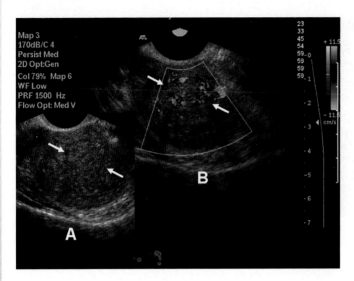

Fig. 25. "Raindrop" vascularity of adeno-myosis. (A) The uterine fundus is globu-larly enlarged and in heterogeneous echogenicity (arrows). (B) Color Doppler image of the same area shows scattered color encoding areas resembling "raindrops."

doppler sonography can be useful in differentiating benign and malignant endometrial lesions; however, endometrial biopsy still remains the gold standard for diagnosing endometrial carcinoma.[1]

Endometrial polyps are intracavitary, pedunculated or broad-based lesions seen in peri- and postmenopausal women, often causing uterine bleeding. The diagnosis of an endometrial polyp is considered when hyperechoic endometrial thickening of greater than 5 mm is observed on

US. Color Doppler or power Doppler imaging enable easy detection of endometrial polyps by demonstrating a single feeding artery known as the "pedicle artery sign."[42] The sensitivity of the pedicle artery sign in diagnosing an endometrial polyp on endovaginal sonography was 76%, the specificity was 95%, and the negative predictive value was 94%.[43]

Gestational trophoblastic disease covers the pathologic spectrum of abnormal trophoblastic

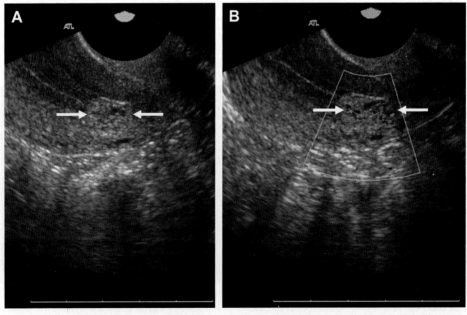

Fig. 26. Endometrial neoplasm. Gray-scale (A) and color Doppler (B) images of a patient with endometrial tumor (arrows), pathologically confirmed as endometrial carcinosarcoma. The tumor is seen as an infiltrative, echogenic endometrial mass in the low part of the uterine corpus (A). Color Doppler demonstrates irregular and randomly dispersed vessels (B).

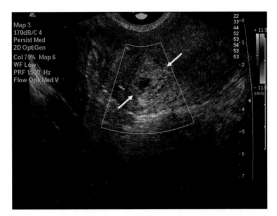

Fig. 27. Gestational trophoblastic disease. Proliferation of the trophoblastic tissue is seen as an echogenic lesion with prominent vascularity (*arrows*) in a patient with elevated β-hCG.

Uterine vascular pathologies such as arteriovenous malformations (AVM) or fistulae (AVF) and uterine artery aneurysms and pseudoaneurysms can readily be diagnosed by CFD imaging. Color Doppler findings of AVM and AVF are more consistent and specific, and include intense multidirectional turbulent flow typified by aliasing.[5,45,46] Spectral analysis characteristically depicts a low-resistance, high-velocity arterial flow with a low RI in the range of 0.25 to 0.55.[47] Peak systolic velocity within the AVM is also usually high in the range of 40 to 100 cm/s.[47–49] Uterine artery aneurysms show the dilatation of the uterine artery with its characteristic arterial flow pattern.[5] Pseudoaneurysms demonstrate a "ying-yang" or "South Korea flag" pattern of color encoding, and to-and-fro waveform spectrum at the neck of the pseudoaneurysm.[49,50]

proliferation including molar pregnancy (partial or complete), invasive mole, choriocarcinoma, and placental site trophoblastic tumors. Proliferation of the trophoblastic tissue demonstrates prominent vascularity with abnormal shunting (**Fig. 27**). Spectral imaging depicts high-velocity, low-impedance flow; the RI usually measures less than 0.4 compared with 0.66 in normal pregnancy.[44]

Retained products of conception is a complication of spontaneous or induced abortion. A focal echogenic mass in the endometrium on gray-scale US is the most useful finding to predict its presence, however such a mass may also represent a blood clot. Depiction of flow in the echogenic mass within the endometrium favors the retained products (**Fig. 28**), excludes a blood clot, and repeated curettage can be avoided.[1]

Ovaries

Ovarian torsion is a gynecologic emergency in which CFD can be used for definitive diagnosis. Completely absent arterial and venous ovarian blood flow are specific for ovarian torsion; however, evidence of flow within the ovary does not exclude ovarian torsion. The dual blood supply to the ovary is responsible for the variable Doppler findings in adnexal torsion. Technical errors with improper settings of the color flow parameters may result in a false-positive diagnosis of torsion.[29]

Ectopic pregnancy is an emergency condition that should be discriminated from the other abdominal emergencies. Sonographically, the presence of an extraovarian thick-walled adnexal mass called the tubal ring is the most common feature of an ectopic preganancy.[51,52] CFD

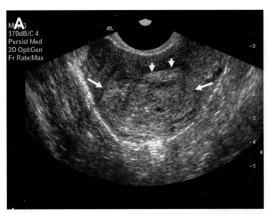
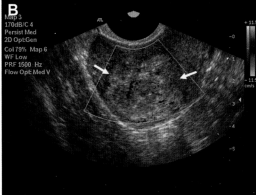

Fig. 28. Retained products of conception. In a patient with recent history of induced abortus and normal level of β-hCG at the time of examination, the gray-scale imaging (*A*) demonstrates an echogenic mass (*arrows*) at the posterior of the endometrium (*arrowheads*). (*B*) Color Doppler image shows increased vascularity in the same area (*arrows*).

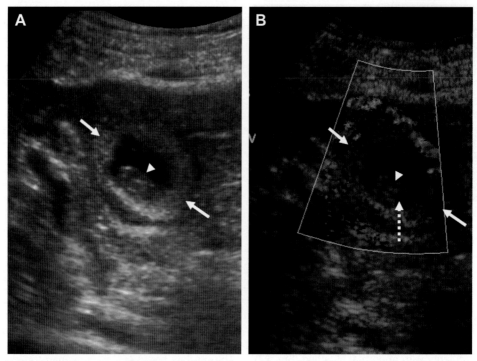

Fig. 29. Tubal ectopic pregnancy. (*A*) Gray-scale image shows the tubal ring (*arrows*) and the embryo (*arrowhead*). (*B*) Color Doppler image demonstrates the peripheral vascularity of the tubal ring (*arrows*) and the cardiac activity (*dotted arrow*) of the embryo (*arrowhead*).

depicts the vascularity of tubal ring. If present, demonstration of cardiac activity of the fetal pole by CFD is pathognomonic (**Fig. 29**).

Ovarian vein thrombosis is seen in the puerperal period and in the right side in 90% of cases, can be diagnosed by demonstration the lack of ovarian vein flow in CFD imaging.[1]

Ovarian malignancies may display certain CFD findings that can be used for correct diagnosis together with the gray-scale findings (**Fig. 30**).[1] These findings include increased vascularization, pulsatility index less than 1.0, resistive index less than 0.4, end diastolic velocity distribution slope (the slope of the mean velocity spectrum at end-diastole) of 1.90 ± 1.33,[53] and shorter uptake and longer washout time of sonographic contrast agent in contrast-enhanced sonography imaging.[54]

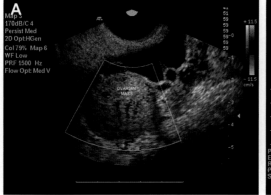
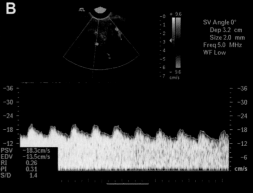

Fig. 30. Ovarian malignancy. (*A*) The solid part of the ovarian tumor displays high vascularity in color Doppler imaging. (*B*) The spectral sampling of the arteries inside of the mass depicts very low resistance.

SUMMARY

CFD imaging is a valuable tool for the diagnosis of various uterine and ovarian pathologies. The transvaginal approach is the best way in suitable patients. Imaging with CFD includes three steps of evaluation of uterus and ovaries: gray-scale, color, and spectral Doppler imaging. For a proper evaluation, the user should be familiar with the technique, the basic Doppler physics including the origin of the artifacts, and how to optimize the use of the operational parameters. Inappropriate use of color and spectral Doppler parameters may lead to false diagnosis because of artifacts. The operator should be aware that the major potential pitfall is the operator himself or herself, working with CFD parameters that are not optimally set.

REFERENCES

1. Bhatt S, Dogra VS. Doppler imaging of the uterus and adnexae. J Clin Ultrasound 2006;1:201–21.
2. Fleischer AC. Color Doppler sonography of uterine disorders. Ultrasound Q 2003;19:179–89.
3. Sheth S, Macura K. Sonography of the uterine myometrium: myomas and beyond. J Clin Ultrasound 2007;2:267–95.
4. Bertolotto M, Serafini G, Toma P, et al. Adnexal torsion. J Clin Ultrasound 2008;3:109–19.
5. Polat P, Suma S, Kantarcý M, et al. Color Doppler us in the evaluation of uterine vascular abnormalities. Radiographics 2002;22:47–53.
6. Bhatt S, Kocakoc E, Dogra VS. Endometriosis: sonographic spectrum. Ultrasound Q. 2006;22:273–80.
7. Joshi M, Ganesan K, Munshi HN, et al. Ultrasound of adnexal masses. J Clin Ultrasound 2007;2:133–53.
8. Brown DL. A practical approach to the ultrasound characterization of adnexal masses. Ultrasound Q 2007;23:87–105.
9. Horrow MM, Rodgers SK, Naqvi S. Ultrasound of pelvic inflammatory disease. J Clin Ultrasound 2007;2:297–309.
10. Bhatt S, Ghazale H, Dogra VS. Sonographic evaluation of ectopic pregnancy. Radiol Clin North Am 2007;45:549–60.
11. Dialani V, Levine D. Ectopic pregnancy: a review. Ultrasound Q 2004;20:105–17.
12. Jain KA. Gynecological causes of acute pelvic pain: ultrasound imaging. J Clin Ultrasound 2008;3:1–12.
13. Holt SC, Levi CS, Lyons FA. Normal anatomy of the female pelvis. In: Callen PW, editor. Ultrasonography in obstetrics and gynecology. 3rd edition. Philadelphia: WB Saunders; 1994. p. 548–68.
14. Taylor K, Burns PN, Wells PN. Ultrasound Doppler flow studies of the ovarian and uterine arteries. Br J Obstet Gynaecol 1985;92:240–6.
15. Ritchie WGM. Ultrasound evaluation of normal and induced ovulation. In: Callen PW, editor. Ultrasonography in obstetrics and gynecology. 3rd edition. Philadelphia: WB Saunders; 1994. p. 569–85.
16. Bonilla-Musoles F, Marti MC, Ballester MJ, et al. Normal uterine arterial blood flow in postmenopausal women assessed by transvaginal color Doppler ultrasonography. J Ultrasound Med 1995;14:491–4.
17. Gomez O, Figueras F, Martínez JM, et al. Sequential changes in uterine artery blood flow pattern between the first and second trimesters of gestation in relation to pregnancy outcome. Ultrasound Obstet Gynecol 2006;28:802–8.
18. Makikallio K, Jouppila P, Tekay A. First trimester uterine, placental and yolk sac haemodynamics in pre-eclampsia and preterm labour. Humanit Rep 2004;19:729–33.
19. Fleischer AC, Brader KR. Sonographic depiction of ovarian vascularity and flow: current improvements and future applications. J Ultrasound Med 2001; 20:241–50.
20. Kruskal JB, Newman PA, Sammons LG, et al. Optimizing Doppler and color flow US: application to hepatic sonography. Radiographics. 2004;24:657–75.
21. Merritt CR. Doppler US: the basics. Radiographics 1991;11:109–19.
22. Rubin JM. Spectral doppler US. Radiographics 1994;14:139–50.
23. Rubens DJ, Bhatt S, Nedelka S, et al. Doppler artifacts and pitfalls. Radiol Clin North Am 2006;44: 805–35.
24. Goldstein A, Madrazo BL. Slice-thickness artifacts in gray-scale ultrasound. J Clin Ultrasound 1981;9: 365–75.
25. Zweibel WJ, Pellerito JS. Basic concepts of doppler frequency spectrum analysis and ultrasound blood flow imaging. Introduction to vascular ultrasonography. Philadelphia: Elsevier Saunders; 2005.
26. Pozniak MA, Zagzebski JA, Scanlan KA. Spectral and color Doppler artifacts. Radiographics 1992; 12:35–44.
27. Nilsson A. Artifacts in sonography and Doppler. Eur Radiol 2001;11:1308–15.
28. Scanlan KA. Sonographic artifacts and their origins. AJR Am J Roentgenol 1991;156:1267–72.
29. Pellerito JS, Troiano RN, Quedens-Case C, et al. Common pitfalls of endovaginal color Doppler flow imaging. Radiographics 1995;15:37–47.
30. Campbell SC, Cullinan JA, Rubens DJ. Slow flow or no flow? Color and power Doppler US pitfalls in the abdomen and pelvis. Radiographics 2004;24:497–506.
31. Schwartz SM. Epidemiology of uterine leiomyomata. Clin Obstet Gynecol 2001;44:316–26.
32. Fleischer AC, Donnelly EF, Campbell MG, et al. Three-dimensional color Doppler sonography before and after fibroid embolization. J Ultrasound Med 2000;19:701–5.

33. Kim JC, Kim SS, Park JY. "Bridging vascular sign" in the MR diagnosis of exophytic uterine leiomyoma. J Comput Assist Tomogr 2000;24:57–60.

34. Kim SH, Sim JS, Seong CK. Interface vessels on color/power Doppler US and MRI: a clue to differentiate subserosal uterine myomas from extrauterine tumors. J Comput Assist Tomogr 2001;25:36–42.

35. Azziz R. Adenomyosis: current perspectives. Obstet Gynecol Clin North Am 1989;16:221–35.

36. Dogan E, Gode F, Saatli B, et al. Juvenile cystic adenomyosis mimicking uterine malformation: a case report. Arch Gynecol Obstet 2008 [Epub ahead of print].

37. Hata T, Hata K, Senoh D, et al. Doppler ultrasound assessment of tumor vascularity in gynecologic disorders. J Ultrasound Med 1989;8:309–14.

38. Chiang CH, Chang MY, Hsu JJ, et al. Tumor vascular pattern and blood flow impedance in the differential diagnosis of leiomyoma and adenomyosis by color Doppler sonography. J Assist Reprod Genet 1999; 16:268–75.

39. Reinhold C, Tafazoli F, Mehio A, et al. Uterine adenomyosis: endovaginal US and MR imaging features with histopathologic correlation. Radiographics 1999;19 Spec No:S147–60.

40. Kurjak A, Kupesic S. Three dimensional ultrasound and power Doppler in assessment of uterine and ovarian angiogenesis: a prospective study. Croat Med J 1999;40:413–20.

41. Alcazar JL, Galan MJ, Jurado M, et al. Intratumoral blood flow analysis in endometrial carcinoma: correlation with tumor characteristics and risk for recurrence. Gynecol Oncol 2002;84:258–62.

42. Jakab A, Ovari L, Juhasz B, et al. Detection of feeding artery improves the ultrasound diagnosis of endometrial polyps in asymptomatic patients. Eur J Obstet Gynecol Reprod Biol 2005;119:103–7.

43. Timmerman D, Verguts J, Konstantinovic ML, et al. The pedicle artery sign based on sonography with color Doppler imaging can replace second-stage tests in women with abnormal vaginal bleeding. Ultrasound Obstet Gynecol 2003;22:166–71.

44. Zhou Q, Lei XY, Xie Q, et al. Sonographic and Doppler imaging in the diagnosis and treatment of gestational trophoblastic disease: a 12-year experience. J Ultrasound Med 2005;24:15–24.

45. Salem S, Wilson SR. Gynecologic ultrasound. In: Rumack CM, Wilson SR, Charboneau JW, editors. 3rd edition, Diagnostic ultrasound, Vol 2. St. Louis (MO): Elsevier, Mosby; 2004. p. 527–87.

46. Kwon JH, Kim GS. Obstetric iatrogenic arterial injuries of the uterus: diagnosis with US and treatment with transcatheter arterial embolization. Radiographics 2002;22:35–46.

47. Ghi T, Giunchi S, Rossi C, et al. Three dimensional power Doppler sonography in the diagnosis of arteriovenous malformation of the uterus. J Ultrasound Med 2005;24:727–31.

48. Huang MW, Muradali D, Thurston WA, et al. Uterine arteriovenous malformations: gray-scale and Doppler US features with MR imaging correlation. Radiology 1998;206:115–23.

49. Henrich W, Fuchs I, Luttkus A, et al. Pseudoaneurysm of the uterine artery after cesarean delivery: sonographic diagnosis and treatment. J Ultrasound Med 2002;21:1431–4.

50. Langer JE, Cope C. Ultrasonographic diagnosis of uterine artery pseudoaneurysm after hysterectomy. J Ultrasound Med 1999;18:711–4.

51. Braffman BH, Coleman BG, Ramchandani P, et al. Emergency department screening for ectopic pregnancy: a prospective US study. Radiology 1994;190: 797–802.

52. Atri M, Leduc C, Gillett P, et al. Role of endovaginal sonography in the diagnosis and management of ectopic pregnancy. Radiographics 1996;16:755–74 [discussion: 775].

53. Shaharabany Y, Akselrod S, Tepper R. A sensitive new indicator for diagnostics of ovarian malignancy, based on the Doppler velocity spectrum. Ultrasound Med Biol 2004;30:295–302.

54. Orden MR, Jurvelin JS, Kirkinen PP. Kinetics of a US contrast agent in benign and malignant adnexal tumors. Radiology 2003;226:405–10.

Index

Note: Page numbers of article titles are in **boldface** type.

A

Abdominal pregnancy, 337
Abortion, spontaneous, 349–350, 352
Abscess
  breast, 279–280
  tubo-ovarian, 373–374
Adenomyosis, uterine, 437, 439, 476–477
Adhesions, uterine, 401, 403, 439
Adnexal masses, **369–389**
  benign, 369–379
  cystadenocarcinoma, 380
  Doppler studies in, 383–387
  endometriosis, 371–372
  hydrosalpinx, 372–373
  in ectopic pregnancy, 331, 333, 357–358, 376–378
  in pregnancy, 382
  malignant, 379–382
  mature cystic teratoma, 374
  metastatic, 380–382
  mimics of, 382–383
  mucinous cystadenoma, 378–379
  nongynecologic, 382
  ovarian cysts, 369–371
  ovarian fibroma, 379
  ovarian remnant syndrome, 378
  paraovarian/paratubal cysts, 374
  pelvic inflammatory disease, 373–374
  peritoneal inclusion cysts, 374–375
  polycystic ovary, 375
  postmenopausal cysts, 375
  serous cystadenoma, 378
  three-dimensional ultrasound in, 383
American College of Radiology Imaging Network, 277
Angiography, in pelvic congestion syndrome, 421–422
Angle, for color flow Doppler imaging, 470–474
Arcuate uterus, 443, 445
Arteriovenous malformations, uterine, 354–355, 439, 479
Aspiration, of breast cysts, 285, 290
Atrophic endometrium, 393, 436

B

Bicornuate uterus, 442–443
Biopsy, breast. *See* Breast masses, biopsy of.
Bladder, endometriosis of, 409
Bladder flap hematoma, 382

Bleeding
  abnormal, sonohysterography in, 431–432, 436
  in ectopic pregnancy, 331
  postmenopausal, **391–397**
  premenopausal. *See* Premenopausal bleeding.
Boundary, of breast mass, 281
Brachytherapy, for breast cancer, 305
Breast, edema of, 304–305
Breast cancer
  conservation surgery for, 295–311
  solid masses, 280–285
  with implants, 324
Breast Imaging Reporting and Data System (BI-RADS), 277, 279
Breast masses, **277–287**. *See also* Breast cancer.
  anatomic considerations in, 277
  biopsy of, **289–294**
    complex, 280
    core needle/vacuum-assisted, 291, 293
    cyst aspiration in, 290
    fine needle, 290–291
    imaging–histologic correlation with, 292–293
    in highly suggestive of malignancy category, 285
    marker placement in, 291–292
    nonpalpable, 291
    preparation for, 289–290
  complex, 279–280
  cysts, 285
    biopsy of, 285, 290
    clustered, 278–279
    complicated, 278
    lipid, 303–304
  highly suggestive of malignancy in, 285
  indications for, 278
  nonpalpable, 278–285, 291
  palpable, 285
  probably benign, 283–284
  solid, 280–285
  surgery for. *See* Breast surgery.
  suspicious abnormality in, 284
Breast surgery, **295–329**
  conservation, for cancer, 295–311
    diffuse changes in, 304–305
    failure of, 305–311
    fat necrosis in, 303–304
    fluid collections in, 298–299
    postoperative monitoring of, 296–298
    preoperative imaging in, 295–296

doi:10.1016/S1556-858X(08)00120-5

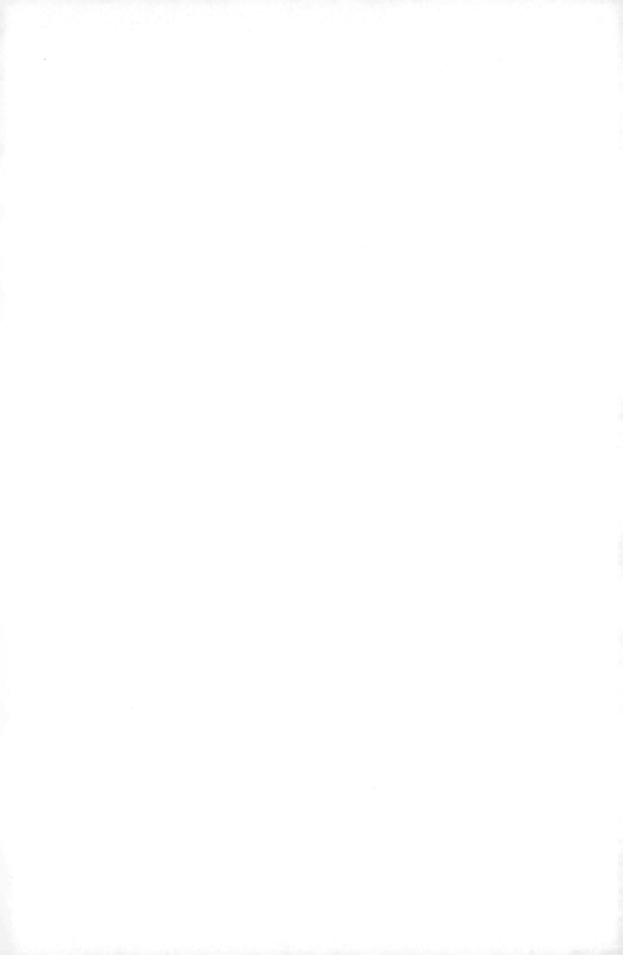